e-Mental Health

Davor Mucic • Donald M. Hilty
Editors

e-Mental Health

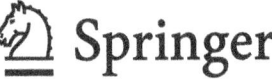 Springer

Editors
Davor Mucic
The Little Prince Psychiatric Centre
Copenhagen
Denmark

Donald M. Hilty
Keck School of Medicine
University of Southern California
Los Angeles, CA
USA

ISBN 978-3-319-37050-7   ISBN 978-3-319-20852-7 (eBook)
DOI 10.1007/978-3-319-20852-7

Springer Cham Heidelberg New York Dordrecht London
© Springer International Publishing Switzerland 2016
Softcover re-print of the Hardcover 1st edition 2016

Printed on acid-free paper

Springer International Publishing AG Switzerland is part of Springer Science+Business Media
(www.springer.com)

Dedicated to Nikola Tesla

Preface

Dear Readers,

This is the book on e-mental health, which is the use of telecommunication and information technologies to deliver mental health services at a distance. The oldest and most comprehensive form of e-mental health is telepsychiatry – videoconferencing in "real-time" (synchronous telemental health). More recently, asynchronous (formerly store-and-forward) telemental health has led to doctor-patient care in many forms: e-mail, video capture of a patient's history and forwarding to a psychiatrist, and other web- or Internet-based methods. All these forms lead to an evaluation and/or treatment that it is *not* in real-time. Officially, telemedicine as a term legal implies synchronous means, though it can be complemented by other means; synchronous visual contact is required for calling it "clinical care," billing companies, and the official term of telepsychiatry, at least in the United States. A broad view of medicine, technology, and telepsychiatry (Chap. 1) extends to specific efforts at prevention (Chap. 3), populations (e.g., addictions Chap. 14), and treatments.

We have discussed telepsychiatry internationally since 1996 at scientific meetings, research forums, clinical conferences, and many other venues – some common misunderstandings abound about telepsychiatry. Professionals (psychiatrists, psychologists, and nurses) at conferences in Denmark (DM) and the United States (DH) wondered: (1) "Does it well as in-person care?" and (2) "Is it just regular care by video or is it something different?" Other folks got confused more literally (e.g., "Is it something about telepathy?") and patients, specifically thought the video would be heard by others (i.e., "Big Brother") or taped and somehow distributed (i.e., put in medical record and other places?) Today, others say, "It is just like Skype, isn't it?"

In spite of the plethora of possibilities for improved patient care through the use of technology, human factors present the greatest impediment to the implementation of new systems [1]. The analogy to Skype, a patient's narrative or other story helps us grasp the tangibles and the intangibles – a key goal in our book in talking about, e.g., telepsychiatry within e-mental health (eMH) – and it becomes much easier to accept and adopt it [2]. There have been many positive and a few negative, unexpected consequences of telepsychiatry (Chap. 2). We take great care in discussing communication and technology as they slightly affect the doctor-patient relationship (Chap. 13). The current younger generations push us forward with social media, which invigorates our work and raises new issues to consider (Chap. 8). We also have to employ technology to serve additional populations, to complement other service delivery models, and to shape the future (Chaps. 6, 7 and 15).

Narratives from daily clinical work may significantly increase the understanding and acceptance of e-mental health among professionals with no e-mental health-related experience or professionals that are still in doubt, so we share the following story with you (DM's case):

> NN is a 28-year-old female, refugee from my Bosnia-Herzegovina, ex-Yugoslavia (home country of DM). In Bosnia, during the war, NN was unfortunately raped several times while her husband was in the army. After immigrating to Denmark, NN was referred to a psychiatrist due to occurred posttraumatic stress disorder symptomatology. As her Danish language abilities were poor, the communication was provided via an interpreter. Consequently, she received psychiatric treatment with medication and psychotherapy via interpreter for around 3 years prior to our first telepsychiatry session. The video equipment was installed at psychiatric department where NN used to come and speak with her psychiatrist in-person. I was in Copenhagen while NN was located 245 km away in outskirts of Denmark. At the first consultation via telepsychiatry, the first question NN asked was, "Can all of Denmark see us now?"

> When assured that no one follows our conversation and that the session will not be recorded, NN replied, "Then I have a secret I would like to disclose" and so she started her story about traumatic events, i.e., rape and torture in home country. NN cried while spoke in a stream without a break except to wipe her tears and blow her nose. She said that it was not possible for her to speak about it with her past psychiatrist as all communication runs via the interpreter. The presence of the interpreter for her changed the dynamic of the interview and more tangibly, it increased the risk that her husband would find out about the rape and consequently divorce her.

> While NN spoke about her painful experiences, the Internet suddenly disconnected. When that happens, the last frame remains on the screen as a frozen picture. So NN could see me as a still image and I could see her frozen in the middle of a movement…and of course we could not hear each other. I panicked, thinking what she would say to this, or fearing that she probably would never come again (i.e., use the video). My technician was in the office next door, so he restored the connection. The break varied about 30 seconds in total, but it felt like much longer. To my surprise, when the connection was restored, I could see and hear NN who spoke in a stream and cried at the same time. She didn't even notice that I was gone for a while.

Personally, it was an experience that shaped the next 15 years of dedicated work on developing of the "cross-cultural telepsychiatry concept" for telepsychiatry, whereby the treatment of ethnic minorities de-emphasized use of interpreters (Chaps. 5, 9, and 10). Further, we realized that telecommunication and information technology has the potential to increase the exchange of expertise across national borders without need for travel (Chap. 12). Gradually, we found out that many colleagues around the globe are interested in the development of various e-mental health (eMH) applications capable of increasing the quality of mental health care, which is why we invited some of them to share their experiences through this book. So this book is aimed to provide mental health workers with substantial knowledge and latest updates within the fastest growing field in psychiatry: *e-mental health*. This includes eMH by video and often augmented by other strategies (Chap. 9).

The strength of this book is that it balances the innovation of a new technology, with a scientific evidence base, and the experience of many talented clinicians (and writers). We wish to thank all contributors that have invested a great deal of time and work in writing the respective chapters.

Special thanks to Prof. Norman Sartorius and Prof. Anita Riecher-Rössler, for their support and useful advice during the book project.

We also thank the many clinicians, researchers, and trainees – including those from a variety of disciplines from medicine, psychiatry, psychology, social science, culture, communication, and other fields.

Finally, our fervent, complimentary, and wide-ranging discussions on how to shape this – along with our time and efforts – have brought us together as colleagues from literally across the world. The relationships we now share through this work are themselves precious extraordinary.

Copenhagen, Denmark	Davor Mucic
Los Angeles, CA, USA	Donald M. Hilty

References

1. Luo JL, Hilty DM, Worley LLM, Yager J. Considerations in change management related to technology. Acad Psychiatry. 2006;30(6):465–9.
2. Casey LM, Joy A, Clough BA. The impact of information on attitudes toward e-mental health services. Cyberpsychol Behav Soc Netw. 2013;16(8):593–8.

Contents

Part I   Introduction
Davor Mucic

**1   Technology, Health, and Contemporary Practice:
How Does e-Mental Health Fit It and What Does It Offer?**   3
Donald M. Hilty and Davor Mucic

**2   Entangled in the Web. Unexpected Events with New
Technologies: Addiction, Consequences on Communication** 29
Agnes Wrobel and Janusz Wrobel

Part II   Prevention, Early Detection and Health Promotion
Donald M. Hilty

**3   e-Mental Health Improves Access to Care, Facilitates
Early Intervention, and Provides Evidence-Based
Treatments at a Distance** 43
Erica Z. Shoemaker and Donald M. Hilty

**4   How to Build, Evaluate, and Increase Your e-Mental
Health Program Efficiency.** 59
Donald M. Hilty, Erica Z. Shoemaker, and Jay Shore

**5   e-Mental Health Toward Cross-Cultural Populations
Worldwide** 77
Davor Mucic, Donald M. Hilty, and Peter M. Yellowlees

**Part III   Clinical Care Models: Stepped Care, Collaborative Care
and Integrated Care By Telepsychiatry**
Donald M. Hilty

**6   The Effectiveness of e-Mental Health: Evidence Base,
How to Choose the Model Based on Ease/Cost/Strength,
and Future Areas of Research** 95
Donald M. Hilty, Peter M. Yellowlees, Kathleen Myers,
Michelle B. Parish, and Terry Rabinowitz

7   How e-Mental Health Adds to Traditional Outpatient
    and Newer Models of Integrated Care for Patients,
    Providers, and Systems..................................... 129
    Donald M. Hilty, Barb Johnston, and Robert M. McCarron

8   Social Media and Clinical Practice: What Stays the Same,
    What Changes, and How to Plan Ahead?...................... 151
    Christopher E. Snowdy, Erica Z. Shoemaker, Steven Chan,
    and Donald M. Hilty

Part IV   New Therapies/Methods/Treatments
          Davor Mucic

9   Web- and Internet-Based Services: Education,
    Support, Self-Care, and Formal Treatment Approaches 173
    Davor Mucic, Donald M. Hilty, Michelle B. Parish,
    and Peter M. Yellowlees

10 Cognitive Behavioural Therapy and Cognitive Bias
    Modification in Internet-Based Interventions for Mood,
    Anxiety and Substance Use Disorders....................... 193
    Matthijs Blankers, Elske Salemink, and Reinout W. Wiers

11 Psychiatric Apps: Patient Self-Assessment,
    Communication, and Potential Treatment Interventions 217
    Steven Chan, John B. Torous, Ladson Hinton,
    and Peter M. Yellowlees

Part V   Consequences, Limits and Risks
         Davor Mucic and Donald M. Hilty

12 Global/Worldwide e-Mental Health: International
    and Futuristic Perspectives of Telepsychiatry and the Future 233
    Peter M. Yellowlees, Donald M. Hilty, and Davor Mucic

13 How Does the Internet Influence the Doctor–Patient
    Relationship?.. 251
    Mark Agius and Helen Stangeland

14 Pathological Use of the Internet.......................... 269
    Vladimir Carli and Tony Durkee

15 From Telehealth to an Interactive Virtual Clinic................. 289
    Michael Krausz, John Ward, and Damon Ramsey

Editors

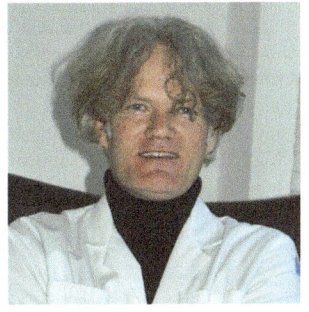

Davor Mucic, born in Former Yugoslavia, educated psychiatrist in Denmark, with special interest in treatment of asylum seekers, refugees, and migrants via their respective mother tongue. Davor Mucic established Little Prince Psychiatric Centre, the only place in Denmark for refugees and migrants from Ex-Yugoslavia, Eastern Europe, the Middle East, and Africa where the therapists speak the same languages as the clients.

The Centre has been frontier in developing of *telepsychiatry* in Denmark since 2000. More information is available on www.denlilleprins.org

In 2011, Davor Mucic launched *Telemental Health Section* within EPA.

In addition, Davor Mucic is a clinical lector on Danish Copenhagen University and reviewer for *Journal of Telemedicine and Telecare* as well as editor on *Edorium Journal of Psychiatry*.

Davor Mucic published a number of articles related to telepsychiatry development in Denmark, e.g., scientific articles about the first international telepsychiatry in the world service as well as the first cross-cultural telepsychiatry service established in 2004 on Island Bornholm, where the service is still functioning, offering its cross-cultural patients mental health service via their own mother tongues.

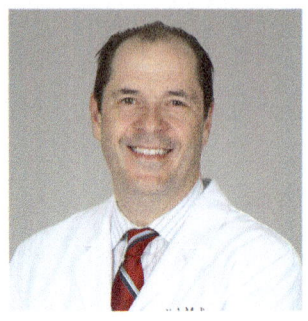

Donald M. Hilty M.D. is Vice-Chair of Education and Director of Telepsychiatry and Distance Education at Keck School of Medicine at USC. His research involves health services, telepsychiatry, models of care, mood disorders, and underserved populations. His telemedicine studies have compared telepsychiatric care to on-site psychiatric care, other specialty care via telemedicine, and mental health care by primary care physicians. He moved on to help providers diagnose, triage, and prescribe per national guidelines in the primary care setting. His randomized trial of the treatment of depression via telemedicine, based on collaborative care, provided disease management care to patients in rural California. He is currently a Co-Investigator of an AHQR RCT comparing synchronous and asynchronous telepsychiatry.

Dr. Hilty's specific educational interests include pedagogy, evaluation, and distance education. He was the Director and Developer of the 5-year MD/MPH UC Davis Rural Program in Medical Education. Dr. Hilty has authored over 180 articles, chapters, book reviews, and/or books and done over 200 peer-reviewed presentations as a member of the Association for Academic Psychiatry, the Academy for Psychosomatic Medicine, the American Telemedicine Association, the American Psychiatric Association (APA), and the American College of Psychiatry. He is writing Treatment Guidelines in a collaborative APA project with the Institute of Medicine.

Part I

Introduction

Davor Mucic

Technology, Health, and Contemporary Practice: How Does e-Mental Health Fit It and What Does It Offer?

1

Donald M. Hilty and Davor Mucic

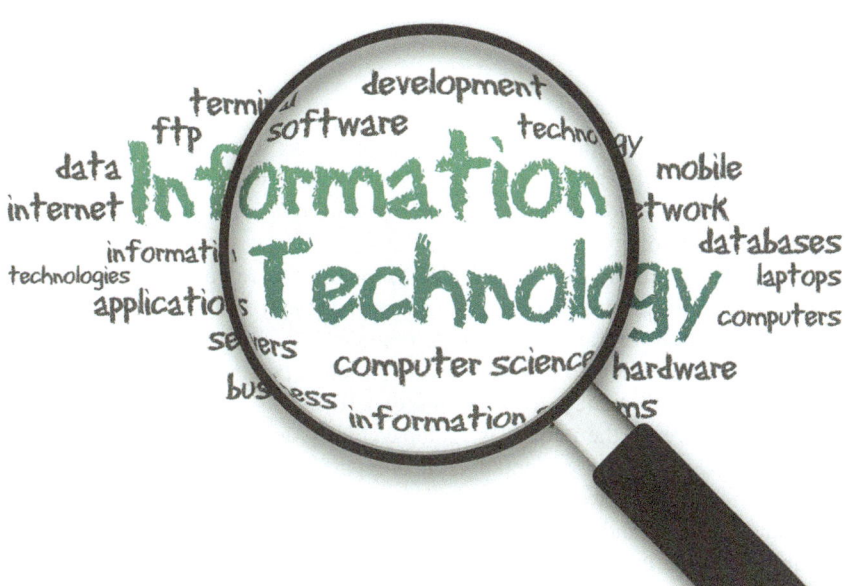

D.M. Hilty, MD (✉)
Keck School of Medicine, University of Southern California,
Los Angeles, CA, USA
e-mail: donh031226@gmail.com

D. Mucic, MD
The Little Prince Psychiatric Centre, Copenhagen, Denmark
e-mail: info@denlilleprins.org,
http://www.denlilleprins.org, http://www.tv-psykiater.dk

© Springer International Publishing Switzerland 2016
D. Mucic, D.M. Hilty (eds.), *e-Mental Health*,
DOI 10.1007/978-3-319-20852-7_1

3

Contents

1.1 Introduction 4
1.2 Current Healthcare Trends in the USA and Worldwide:
    A Historical Perspective and the Platform of Technology 6
1.3 History of Technology, Telemedicine, and eMH 13
    1.3.1 What We Know So Far: An Overview on eMH 13
    1.3.2 Digital Communication: E-Mail, Messaging Services, and Online Options 17
    1.3.3 Social Media Communication 18
    1.3.4 Program and Administration Approaches to Evaluation,
          Legal Issues, and Reimbursement Issues 19
1.4 eMH Benefits to Patients, Providers, and Systems of Care:
    Access, Versatility, and Empowerment 20
    1.4.1 Patient Benefits 20
    1.4.2 Provider Benefits 20
    1.4.3 Healthcare Systems and Administration 21
1.5 Discussion and Conclusion 22
References 22

Abstract

Patient- or person-centered healthcare confronts us with questions on how to deliver quality, affordable, and timely care in a variety of settings. The international history of medicine, patient-centered care models, healthcare financing, and use of technology frame how e-mental health (eMH) develops, is employed, and positively influences outcomes. Models of care and patient-centered approaches are steering eMH services forward from in-person to videoconferencing to online formats—technology complements existing traditional medical approaches. Telemedicine empowers patients, personalizes care, increases administrative efficiency, and ensures expertise gets to the place it is most needed—wherever the patient is. Telepsychiatry, as the oldest eMH application, is effective, well accepted, and comparable to in-person care. As we employ technology, we must maintain high-quality clinical care and professional standards and be sensitive to differences in participants. Good care requires evaluation and attends to clinical, legal, reimbursement about the technological issues. eMH may soon reshape healthcare service delivery particularly as telepsychiatry appears better for some disorders and in some models of care than traditional in-person approaches; online services will boost this shift even more. Mental health providers may soon practice in-person, virtually, or both.

1.1 Introduction

Patient-centered healthcare—suggested as far back as 2001 [1]—focuses on quality, affordable, and timely care [2], and person-centered healthcare has been reinvigorated to know the whole person or person behind the patient [3, 4]. Regulatory divergences (the USA versus Europe, Australia, the Middle East, and the rest of the world) determine how quickly regulatory decisions are reached and consequently result in huge differences in current state of the eMH development and adoption around the globe. Our view of eMH, like our view of medicine, has changed over time with social, political, and scientific roots. Its path has been summarized as a social science, the germ theory of disease, healthcare as a battleground (or the war metaphor), managing healthcare resources (or the market metaphor), Health for All (the social justice model), evidence-based medicine, and ObamaCare (the ACA) [5]. Placing the individual and his/her needs at the center (the attractor for the health system) of our thinking, as emphasized by the World Health Organization's International Classification of Function framework and the European Society of Person-Centered Healthcare, may provide the frame to refocus health and health-care as interdependent experiences across individual, community, and societal domains. Two of the significant trends are in the USA and Europe, though the World Health Organization, too: surveying on telemedicine opportunities and developments in member states [6]. The patient-centered medical home (PCMH) is one such specific movement—along with the affordable care act (ObamaCare; ACA) in the USA—which involves a deceptively simple set of key structural practice features that have been proposed to result in enhanced access for routine primary care, improved delivery of preventive services, high-quality chronic disease management, and reduced emergency department and hospital utilization [7, 8]. The approaches or tools for the changing environment are PCMH, collaborative or integrated care, stepped care, and still more innovative models. The crucial initiative of the European Commission is ROAMER (roadmap for mental health research and well-being in Europe), which is aimed at gaining more insight into the gaps in care and needs for mental health services. Blended eHealth/mental health decision aids/guidance tools are suggested to help the clinician to choose between various treatment modalities and hopefully result in increased efficacy and impact across Europe. Finally, the experts stressed the importance of creating funding and coordinated networking as essential action needed in order to target the variety of challenges in clinical mental health research [9].

Internationally, countries present a kaleidoscope of funding models, from tax-funded national health systems to national insurance systems with competing regulated private health insurance plans, some operating through so-called health insurance marketplaces or their equivalent. The extent to which the nations meet the needs of their most vulnerable populations varies with benefit design, cost-sharing thresholds and exemptions, and subsidies [10]. A critical characteristic of these many healthcare systems is a skewed distribution of healthcare utilization across the population (e.g., about 25 % of all medical care is consumed by 1 % of the patient population and nearly half by just 5 %) [11]. eMH—or more broadly e-service delivery—is in the thick of things due to its versatility and leveraging of essential resources [12, 13] at multiple points of service [13, 14]. Indeed, eMH providers' input to the primary care provider has improved patient care, is convenient, and is less costly with desk-mounted video systems [12, 15, 16]. eMH also leverages inter-disciplinary team members' clinical, administrative, and other care coordination expertise [17].

eMH—using a broad, inclusive definition for online services, too—is in the thick of things for several other reasons. First, it adds to what we do by giving us a ton of new options for communication (Chap. 2), improving access to the best treatments (Chap. 3), and disseminating culturally sensitive care (Chap. 5). Second, eMH provides clinicians more virtual options by way of the Internet or web (Chaps. 9 and 10). On one hand, they are adapting, but on the other hand, many feel eMH is changing what they do or shifting clinical practice (Chap. 11). Newer generations embrace these changes but also have to learn the basics of doctor-patient relationship and how eMH affects it (Chaps. 8 and 13). Third, clinicians and administrators need an approach to develop a program (Chap. 4), assess effectiveness (Chap. 6), and use it for patient-centered and integrated care movements (Chap. 7). Having a plan in advance is needed, in and of itself, but also to guide others on hot topics like addiction on the Internet (Chap. 14) and dealing with social media in patient care (Chap. 8). Clinicians and patients not surprisingly wonder if the future will be mostly virtual in terms of service delivery (Chap. 15), based on worldwide trends (Chap. 12).

The Internet and World Wide Web—technology, in general—have complemented regular mental health (MH) care, added user-friendly additional care, greater access, and additional customization/ personalization. So the "content" or ranges of services for care are broader—and "process" toward access to services is more variable. Patients' preferences for help seeking, education, and treatments are becoming better known—at least to providers who evolve with practice trends and the new applications of technology. MH providers must meet the challenges and requirements that are emerging to fulfill the care-related requests. While the buffet of informal or self-directed services is increasing, one question is, "If the person or patient is in care, should this be overseen by a professional, and if so, how?" While the options have grown (e.g., in-person or eMH "traditional" services to informal spectrum above), another question arises, which is, "Can we assume the person or patient will plug in and get where they need to go or find the best service for them?" In banking, people migrated to ATMs based on simple task completion and used tellers as necessary—is it that simple for MH issues, symptoms, and disorders?

This chapter will help the reader to: (1) Understand the history of telemedicine and eMH (2) See how eMH, technology, and online options have become part of and shaped current healthcare trends, in the USA and worldwide (3) Apply telehealth to realize benefits of new technology to patients (access to care, innovative treatment), providers, systems, and global communities (e.g., empowerment, more versatile approaches to care, and "better" care)

1.2   Current Healthcare Trends in the USA and Worldwide: A Historical Perspective and the Platform of Technology

We might begin by looking at how medicine and eMH are framed, conceptually, and in other dimensions. To "frame" is to select some aspects of a perceived reality and make them more salient in a communicating text, in such a way as to promote a particular problem definition, causal interpretation, moral evaluation, and/or treatment recommendation for the item described [18]. The focus of these frames is causal, instrumental, political/economic, or social in nature. All remain relevant but recycling individual past frames in response to current problems will not achieve the outcomes we seek. Frames "organise everyday reality by providing meaning to an unfolding strip of events and promoting particular definitions and interpretations" [19]. Of note, framing the same issue through positive or negative reference points [20] provides differing contexts that influence our perception and decision-making, that is, advances different cognitive and motivational consequences [21] (Table 1.1).

Australia has been progressive in the use of eMH and e-platforms, particularly for rural and remote communities to improve access to specialists, quality care, decision support/supervision, and therapies [22–24, 56]. Telepsychiatry is proving successful through a number of programs to service rural Australian regions (e.g., Wagga Wagga, Dubbo, Western Australia, and South Australia) across different psychiatric services. The Mental Health Emergency Care-Rural Access Program (MHEC-RAP), which is a telehealth solution, provides specialist emergency mental health care to rural and remote communities across western NSW, Australia, since 2008, and provides timely information and support, emergency telephone triage assessments, and video assessments. Benchmarks for efficient service delivery and information about the development of similar telehealth programs are needed both in Australia and overseas [25]. Due to accessibility, the telephone has become a standard tool for Australian psychiatrists in scheduling, consultation, payment, and crisis management.

The most popular current "frame" for taking action in healthcare appears to be the PCMH in the USA and a hybrid of patient-centered, stepped, and/or collaborative care worldwide. The PCMH is founded on the absence of adequate treatment or access to it in primary care [57]. It is believed to be efficient in a high-performing, cost-effective healthcare system [7]—though frankly other models, approaches, or tools function better in that context, too. Indeed, integrated care and stepped care models provide efficient expertise to the point of service. The core characteristics of integrated care are (1) responsibility, decision-making, and oversight of patient care; (2) co-location of services, both literally and virtually, that applies to both inpatient and outpatient sector care; (3)–(5) integrated funding, evaluation, and outcome measurement; (6) an e-platform; and (7) reimbursement, preferably aligned (e.g., a capitated or sole "Medicare" population) rather than unaligned (i.e., mixed populations). Stepped care models may be the most cost-effective models in health system where the effectiveness of the intervention is maximized by making the best use of resources adequately available at the right time [58, 59].

E-platforms have traditionally distributed academic networks of like-minded researchers and clinicians into regional health information organizations (RHIOs) [60]. These RHIOs empower consumers and clinicians in day-to-day healthcare delivery by improving access to evidence-based information at the point of care; facilitate the delivery of a wider range of health services, particularly to primary and community care; provide accurate data to support research and clinical policy and governance arrangements; and ensure a sustainable, secure, reliable electronic environment, underpinned by strong, policy-driven privacy protection [60]. Previously, the single most important technical innovation was broadband distribution, which enables high-quality videoconferencing, multimedia-based applications, and other options, particularly doctor's desk. The contemporary e-platform adds the electronic medical record (EMR), integration of

Table 1.1 Technology, telemedicine, and e-mental health/telepsychiatry history: evolution and selected key events

Decade	Technologies	Event(s)	Comment(s)
Pre-1950s	Analog wave radio Modem (*modulator-demodulator*)	Communication (military, ship) Modulates signals to encode digital information and demodulates signals to decode the transmitted information	IBM, 1942, 25 bits per second (BPS) Amplitude modulation (AM) or FM (frequency modulation)
1950s	Endec (precursor to coder-decoder or CODEC) CODEC Telephone	Pulse code modulation	Converts between different signal formats
1960s	Prototypes of the Internet Video 32–56 KBPS[a] Store and forward prototype?	US military, 1960 Nebraska Psychiatric Institute and Norfolk State Hospital, 1964 MGH and Logan Airport, 1964 Plain old telephone service; POTS NASA biosensor harnesses, 1968	Two-way linkage via NIH $ Occupational health with nurses Poor image, color, and other characteristics
1970s	128 KBPS Handheld phone, USA, Motorola, 1973 New service Automated network	NPI with Omaha Veterans' Administration NASA, 1973 TMH consultation via interactive TV, 1973 Intercity TMH, 1976 Japan, 1979	Test of group therapy with 26 sites linked using four receivers and two-way videoconferencing Routine biomedical research; data transfer in time for adjustments
1980s	Handheld on market Developments: Facsimile/fax 1G network ISDN[b] Modern Internet Personal digital assistant (PDA) NASA space bridge	DynaTAC8000x, Motorola Mid 1980s Ditto Ditto Ditto, USA, Europe, and others Psion, 1984 and Palm, 1996 To Russia for clinical services, 1988	Phased out in 2010 with smartphone evolution Infectious disease; space, internal, emergency, preventative, and hyperbaric medicine; cardiology; surgery; cancer treatment

1990–94	128 KBPS and whiteboard and shared databases Developments: 2G network SIM card SMS (short message service) texting First report of "new" service; probably done before then Store and forward (later asynchronous)	MedTAC and Dominican Republic Samana Hospital, 1991 Germany, 1991 Finland, 1993 Rural telepsychiatry paper, 1992 Clinical reports, 1994 (dermatology)	Physicians at the Virginia Commonwealth University
1995–99	18–384 KBPS Legislation Media content Communication Reimbursement New services	Mid 1990s Telemedicine development act in California, 1996 Finland, 1998 Social presence by TMH, 1998 Medicare and medical coverage, 1999 Tele-ultrasound report, 1996 TMH consultation to primary care, 1999 TMH cultural consultation, 1999	Senate Bill 1665
2000–04	3G network PDA iPhone	2001 PDA used for clinical care, 2001 First on the market	
2005–09	Internet-paid media content Electronic health record New services	2006 2005? STP[c] comparable to in-person ATP[d], U.S., 2008	Also known as EPR (electronic patient record) and EMR (electronic medical record)
2010	Top Events	Most read articles	Healthcare via Cell Phones: A Systematic Review, Krishna et al., 2009 Practice Guidelines for Videoconferencing-Based Telemental Health, Yellowlees et al., 2010

(continued)

Table 1.1 (continued)

Decade	Technologies	Event(s)	Comment(s)
2011		Most read articles 2011	Effectiveness of Home Telehealth for Diabetes and Hypertension: A TCT, Wakefield et al., 2011 Evidence-Based Practice for TMH, Grady et al., 2011
2012	Top Events	Most read article 2012	Diabetes Management via Mobile Phones: A Systematic Review, Holtz et al., 2012 Chronic Diseases Social Groups on Facebook and Twitter, de la Torre-Diez et al., 2012
2013	Top Events	TMH Special Edition in *Tele-Health*	Top paper: Obstacles and overcoming them, Brooks et al. Videoconferencing-Based TMH Guidelines, TMH IG TMH is effective, Hilty et al.
2014	Top Events	Psych apps, wearables, and embedded sensors Reimbursement in the USA	mHealth predictions: technology integrated into patient care… prescribed apps to come shortly? Center for Medicare (CMS) services covered and includes patient-doctor communication expectation
2015	ATA	Annual Meeting 20th Anniversary	

Footnotes

[a]*KBPS* kilobits per second

[b]*ISDN* Integrated Services for Digital Network

[c]*STP* synchronous telepsychiatry

[d]*ATP* asynchronous telepsychiatry (or store and forward telepsychiatry)

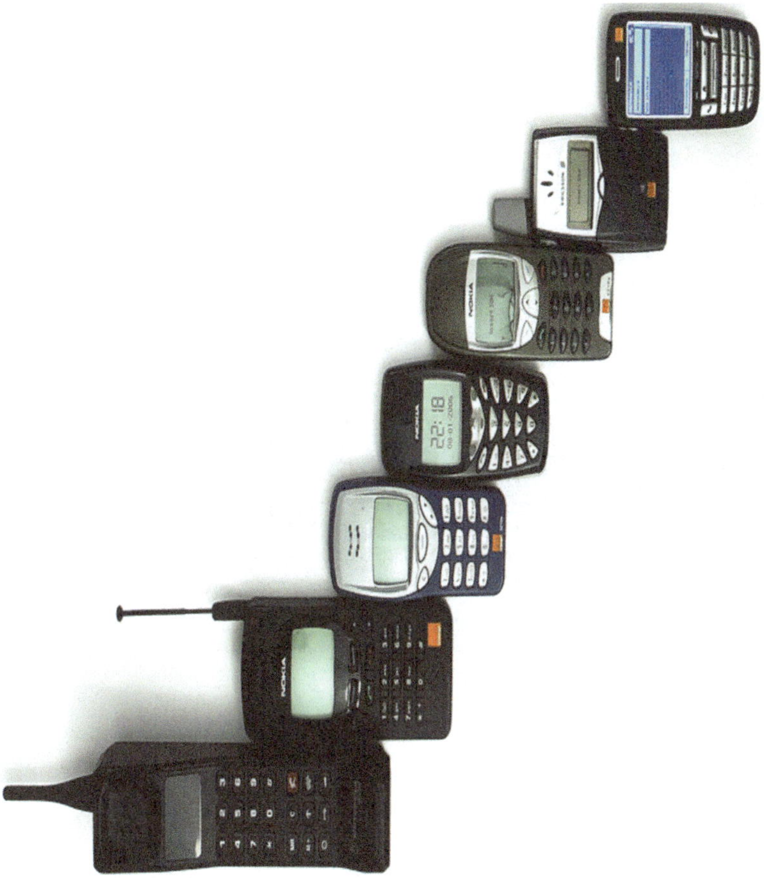

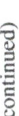

(continued)

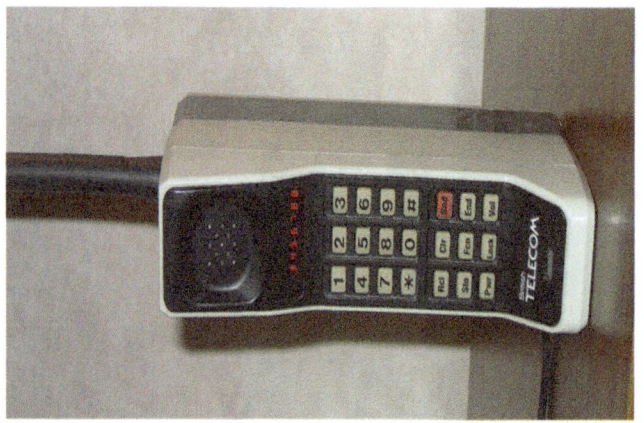

Table 1.1 (continued)

in-person and eMH care administration (i.e., scheduling, documentation, payment, and others), enhanced patient to doctor or system engagement/communication (e.g., HIPAA[1] compliant e-mail "into" the EMR (e.g., Relay Health), and leveraging the expertise at a distance (phone, e-mail, video, asynchronous and other methods).

Another movement is the participatory medicine and patient-centered care, in the form of the personal health record (PHR). Participatory medicine is defined as "movement in which networked patients shift from being mere passengers to responsible drivers of their health, and in which providers encourage and value them as full partners" [61], and this may include patient-driven research (PDR) [62]. The patient-centered PHR (PCPHR) is moving forward, but its uptake is limited partly due to patient characteristics like comorbid illness, culture/ethnicity, and age [63]. Involving patients in personal healthcare decisions may use decision aids for shared decision-making between patients and their clinicians by presenting relevant scientific information in balanced, understandable ways, helping clarify patients' goals, and guiding decision-making processes. International standards stipulate that patients and clinicians should be involved in decision aid development [64]. The patient-reported outcome (PRO) is a standardized method for measuring patients' views of their health status. Our international study showed that experts in clinical practice and performance measurement supported the integrated collection of PRO data for use in both clinical care and performance measurement [65].

The broader theme on the PCPHR is shared medical decision-making. Complex situations require partnership with patients/learners to reach the best outcome. Shared decision-making equalizes the informational and power symmetry between doctors and patients—both parties share information and develop consensus in a decision [66]. Psychiatry is a good model of early and contemporary shared decision-making. When patients were allowed to choose between different treatment options for depression rather than being randomly allocated to treatment groups, patients chose psychotherapy more often than pharmacotherapy with no significant difference in patient satisfaction or outcomes. A study about continuation or discontinuation of an antipsychotic depot medication in patients with schizophrenia led to 87 % of 96 patients continuing medication—a very high rate [66].

1.3 History of Technology, Telemedicine, and eMH

1.3.1 What We Know So Far: An Overview on eMH

The American Telemedicine Association (ATA) Videoconferencing Guidelines [67] review organizations' technical responsibilities to ensure the equipment readiness, safety, effectiveness, security of data, connectivity, and compliance with legal/regulatory guidelines. An Overview on eMHs history worldwide is shown in Table 1.2.

---

[1] HIPAA is the US Federal Health Insurance Portability and Accountability Act of 1996. The primary goal of the law is to make it easier for people to keep health insurance, protect the confidentiality and security of healthcare information, and help the healthcare industry control administrative costs.

Table 1.2 e-Mental Health Worldwide trends in 2015

Country	Description	Comment(s)/planning
Australia	Australia has been progressive in the use of eMH and e-platforms, particularly for rural and remote communities to improve access to specialists, quality care, decision support/supervision, and therapies [22–24]. Telepsychiatry is proving successful through a number of programs to service rural Australian regions (e.g., Wagga Wagga, Dubbo, Western Australia, and South Austral) across different psychiatric services. Benchmarks for efficient service delivery and information about the development of similar telehealth programs are needed both in Australia and overseas [25] The Mental Health Emergency Care-Rural Access Program (MHEC-RAP), which is a telehealth solution, provides specialist emergency mental health care to rural and remote communities across western NSW, Australia, since 2008, and provides timely information and support, emergency telephone triage assessments, and video assessments	Due to accessibility, the telephone has become a standard tool for Australian psychiatrists in scheduling, consultation, payment, and crisis management [26]. The telephone has also been widely used for psychotherapy (e.g., free, confidential, and anonymous, telephone counseling service for young people aged between 5 and 25). Counselors respond to more than 10,000 phone calls each week about issues ranging from relationship breakdown and bullying to sexual abuse, homelessness, suicidal thoughts, and drug and alcohol usage. Since 1991 more than 5.2 million telephone and online chat sessions (audio and visual) [27]
Canada	eMH has been widely adopted in Canada, particularly outside of Ontario, near Alberta, and for Native American (e.g., Nunavut), geriatric, and child and adolescent populations [28–31]	Canada has led in terms of some education models in child and adolescent psychiatry, as well as the call for objectives, goals, and curricula [32, 33]
Middle East	The Middle East (ME) and eMH use may be a good example of some of the main struggles of programs across the world. The ME is a heterogeneous part of the world with certain variations in mental health services. The spectrum includes countries that have very good (e.g., Israel), fair (e.g., Turkey, Iran, Saudi Arabia), or poor (e.g., Iraq, Syria) services. Given the disparities, there is a need to implement eMH in the ME, but there are only three reports of randomized controlled trials related to eMH, which were done in Turkey, Israel, and Iraq, which focus on effectiveness, psychoeducation and the doctor-patient working alliance [34–36] As telemedicine is not an integrated part of health systems in the ME, there are no regulations or legislations that guide such practices. Fear of political persecution is a threat unique to, and commonly seen in, the ME, and it may also impact patients' acceptance to eMH [37, 38]	Four main barriers to implement eMH in the ME are frequently observed: cultural, technical, financial, and regulatory barriers The process of building an eMH in the ME would require a parallel reconstruction of the medicolegal system to allow for more considerate approach to sensitive ethical concepts such as confidentiality, informed consent, and liability. Countries in the ME also vary in their readiness to adopt the technology and built eMH systems

European Union (EU)	The EU has supported the project MasterMind [39], which treats depression in the home in Southern Denmark so that developing the methods for treatment can be continued and the experiences can be shared with other EU countries. The MasterMind consortium consists of 23 partners from different European countries (Denmark, Greenland, Scotland, Wales, The Netherlands, Germany, Estonia, Belgium, Spain, Italy, Turkey, and Norway)	Similar situation is with other European countries where the use of videoconference in assessment and/or treatment has not been grounded yet while Internet-based approaches have
Denmark	The Little Prince Treatment Centre in Copenhagen and augmented individual efforts in development and promotion of various telepsychiatry services since 2004. Clinicians from the center have conducted several pilot projects supported by the Ministry of Health, Ministry of Internal Affairs, and private grants (e.g., Egmont Foundation)	Cross-cultural, shared care within general practice, vocational rehabilitation, and finally international telepsychiatry services are some of the most important projects, which helped pave the way for today's eMH expansion in Denmark [40, 41]
Canary Islands	The Canary Islands telepsychiatry program in Spain provides psychiatric service to rural regions. From the same program in the Canary Islands, a randomized control trial demonstrated that telepsychiatry treatment has equivalent efficacy to face-to-face consultation in psychiatric treatment [42]	
UK	The use of videoconferencing has proved its potential to enhance psychiatric services within the UK especially for those patients who live in rural areas [43] The integration of an eMH service into rural primary medical care is an obvious way to improve assessment and treatment of mild mental health. UK psychiatrists have achieved more than the rest of Europe within this task, followed by the development of forensic telepsychiatry [43–46]	Unfortunately, lack of training and experience, inadequate access to equipment, and insufficient technical support have all limited the take-up of this technology in the UK [47]
Sweden	Sweden is one of Scandinavian countries that invested in equipment in the 1990s but has not used it on a large scale. Few telepsychiatry projects have been done, but videoconferencing is used for staff communications in Northern part of the country. Internet-delivered cognitive behavioral therapy (ICBT) has been well accepted and adopted by both patients and professionals [48]	
France	In France, eMH is still not widely developed, but applications are of supportive character, i.e., staff meetings via videoconference while patient-centered service is described within the autistic spectrum [49]	

(continued)

Table 1.2 (continued)

Country	Description	Comment(s)/planning
Netherlands	In Netherlands there are a number of eMH-related activities, primarily web-/mobile-based applications, where cognitive therapy in different settings leads [50, 51]	
Others	Developing countries are far behind despite a numbers of clinical, economical, and other benefits that eMH offers India: the Society for Administration of Telemedicine and Healthcare Informatics (SATHI) offered telepsychiatry services to tsunami-affected persons in Nagapattinam district in the state of Tamil Nadu [52] Pakistan: training and education of existing staff in Pakistan from a distance [53] South Africa: a pilot project within forensic telepsychiatry is on its way [54, 55]	

Evaluation of telepsychiatry has gone through three phases [12]. First, it was found to be effective in terms of increasing access to care, acceptance, and good educational outcomes [12]. Second, it was noted to be valid and reliable as compared to in-person services [67]. In addition to comparison (or "as good as") studies, telepsychiatric outcomes are not inferior to in-person care (i.e., non-inferiority studies). Third, frameworks are being used to approach complex themes like costs and models [67–69].

eMH models of clinical care and education have pros and cons [12, 69, 70] including their level of overall intensity, cost, feasibility, and depth of the relationship between the eMH provider, the PCP, and the patient. *Low-intensity* models include tele-education, formal case review, and in-person, telephone, or e-mail doctor-to-doctor "curbside" consultations. A systematic approach was a multispecialty phone and e-mail teleconsultation system for adults and children with developmental disabilities [71]. *Moderate-intensity* models include an integrated program of mental health screening, therapy on site, and telepsychiatric consultation (phone, e-mail, or video), with continuing medical education (CME) and training on screening questionnaires [72] or asynchronous telepsychiatry (ATP) to primary care in English- and Spanish-speaking patients in primary care [73]. *High-intensity* models are typically the ones previously mentioned involving collaborative care [74–76].

The traditional models of care have been in-person, synchronous telepsychiatry (STP), and more recently ATP—that is really only the beginning and emerging models are sprouting quickly. On general, it is how technology affects basic clinical practice. Its impact on clinical boundaries, communication, and engagement has been under review [77]. The American Psychiatric Association (APA) has a guideline on e-prescribing [78]. The effect on professionalism and education/training of the next generations has been explored [79]. Telepsychiatry can extend beyond videoconferencing modalities to other mechanisms: (1) New digital communication from one user to another user using standard protocols: e-mail, SMS text messaging, MMS messaging, and instant messaging (2) New digital communication from one user to another user using proprietary networks: Twitter direct messages, Facebook Messenger, Epic MyChart electronic medical record messaging, and My HealtheVet electronic medical record messaging (3) New social media communication platforms that transmit from one to many users: Internet forums, Facebook pages and profiles, and Twitter streams.

1.3.2 Digital Communication: E-Mail, Messaging Services, and Online Options

Online digital information is an important source of information for today's online user. As of January of 2014, 90 % of adults have a cell phone and 58 % have a smartphone [80]. In the public health space, 35 % of US adults have gone online to research health information and learn from other patients' experiences [81]. Aside from entertainment purposes, those aged 13–54 years in the USA use a majority of their smartphone time to socialize and interact with others, manage themselves including their health, and research information [82].

These developments have implications for psychiatrists. First, online messaging is required for providers caring for Medicare and Medicaid patients under federal electronic medical record guidelines as required by meaningful use stage 2 by 2014 [83]. In fact, the government's financial incentives and penalties program requires more than 5 % of unique patients to be sending secure messages to clinicians, thus incentivizing use of messaging. Although the general public may use e-mail, short-messaging service (SMS), and multiple-messaging service (MMS), these do not, by default, provide HIPAA-compliant encryption. Another surprising turn of events is the use of patient-centered Googling (PTG) and other Internet searches, in general, to resolve emergencies and to aid in forensic psychiatric evaluations [84]. Providers must weigh the value or risk for treatment [85]. Indeed, the patient's best interests must be kept in mind.

MH-related Internet-based services may be characterized in several categories: (1) Health information via sites (2) Support groups (i.e., general or specific topic) or participation in a "community" (3) Formal materials for patients (psychoeducation) and providers (professional education) (4) Tools for self-directed assessment and lifestyle (e.g., good habits/health promotion, disease prevention) (5) Decision-making on an illness or its management (e.g., diabetes, depression), one-time medical advice/consultation or general advice in a group led by a professional, self-directed formal treatment (e.g., Internet- or application-based follow-up assessment and engagement of treatment), and MH services with professionals (Internet-based CBT (ICBT)). The Internet may provide resources, connections, and meaningful activities for people with particular obstacles: geographic distance from services, those with special needs (i.e., autism-spectrum, sensory, and motor disabilities), the housebound (i.e., physical or MH like panic disorder or phobias), and of particular generations (i.e., teenagers).

1.3.3   Social Media Communication

The advantages for social media are disseminating health information and connecting healthcare with the general public. Child and adolescent populations—known as digital natives—are more adept at using social media, and this may destigmatize mental health issues. Users seek credible sources of reliable information that are personalized and maintain their anonymity and confidentiality. More treatments are being done by mobile phones [86]. Social networks also enhance social connectedness: cancer survivors [87], new mothers' well-being [88], and older adult users and the elderly with family and friends [89]. Social networks also provide an access point for those reluctant to seek help in person. For instance, 33 % of soldiers unwilling to speak to an in-person counselor were willing to use technology-based social networks for mental healthcare [90]. Of young college students, 68 % indicated they would use the Internet for mental health support and 94 % of participants with mental illnesses used social networking sites [91].

Caution with social media is also in order. A patient's expression of suicidal intent may be left otherwise unannounced as a post on a provider's "wall" or in an inbox of e-mails. Literature is limited, but some preliminary guidelines discuss concerns about patient privacy, confidentiality, and expectations (e.g., Facebook or other visits between appointments) and providers' professionalism (e.g., friending on Facebook, use of texting) [77, 92–96]. The timing (i.e., e-mails should be sent during regular working hours to attend to expectation and boundary issues) and the style (e.g., synchronous written or e-mail language does not have verbal pitch modulations, change in volume, ability to pause, and nonverbal information) of communication are delicate [77].

International and US guidelines have emerged for use of social media. The American College of Physicians released a comprehensive overview of physician online professionalism, including the following recommendations [96], focusing on communication with patients, gathering information, online education, and other topics. Overall, providers should maintain professionalism, follow institutional policies, assume that all information exchanged is public, enhance informed consent, pay attention to how people interact, and enable and empower others [97]. Guidelines are available for addressing youth patients and addressing privacy issues. Additional ethics codes from the American Medical Association, American Psychological Association, American Counseling Association, and the American Psychiatric Association are available.

1.3.4 Program and Administration Approaches to Evaluation, Legal Issues, and Reimbursement Issues

Organizational leadership and program evaluation has become increasingly important to meet program, patient, provider, and externally driven (e.g., Joint Commission, reimbursement) needs—it is key to preserve the standard of care and employ best practices. Assessment typically includes satisfaction, technology, cost, clinical measures, and process of care with an iterative feedback loop for quality improvement. Programs must contend with more basic issues in the USA and other countries with similar economies—credentialing, licensing, confidentiality, privacy, malpractice, and reimbursement.

Financial feasibility is key for those countries with more stability, socialized or capitalized healthcare, and an electronic platform—usually assessed based on technical cost, patient volume, appointment adherence, payment model (e.g. payment for time, whether one shows or not), patient mix in terms of complexity, payer(s) mix, and other issues. Studies are now being conducted using economic modeling, clinical encounter costing and data sets, healthcare reform, healthcare costs with changes in health risks among employers of all sizes, and prototypes of existing health systems (e.g., Veterans Affairs).

The use of eMH in the Middle East (ME) may be a good example of some of the main struggles of programs across the world. The ME is a heterogeneous part of the world with certain variations in MH services. The spectrum includes countries that have very good (e.g., Israel), fair (e.g., Turkey, Iran, Saudi Arabia), or poor (e.g., Iraq, Syria) services. Given the disparities, there is a need to implement eMH in the ME, but there are only 3 reports of randomized controlled trials related to eMH, which were done in Turkey, Israel, and Iraq, which focus on effectiveness, psychoeducation, and the doctor-patient working alliance [34–36].

1.4   eMH Benefits to Patients, Providers, and Systems of Care: Access, Versatility, and Empowerment

1.4.1   Patient Benefits

eMH has had four primary impacts for patients: (1) better access (many sites including home and primary care); (2) evidence-based psychosocial treatments per their preference; (3) empowerment, in the form of choice, access, and incentive to participate; and (4) ability to engage providers, clinics, or systems more directly (e.g., web based, texting, Relay Health). Service points are theoretically limitless: clinics, emergency rooms, patients' homes, nursing homes, homeless shelters, hospices, schools, forensic facilities, and at the battlefront. For example, one significant advantage of telepsychiatry has been improved access to psychiatric care in rural, suburban, and urban areas [70]. Indeed, eMH sometimes is better than in-person care as previously mentioned [13]. Child and adolescent [98] and other populations have been greatly served, including with asynchronous telepsychiatry [99].

Important questions remain—some of these are acutely sensitive to MH issues. While the buffet of informal or self-directed services is increasing, one question is, "If the person or patient is in care, should this be overseen by a professional, and if so, how?" "Can we assume the person or patient will plug in and get where they need to go or find the best service for them?" For persons with MH issues, symptoms, and disorders, a key question is, "What if someone's awareness/perspective is diminished or "lost" (in formal psychiatric wording, capacity; in legal wording, competence) such that insight on the what, how, when, and why components of decision-making suggests additional informal (i.e., family, Internet) or formal (i.e., primary care or MH clinician) advice and direction?"

1.4.2   Provider Benefits

Providers in primary care have had better access to telespecialists, including telepsychiatrist by phone, e-mail, texting, and consultation by STP or ATP. This has facilitated matching patients to specific treatments (e.g., psychotherapy instead of meds, medication augmentation) and correct diagnosis (one study changed it 91 % of the time, and with medication changes in 57 % of the time, significant clinical improvements occurred in 56 % of the patients) [70]. Furthermore, provider knowledge and skills improve over time [100] particularly in rural PCPs [101, 102]—this impact is direct to the provider for the patient seen and indirect to the population that the provider serves. Telemedicine has also offered formal training (e.g., guided laryngoscopic evaluation with the specialist at distance) and "on the fly" (e.g., pediatric intensivist helps a rural provider with a code when there is inadequate time to transfer even with helicopter). A review of effectiveness of video-based tele-education showed high satisfaction and that it is equivalent or better than in-person education, in terms of knowledge acquisition and integration [103]. Coaching via telehealth [104] and clinical procedural assistance is on the rise [105].

Medical and nursing education continues to evolve in terms of skills, competencies, attitude, and other foci in addition to knowledge [106]. Aside from the "core" nursing training, there may be a need for additional training in technology, teamwork, healthcare systems, and changing roles/"hats," depending on what is "needed." Technology is already a target area for skill development—both using and being a leader in implementation—using simulated patients at a distance to teach general nursing skills, how to work as part of a team, how to gain experience in work settings previously unfamiliar to them, and how to get on the same page across disciplines (i.e., how to develop shared mental models) for the care of a patient [105]. This reduces potential misunderstanding among large teams and creates a shared mental model of expectation, roles, and outcomes [107]. Shared mental models will also enhance team performance by their organizing knowledge structures, concepts, and associations around education [108].

Finally, we may be at a tipping point in two dimensions. First, eMH may change our clinical framework and approach to healthcare to a new way to practice—one with in-person, Internet-based, and other virtual care [109], particularly if care for depression and attention deficit/hyperactivity disorder [76, 110] is better at a distance than usual care. Second, will there be a new standard of practice? Patients are getting health information, using support groups, going through formal training, use tools for care, self-manage their condition, and use Internet- or application-based treatment. So again, with the buffet of services increasing, the question is, "If the person or patient is in care, should this be overseen by a professional, and if so, how?"

1.4.3 Healthcare Systems and Administration

Healthcare is being confronted with questions on how to deliver quality, affordable, and timely care to patients in a variety of settings [111]. Increased clinical operating efficiency gets the clinician with expertise to the point of service and emphasizes teamwork for clinical, administrative, and informal care coordination. Specifically, this involves many disciplines working at the "top of one's license." For psychiatry, this is facilitated by having non-MD MH professionals seeing the less complex cases and reserving the psychiatrist's direct clinical time judiciously; this may include management of more complicated cases or providing clinical oversight and review of cases seen by others.

eMH may soon reshape healthcare service delivery, particularly as telepsychiatry appears better for some disorders and models of care are better than traditional in-person or usual care approaches (e.g., depression and attention deficit/hyperactivity disorder) [76, 110]. Clinicians are already adapting to "hybrid" models of care with in-person and virtual assessment and treatment [109, 112]. New "hybrid care models" employ in-person and technology-based care [109, 112] and, by implication, multiple levels of technological complexity (i.e., from low-intensity e-mail and phone to high-intensity videoconferencing).

1.5   Discussion and Conclusion

Patient- or person-centered healthcare confronts us with questions on how to deliver quality, affordable, and timely care—around the globe. Telemedicine empowers patients, increases administrative efficiency, and ensures expertise gets to the place it is most needed—the patient. Telepsychiatry is effective, well accepted, and comparable to in-person care. As we employ technology, we must maintain high-quality clinical care and professional standards and be sensitive to differences in participants. Good program evaluation attends to clinical, legal, reimbursement, and the variable technological issues. Models of care, patient-centered approaches, and an e-platform for services are steering eMH services forward from in-person to videoconferencing to other ways of digital engagement. Online innovation disseminates more information, facilitates traditional treatments, and may add opportunities for new treatments.

Regulatory divergences (the USA versus Europe, Australia, the Middle East, and the rest of the world) determine how quickly regulatory decisions are reached and consequently result in huge differences in current state of the eMH development and adoption around the globe. Four main barriers to implementation are cultural, technical (e.g., electricity and Internet access), financial, and regulatory [37]. There are no regulations or legislations that guide such practices, and fear of political persecution is a unique threat to eMH in general and patients' acceptance of it [38]. The process of building an eMH there would require regulation, legislation, and a parallel reconstruction of the medicolegal system to allow for more considerate approach to sensitive ethical concepts such as confidentiality, informed consent, and liability.

Finally, we may be at a tipping point in two dimensions. First is the hybrid model of in-person, Internet-based, and other virtual care [109]. Second, will there be a new standard of practice? Patients are getting health information, using support groups, going through formal training, use tools for care, self-manage their condition, and use Internet- or application-based treatment. So again, with the buffet of services increasing, the question is, "If the person or patient is in care, should this be overseen by a professional, and if so, how?" This would require new terminology relative to the following areas: (1) PCMH would apply in part, but it denotes a patient (not a person) and a central contextualization of disease and traditional healthcare services; (2) mobile health would apply in part, but it is defined as the practice of medicine and public health supported by mobile devices; and (3) connected care may apply in part but is defined as the real-time, electronic communication between a patient and a provider, including telehealth, remote patient monitoring, and secure e-mail communication.

References

1. Institute of Medicine. 28 Feb 2015. At: http://www.iom.edu/~/media/Files/Report%20 Files/2001/Crossing-the-Quality-Chasm/Quality%20Chasm%202001%20%20report%20 brief.pdf.
2. Council LS, Geffken D, Valeras AB, et al. A medical home: changing the way patients and teams relate through patient-centered care plans. Fam Syst Health. 2012;30:190–8.

3. Miles A, Mezzich J. The care of the patient and the soul of the clinic: person-centered medicine as an emergent model of modern clinical practice. Int J Pers Centered Med. 2011;1(2):207–22.
4. Ekman I, Swedberg K, Taft C, et al. Person-centered care—ready for prime time. Eur J Cardiovasc Nurs. 2011;10(4):248–51.
5. Sturmberg JP, et al. Health care frames – from Virchow to Obama and beyond: the changing frames in health care and their implications for patient care. J Eval Clin Pract. 2014;20(6): 1036–44.
6. World Health Organization. Telemedicine opportunities and developments in member states. Results of the second global survey on eHealth. Geneva: WHO Press; 2011.
7. Crabtree BF, Nutting PA, Miller WL, et al. Summary of the National Demonstration Project and recommendations for the patient-centered medical home. Ann Fam Med. 2010;8 Suppl 1:80–90.
8. Jackson GL, Powers BJ, Chatterjee R, et al. The patient-centered medical home: a systematic review. Ann Intern Med. 2013;158(3):169–78.
9. Elfeddali I, van der Feltz-Cornelis CM, van Os J, et al. Horizon 2020 priorities in clinical mental health research: results of a consensus-based ROAMER expert survey. Int J Environ Res Public Health. 2014;11(10):115–39.
10. Osborn R, et al. International survey of older adults finds shortcomings in access, coordination, and patient-centered care. Health Aff (Millwood). 2014;33(12):2247–55.
11. Cohen S, Yu W. The concentration and persistence in the level of health expenditures over time: estimates for the US population, Agency for Healthcare Research and Quality, 2008–2009 [Statistical Brief No. 354]. 28 Feb 2015. At: http://meps.ahrq.gov/mepsweb/data_files/publications/st354/stat354.pdf.
12. Hilty DM, Ferrer D, Callahan EJ, et al. The effectiveness of telemental health: a 2013 review. Telemed J E Health. 2013;19(6):444–54.
13. Hilty DM, Yellowlees PM, Chan S, et al. Telepsychiatry: effective, evidence-based and at a tipping point in healthcare delivery. Psych Clin N Am. In Press.
14. Davis MH, Everett A, Kathol R, et al. American Psychiatric Association ad hoc work group report on the integration of psychiatry and primary care, 2011. 28 Feb 2015. At: http://naapimha.org/wordpress/media/Integration-of-Psychiatry-and-Primary-Care.pdf.
15. Hollingsworth JM, et al. Specialty care and the patient-centered medical home. Med Care. 2011;49(1):4–9.
16. Cluver JS, Schuyler D, Frueh BC, et al. Remote psychotherapy for terminally ill cancer patients. J Telemed Telecare. 2005;11:157–9.
17. Hilty DM, Green J, Nasatir-Hilty SE, et al. Mental healthcare to rural and other underserved primary care settings: benefits of telepsychiatry, integrated care, stepped care and interdisciplinary team models. J Nursing Care. In Press.
18. Entman RM. Framing: toward clarification of a fractured paradigm. J Commun. 1993;43(4): 51–8.
19. Chong D, Druckman JN. Framing theory. Ann Rev of Political Sci. 2007;10:103–26.
20. Tversky A, Kahneman D. Loss aversion in riskless choice: a reference-dependent model. Q J Econ. 1991;106(4):1039–61.
21. Levin IP, Schneider SL, Gaeth GJ. All frames are not created equal: a typology and critical analysis of framing effects. Organizational Behav Human Decis Proc. 1998;76(2):149–88.
22. Rajkumar S, Hoolahan B. Remoteness and issues in mental health care: experiences from rural Australia. Epideniologia Psichiatr Soc. 2004;13:78–82.
23. Moffatt JJ, Eley DS. The reported benefits of telehealth for rural Australians. Aust Health Rev. 2010;34:276–81.
24. Griffiths L, Blignault I, Yellowlees P. Telemedicine as a means of delivering cognitive-behavioural therapy to rural and remote mental health clients. J Telemed Telecare. 2006;12(3):136–40.
25. Saurman E, et al. Assessing program efficiency: a time and motion study of the mental health emergency care - rural access program in NSW Australia. Int J Environ Res Public Health. 2014;11(8):78–89.

26. Mallen JM, Vogel DL, Rochlen AB, et al. Online counseling: reviewing the literature from a counseling psychology framework. Counsel Psychol. 2005;33(6):819–71. At http://www. researchgate.net/...Counseling/.../00b7d53c017b765594000000.pdf.
27. Kids Help Line, 1-800-551-1800, Mass Media Studio, Australia. 28 Feb 2015. At: http://www.kidshelp.com.au.
28. Urness D, Wass M, Gordon A, et al. Client acceptability and quality of life–telepsychiatry compared to in-person consultation. J Telemed Telecare. 2006;12(5):251–4.
29. Simms DC, Gibson K, O'Donnell S. To use or not to use: clinicians' perceptions of telemental health. Can Psychol Psychologie Canadienne. 2011;52(1):41–51.
30. Volpe T, Boydell KM, Pignatiello A. Mental health services for Nunavut children and youth: evaluating a telepsychiatry pilot project. Rural Remote Health. 2014;14(2):2673.
31. Statistics Canada. Mortality rates among children and teenagers living in Inuit Nunangat, 1994 to 2008. 28 Feb 2015. At: http://www.statcan.gc.ca/pub/82-003-x/2012003/article/11695-eng.htm.
32. Pignatiello A, Boydell KM, Teshima J, et al. Transforming child and youth mental health via innovative technical solutions. Healthc Q. 2011;14(2):92–102.
33. Sunderji N, Crawford A, Jovanovic M. Telepsychiatry in graduate medical education: a narrative review. Acad Psychiatry. 2015;39(1):55–62.
34. Modai I, Jabarin M, Kurs R, et al. Cost effectiveness, safety, and satisfaction with video telepsychiatry versus face-to-face care in ambulatory settings. Telemed J E Health. 2006;12:515–20.
35. Ozkan B, et al. Effect of psychoeducation and telepsychiatric follow up given to the caregiver of the schizophrenic patient on family burden, depression and expression of emotion. Pak J Med Sci. 2013;29:1122–7.
36. Wagner B, Brand J, Schulz W, et al. Online working alliance predicts treatment outcome for posttraumatic stress symptoms in Arab war-traumatized patients. Depress Anxiety. 2012;29:646–51.
37. Jefee-Bahloul H. Telemental health in the Middle East: overcoming the barriers. Front Public Health. 2014;2:86.
38. Jefee-Bahloul H, et al. Pilot assessment and survey of Syrian refugees' psychological stress and openness to referral for telepsychiatry (PASSPORT Study). Telemed J E Health. 2014;20(10):977–9.
39. Mastermind. 28 Feb 2015. At http://www.southdenmark.com/showcases/terapi-hjemme-i-dagligstuen.aspx/.
40. Mucic D. Telepsychiatry in Denmark: mental health care in rural and remote areas. J E Health Technol Appl. 2007;5(3):426. 28 Feb 2015. At: http://dx.doi.org/10.1016/j.eurpsy.2007.01.1163.
41. Mucic D. International telepsychiatry: a study of patient acceptability. J Telemed Telecare. 2008;14:241–3.
42. De Las CC, Arredondo MT, Cabrera MF, et al. Randomized clinical trial of telepsychiatry through videoconference versus face-to-face conventional psychiatric treatment. Telemed J E Health. 2006;12(3):341–50.
43. Norman S. The use of telemedicine in psychiatry. J Psychiatr Ment Health Nurs. 2006;13(6):771–7.
44. Bose U, McLaren P, Riley A, et al. The use of telepsychiatry in the brief counselling of non-psychotic patients from an inner-London general practice. J Telemed Telecare. 2001;7 Suppl 1:8–10.
45. McLaren P, Ahlbom J, Riley A, et al. The North Lewisham telepsychiatry project: beyond the pilot phase. J Telemed Telecare. 2002;8 Suppl 2:98–100.
46. Harley J. Economic evaluation of a tertiary telepsychiatry service to an island. J Telemed Telecare. 2006;12(7):354–7.
47. Saleem Y, Taylor MH, Khalifa N. Forensic telepsychiatry in the United Kingdom. Behav Sci Law. 2008;226(3):333–44.
48. Andersson G, Hesser H, Veilord A, et al. Randomised controlled non-inferiority trial with 3-year follow-up of internet-delivered versus face-to-face group cognitive behavioural therapy for depression. J Affect Disord. 2013;151(3):986–94.

49. Saint-Andre S, Neira Zalentein W, Robin D, et al. La telepsychiatrie au service de l'autisme (Telepsychiatry at the service of autism). Encéphale. 2011;37(1):18–24.
50. Kok G, Bockting C, Burger H, et al. Mobile cognitive therapy: adherence and acceptability of an online intervention in remitted recurrently depressed patients. Internet Interv. 2014; 1(2):65–73.
51. Riper H, Blankers M, Hadiwijaya H, et al. Effectiveness of guided and unguided low-intensity internet interventions for adult alcohol misuse: a meta-analysis. PLoS One. 2014;9(6), e99912. doi:10.1371/journal.pone.0099912.
52. Majumdar AK. Advances in telemedicine and its usage in India. 15th international conference on advanced computing and communications, IEEE. 2007. 28 Feb 2015. At: http://ieeexplore.ieee.org/xpl/articleDetails.jsp?reload=true&arnumber=4425958.
53. Rahman A. E-Mental health in Pakistan: a pilot study of training and supervision in child psychiatry using the Internet. Psychiatr Bull. 2006;30:149–52.
54. Mars M, Ramlall S, Kaliski S. Forensic telepsychiatry: a possible solution for South Africa? Afr J Psychiatry. 2012;15:244–7.
55. Wynchank S, Fortuin J. Telepsychiatry in South Africa – present and future. S Africa J Psychiatry. 2010;16(1). 28 Feb 2015. At http://www.ajol.info/index.php/sajpsyc/article/view/68822.
56. Buist A. Telepsychiatry in Australia. In: Wootten R, Yellowlees PM, McLaren P, editors. Telepsychiatry and e-mental health. Royal Society of Medicine Press, Ltd; London, UK. 2002.
57. Rosenthal TC. The medical home: growing evidence to support a new approach to primary care. J Am Board Fam Med. 2008;21(5):427–40.
58. Haaga DA. Introduction to the special section on stepped care models in psychotherapy. J Consult Clin Psychol. 2000;68:547–8.
59. van't Veer-Tazelaar N, van Marwijk H, van Oppen P, et al. Prevention of anxiety and depression in the age group of 75 years and over: A randomized controlled trial testing the feasibility and effectiveness of a generic stepped care program among elderly community residents at high risk of developing anxiety and depression versus usual care. BMC Public Health. 2006;1:186.
60. Yellowlees PM, Hogarth MA, Hilty DM. The development of distributed academic networks in America. Acad Psychiatry. 2006;30(6):451–5.
61. Frydman GJ. Patient-driven research: rich opportunities and real risks. J Participat Med. 2009;1(1):e12. 28 Feb 2015. At: http://ojs.jopm.org/index.php/jpm/article/view/28/18.
62. Frydman GJ. A patient-centric definition of participatory medicine, 2010. 28 Feb 2015. At: http://e-patients.net/archives/2010/04/a-patient-centric-definition-of-participatory-medicine.html.
63. Krist AH, et al. Engaging primary care patients to use a patient-centered personal health record. Ann Fam Med. 2014;12(5):418–26.
64. Whitteman HO, et al. User-centered design and the development of patient decision aids: protocol for a systematic review. Syst Rev. 2015;4(1):11.
65. Der Wees V, et al. Integrating the use of patient-reported outcomes for both clinical practice and performance measurement: views of experts from 3 countries. Milbank Q. 2014;92(4):754–75.
66. Hamann J, Leucht S, Kissling W. Shared decision making in psychiatry. Acta Psychiatr Scand. 2003;107(6):403–9.
67. Yellowlees PM, Shore JH, Roberts L, et al. Practice guidelines for videoconferencing-based telemental health. Telemed J E Health. 2010;16(10):1074–89.
68. Shore JH, Mishkind MC, Bernard J, et al. A lexicon of assessment and outcome measures for telemental health. Telemed J E Health. 2013;3:282–92.
69. Hilty DM, Yellowlees PM, Nasatir SEH, et al. Program evaluation and practical, step-by-step program modification in telemental health. Behavioral telehealth series volume 1- clinical video conferencing: program development and practice. Springer Press: New York, NY; 2014. pp. 105–134.
70. Hilty DM, Marks SL, Urness D, et al. Clinical and educational applications of telepsychiatry: a review. Can J Psychiat. 2004;49(1):12–23.
71. Hilty DM, Ingraham RL, Yang RP, et al. Multispecialty phone and email consultation to primary care providers for patients with developmental disabilities in rural California. Telemed J E Health. 2004;10:413–21.

72. Yellowlees PM, Marks SL, Hilty DM, et al. Using e-health to enable culturally appropriate mental health care in rural areas. Telemed J E Health. 2008;14(5):486–92.
73. Yellowlees PM, Odor A, Iosif A, et al. Transcultural psychiatry made simple: asynchronous telepsychiatry as an approach to providing culturally relevant care. Telemed J E Health. 2013;19(4):1–6.
74. Fortney JC, Pyne JM, Mouden SP, et al. Practice-based versus telemedicine-based collaborative care for depression in rural federally qualified health centers: a pragmatic randomized comparative effectiveness trial. Am J Psychiatr. 2013;170(4):414–25.
75. Richardson L, McCauley E, Katon W. Collaborative care for adolescent depression: a pilot study. Gen Hosp Psychiatr. 2009;31:36–45.
76. Myers KM, van der Stoep A, Zhou C, et al. Effectiveness of a telehealth service delivery model for treating attention-deficit hyperactivity disorder: results of a community-based randomized controlled trial. J Am Acad Child Adolesc Psychiatry. 2015;54(4):263–74.
77. Hilty DM, Belitsky R, Cohen MB, et al. Impact of the information age residency training: the impact of the generation gap. Acad Psychiatry. 2015;39(1):104–7.
78. APA Electronic Prescribing Guideline. 28 Feb 2015. At: http://www.psych.org/practice/managing-a-practice/electronic-prescribing.
79. DeJong SM, Benjamin S, Anzia JA, et al. Professionalism and the internet in psychiatry: what to teach and how to teach it. Acad Psychiatry. 2012;36(5):356–62.
80. Pew Research Center, 2013. 28 Feb 2015. At (Internet survey): http://www.pewinternet.org/~/media//Files/Reports/PIP_HealthOnline.pdf (or smart phone).
81. Fox S, Maeve D. Health online 2013. 28 Feb 2015. At: https://www.evernote.com/shard/s277/nl/36107944/281a93a5-fc31-4de9-a1df-76cfc7d2d33f/.
82. Harvard Business Review. How people really use mobile. 2013;91(1):30–31.
83. HealthIT.gov. Meaningful use definition & objectives. EHR incentives & certification, 2014. 28 Feb 2015. At: http://www.healthit.gov/providers-professionals/meaningful-use-definition-objectives.
84. Mossman D, Farrell HM. Facebook: social networking meets professional duty. Curr Psychiatry. 2012;11(3). 28 Feb 2015. At: http://www.currentpsychiatry.com/index.php?id=22661&tx_ttnews[tt_news]=176674.
85. Clinton BK, Silverman BC, Brendel DH. Patient-targeted googling: the ethics of searching online for patient information. Harv Rev Psychiatry. 2010;18(2):103–12.
86. Seko Y, Kidd S, Wiljer D, et al. Youth mental health interventions via mobile phones: a scoping review. Cyberpsychol Behav Soc Netw. 2014;17(9):591–602.
87. McLaughlin M, Nam Y, Gould J, et al. A videosharing social networking intervention for young adult cancer survivors. Comput Hum Behav. 2012;28(2):631–41.
88. McDaniel BT, et al. New mothers and media use: associations between blogging, social networking, and maternal well-being. Matern Child Health J. 2012;16(7):1509–17.
89. Sundar SS, Oeldorf-Hirsch A, Nussbaum J, et al. Retirees on Facebook: can online social networking enhance their health and wellness? In: CHI'11 extended abstracts on human factors in computing systems. ACM; 2011. pp. 2287–92.
90. Wilson JA, Onorati K, Mishkind M, et al. Soldier attitudes about technology-based approaches to mental health care. Cyberpsychol Behav. 2008;11(6):767–9.
91. Horgan A, Sweeney J. Young students' use of the internet for mental health information and support. J Psychiatr Ment Health Nurs. 2010;17(2):117–23.
92. Silk KR, Yager J. Suggested guidelines for E-mail communication in psychiatric practice. J Clin Psychiatry. 2003;64(7):799–806.
93. Frankish K, Ryan C, Harris A. Psychiatry and online social media: potential, pitfalls and ethical guidelines for psychiatrists and trainees. Australas Psychiatry. 2012;20:181–7.
94. Kane B, Sands DZ. Guidelines for the clinical use of electronic mail with patients. J Am Med Inform Assoc. 1998;5(1):104–11.
95. Koh S, Cattell GM, Cochran DM, et al. Psychiatrists' use of electronic communication and social media and a proposed framework for future guidelines. J Psychiatr Pract. 2013;19(3):254–63.
96. Farnan JM, Snyder Sulmasy L, et al. Online medical professionalism: patient and public relationships: policy statement from the American College of Physicians and the Federation of State Medical Boards. Ann Intern Med. 2013;158(8):620–7.

97. Grajales FJ, Sheps S, Ho K, et al. Social media: a review and tutorial of applications in medicine and health care. J Med Internet Res. 2014;16(2), e13.
98. Myers KM, Vander Stoep A, McCarty CA, et al. Child and adolescent telepsychiatry: variations in utilization, referral patterns and practice trends. J Telemed Telecare. 2010;16:128–33.
99. Yellowlees PM, Odor A, Patrice K, et al. PsychVACS: a system for asynchronous telepsychiatry. Telemed J E Health. 2011;17(4):299–303.
100. Hilty DM, Yellowlees PM, Cobb HC, et al. Models of telepsychiatric consultation-liaison service to rural primary care. Psychosomatics. 2006;47(2):152–7.
101. Hilty DM, Yellowlees PM, Nesbitt TS. Evolution of telepsychiatry to rural sites: change over time in types of referral and PCP knowledge, skill, and satisfaction. Gen Hosp Psychiatry. 2006;28(5):367–73.
102. Hilty DM, Nesbitt TS, Kuenneth TA, et al. Telepsychiatric consultation to primary care: rural vs. suburban needs, utilization and provider satisfaction. J Rural Health. 2007;23(2):163–5.
103. Chipps J, et al. A systematic review of the effectiveness of videoconference-based tele-education for medical and nursing education. Worldviews Evid Based Nurs. 2012;9(2):78–87.
104. Young H, et al. Sustained effects of a nurse coaching intervention via telehealth to improve health behavior change in diabetes. Telemed J E Health. 2014;20(9):828–34.
105. Rutledge CM, Haney T, Bordelon M, et al. Telehealth: preparing advanced practice nurses to address healthcare needs in rural and underserved populations. Int J Nurs Educ Scholarsh. 2014;11(1):1–9.
106. Armstrong EG, Mackey M, Spear SJ. Medical education as a process management problem. Acad Med. 2004;79(8):721–8.
107. Ross S, Allen N. Examining the convergent validity of shared mental model measures. Behav Res. 2012;44:1052–62.
108. Langan-Fox J, Code S, Langfield-Smith K. Team mental models: techniques, methods, and analytic approaches. Hum Factors. 2000;42:242–71.
109. Hilty DM, Yellowlees PM. Collaborative mental health services using multiple technologies – the new way to practice and a new standard of practice? J Am Acad Child Adolesc Psychiatry 2015 Apr;54(4):245-6. doi: 10.1016/j.jaac.2015.01.017.
110. Fortney JC, et al. Telemedicine-based collaborative care for posttraumatic stress disorder: a randomized clinical trial. JAMA Psychiatry. 2015;72(1):58–67.
111. Akinci F, Patel PM. Quality improvement in healthcare delivery utilizing the patient-centered medical home model. Hosp Topics. 2014;92(4):96–104.
112. Yellowlees PM, Nafiz N. The psychiatrist-patient relationship of the future: anytime, anywhere? Harv Rev Psychiatry. 2010;18(2):96–102.

Entangled in the Web. Unexpected Events with New Technologies: Addiction, Consequences on Communication

2

Agnes Wrobel and Janusz Wrobel

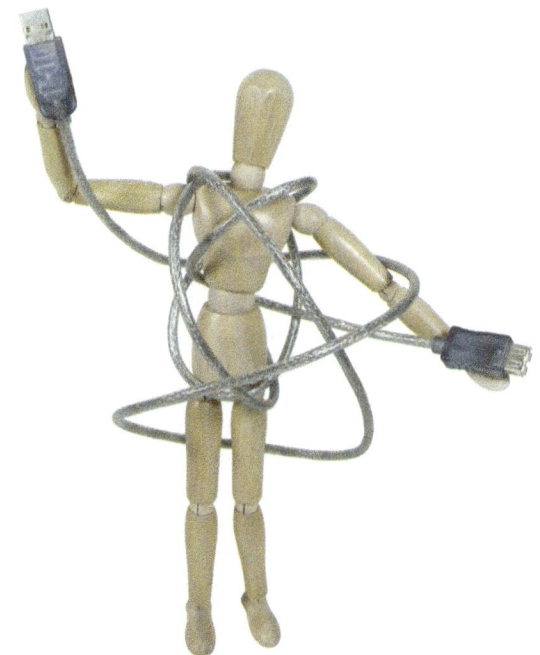

A. Wrobel, MD
Department of Psychiatry, John D Dingell VA Medical Center, Detroit, MI, USA

Wayne State University, Detroit, MI, USA
e-mail: agawrobel@yahoo.com

J. Wrobel, PhD (✉)
Department of International Studies, Balance & Harmony Counseling, LLC, Troy, MI, USA

Oakland University, Rochester, MI, USA
e-mail: obtainbalance@yahoo.com

© Springer International Publishing Switzerland 2016
D. Mucic, D.M. Hilty (eds.), *e-Mental Health*,
DOI 10.1007/978-3-319-20852-7_2

Contents

2.1 Introduction 30
2.2 Technology: Brings Us Together and Life to Our Fingertips? 31
2.3 Science, Education, and Technology 32
2.4 Internet: Pitfalls and Cautions 34
    2.4.1 When Technology Fails 34
    2.4.2 We Save Time (or Not Really?) 34
    2.4.3 Anonymity 35
    2.4.4 Communication Without Context 35
    2.4.5 Technology "Changes" the "What" and "How" 36
    2.4.6 "Orwell's 1984" Revisited 37
2.5 Discussion 37
    2.5.1 Hazards That Affect Mental Well-Being 38
Conclusions 39
2.6 Summary 39
References 40

Abstract

About 20 years ago, the idea of instant communication on massive scale became a reality. Today, the Internet is one the most powerful instruments in the hands of human race that is crucial in fulfilling vital elements of our daily tasks. The Internet created unthinkable opportunities, of which the phenomenon of telepsychiatry (the topic of this book) is one of the examples. It is ironic, however, that such web-based kind of treatment can be used in treating one of the dangerous side effects of applying this new technology, namely, the Internet addiction. *OBJECTIVES*: (1) Discussion of the advantages of the Internet. (2) Exploration of the negative social consequences of malicious misuse of the Internet. (3) Examination of physiological and psychological negative side effects of abuse of the Internet. *RESULTS*: Ad (1) The following are the advantages of the use of the Internet: revolutionary increase in opportunities to disseminate, share, obtain, accumulate, and store information and interpersonal contacts. Ad (2) The major disadvantages of the use of the Internet are deception (scams, cyber crimes, and smearing), manipulation of the public opinion, and the phenomenon of socially accepted and expected compromise of privacy to the point of exhibitionism. Ad (3) When it comes to physiological and psychological negative side effects of abuse of the Internet, the following are mentioned: atrophy of certain brain activities, submissiveness toward "tyranny of tiny tasks," and gradual decrease in face to face interpersonal communication which is being replaced by virtual anonymity.

2.1 Introduction

It was to be fast, effective, and practical; at least such hopes were triggered by the invention of the Internet – and it is. Thanks to the keyboard, writing an e-mail takes much less time than preparing a stationery, a pencil, an envelope, addressing it after finding information on the receiver's location, and putting a stamp. Additional precious minutes are saved because we do not have to make a trip to the mailbox nor post office. What is astonishing as well is the fact that later we do not have to wait for days or weeks in order for the person we sent it to, to receive it, and another chunk of time before we get the answer. Sure, there were telegrams available – in fact, we have checked how it works today. There is the American Telegram's Delivery Company which offers the next day hand delivery of telegrams. In the USA and Canada, the fee for the service is $22.95 plus .79¢ per word.

Now, in the free of charge Skyping era, it will be difficult for our younger readers to imagine that in the 1980s, in order to make a call from Poland to the USA, it had be arranged in advance with the local post office, which would contact the person in the USA to set up time for the conversation. When the day had come, we had to arrive to the post office where we would hear the public announcement: "America, the telephone booth number 7." Later, already during the conversation, we would be interrupted from time to time by the post office clerk who was asking in your telephone receiver: "Still talking? Still talking?" In the 1990s, it was already easier because it was possible to make overseas calls from the home telephone or even from the public telephone booth, but such a pleasure cost at least .50¢ per minute. Then the telephone cards "epoch" followed, which could be bought in many places, and thanks to that, the cost of international telephone connections was drastically lowered. Later yet, the cellular phones appeared. Finally, the Internet made the existence of *Skype* possible which not only is free, but also allows seeing the person with whom you are talking. In order to fully understand how revolutionary this progress is (from the necessity of visiting the post office in order to call somebody to watching him or her on the computer monitor or at the cellular phone) let us imagine that during the future *Skype*-like conversation we maybe will be able to touch and feel the smell of our telephone interlocutor – in other words, be physically present with such a person.

In this chapter, the reader will learn about:

1. The advantages of the Internet
2. The negative social consequences of malicious misuse of the Internet
3. Physiological and psychological negative side effects of abuse of the Internet

2.2 Technology: Brings Us Together and Life to Our Fingertips?

First radio, then later the TV possessed the unimaginable power of simultaneous reaching uncountable masses of the listeners or watchers at the same moment. Those who on the Halloween day in October 1938 were listening to the radio drama based on the book by Orson Welles *The War of the Worlds* experienced how powerful this ability was. The use of the radio and television created an opportunity of disseminating knowledge, delivering entertainment, but also issuing important messages, warnings, and emergency alerts. Today's users of *Twitter* (especially more popular politicians) have the opportunity to inform impressive number of people who are using the cell phones about important events at the moment when they are taking place.

The existence of social networks allows ill people to blog their fights against diseases, which became significant inspiration for others who experience the similar conditions. This led to creation of virtual support groups for people who have to deal with different types of challenges in their lives (i.e., the parents raising children with autism). In not as serious everyday life dimension, when we need to obtain some information (how to get rid of red wine spot on the white table cloth or effectively challenge ants in the kitchen), the most obvious thing to do, just after asking a grandmother about it, would be googling the answer.

For those who produce something, the use of the network opened the unknown potential of advertising different types of products. For those who are looking for them, it became an excellent source of finding them and an opportunity for looking for the best prices. For those who need things or services or have something to offer it created an unlimited platform of letting others know about it. For the charitable institutions, it gave a great chance for publicizing benevolent purposes and collecting resources for achieving them.

Today's lucky tourist, thanks to digital technology and the Internet, is able to share a link to Eiffel Tower pictures with hundreds of *Myspace* contacts by sending it directly from a Parisian bistro by an iPad instead of going through the time (and money) consuming process of developing pictures, printing them, and mailing out to the friends in order to share happy vacation's moments. Photographic documentation of important and less essential occasions is available without time and space limits on the social networks. Thanks to the common access to the Internet, the girl who was kidnapped 10 years ago (she was fifteen at that time) has been recently recognized on *Facebook* by her sister what finally led to the end of the suffering of the victim. Talking about criminal activities, let us mention about the computer registration of the perpetrators, which makes easier the policemen's job, because in their cars they have an access to the registry data with information content more impressive than those of the biggest traditional archives.

The new technologies do a good job serving society with navigation issues too. From time to time, our family would get lost during car trips despite the use of quite accurate maps. It took a child to come up with the idea of presenting us with the GPS to solve the problem. Us, the former skeptics, when it came to the use of the satellite type guidance, now cannot imagine traveling without it.

2.3 Science, Education, and Technology

It is really difficult to overestimate the benefits of the Internet in the domain of science. The Internet library available for everybody with an access to the net created the opportunity of entering not only very impressive data, research results, books, and articles, but also quite rare publications which in the past could be only reached in designated places in the form of microfilms.

The exchange of information and research effects does not require the physical presence anymore. We can attend overseas conferences from our homes thanks to the use of *Skype*. Teachers are able to teach the students online and share links with them illustrating the most recent progress in particular field. Students can watch the lectures, submit their assignments, interact with fellow students, and take quizzes and exams from their homes. The Internet breaks the barriers of a traditional teaching environment which requires all participants of the learning process to comply with the "HERE and NOW" requirement (synchronous type of education). The asynchronous communication allows instructors to reach learners who might be hundreds of miles away; creates a platform in which students are able to participate in forums devoted to particular topics by adding their own posts and/or commenting on others' submissions at different, convenient times; permits the teacher to devote individual attention to each student's needs, concerns, and questions. When one of the authors of this chapter participated in a training preparing him to teach his courses in an online setting, he was not only scared, but skeptical as well. It was difficult for him to imagine not facing the students in the class; he had concerns over effectiveness of his teaching, and worried about the value of the "open-book" exams. The practice of the web-teaching has changed his mind to the point in which when it comes to homework assignments for the students who are taught on campus, they are expected to be submitted on Moodle (e-teaching system used at Oakland University) what makes evaluating them much easier, and allows students to check their grades at any time. Interestingly enough, his concerns over testing students proved to be ungrounded – the average final grade for the same course taught online and on campus is similar.

When it comes to scholars, the Internet creates an unparalleled chance of the worldwide exchange of the creative thoughts and, related to them, hope for the acceleration of the positive effects of attempts to deal with many plagues which haunt us, including finding cures for illnesses. On the micro-scale level, computerization of the patient data allows the ER doctor immediate access to the history of the disease and results of many tests and exams of the patient who comes there in the middle of the night. As Chap. 3 of this book stresses, the telemental health model creates numerous opportunities for the improvement of the health care which relates to expanding accessibility to it, promoting prevention and when it comes to behavioral health allowing "Cadillac treatment" at a distance. As Hilty et al. indicated [1]:

> One significant advantage to telepsychiatry has been improving access to psychiatric care in urban, suburban, and rural areas, often by providing academic specialists to areas with provider shortages.

The results of a study of 200 telepsychiatric consultations [2] showed a high level of satisfaction among psychiatrists who performed them; the average level of positive experience was 6.6 on a scale of 1 to 8 (the highest score).

The Internet removes work barriers created by inability of physical reach of an office, a store, or the bank. The life of those who are able to use this opportunity is much easier – they can buy, return taxes, do banking, including making payments by the use of the computer. Thanks to the communicative net, many people can work or look for a job from home, and can use it for entertaining purposes such as watching shows and movies from all around the world. They are also able to establish contact with the unknown people or even, with the use of dating portals, find candidates for husbands or wives.

Those are only few out of many more positive aspects of the use of the technological revolution in the field of communication. Let us now take a closer look at the price that we have to pay for the described above benefits.

2.4   Internet: Pitfalls and Cautions

It was to be fast, effective, and practical; at least such hopes were triggered by the invention of the Internet whereas we found out that despite incredible opportunities, the use of the net may lead to many serious inconveniences, or even dangers. The following is the review of some of them.

2.4.1   When Technology Fails

Let us start with writing letters. In the past, writing one was a time-consuming chore; today, preparing it and sending in an electronic form takes couple of minutes or even less. However, as Wu [3] aptly noticed in his article *The Problem with Easy Technology* it does not always work for us:

> Our technologies may have made us prosthetic gods, yet they have somehow failed to deliver on the central promise of free time. The problem is that, as every individual task becomes easier, we demand much more of both ourselves and others. Instead of fewer difficult tasks (writing several long letters) we are left with a larger volume of small tasks (writing hundreds of e-mails). We have become plagued by a tyranny of tiny tasks, individually simple but collectively oppressive.

2.4.2   We Save Time (or Not Really?)

In reality, saving time became an illusion. Instead of accumulating it, we spend more of it, when compulsively, several times per day, we first check than respond to dozens of e-mails. The proud owner of an e-mail address may expect to receive enormous amount of e-mail letters daily of which the majority of them are advertisements (*spam*). From time to time, we can get an electronic chain letter sent to us by the horrified friend (*Tim Smith has not sent this letter immediately to fifteen persons, so on the third day his right leg was amputated, and after 14 days he died*). Sometimes a good soul would warn us about the message encouraging *see the attached birthday card sent to you by your friend*, which in fact carries a virus that just in a moment may damage all the data on the hard disk. These are just a few among many possible scenarios.

2.4.3 Anonymity

Distant communication, without personal contact, creates a new quality of discourse in which its participants, or the sender and receiver of the message, may but not have to reveal their true identity. Anonymity, a possibility of claiming a false name, age, or gender, or using a virtual avatar is used in the net by people who want to achieve their dishonest, vile, or malicious goals. Too many times a young girls' cyber friend, who she believes is a teenage boy, is in reality an adult man with foul intentions. One of the mechanisms preventing people from acting on their repugnant impulses or temptations is the fear of being recognized, and in consequence, being punished or at least publicly stigmatized. Hiding behind the mask or even using several different individualities leads to a situation in which such a person does not feel like taking responsibility for his/her actions (because it is not him/her, etc).

When we really think about the nature of the Internet communication, we come to the conclusion that when reading an e-mail message, theoretically we cannot be fully sure who sent it to us. The same uncertainty is true when it comes to the person who is a receiver of our messages. It only takes hacking of our user profile in order for somebody being able on our behalf to send a request for a financial assistance to all our contacts under the pretext of us being allegedly in a dramatic situation. Examples include allegedly losing our wallet, having passport and our credit card stolen during the trip abroad. In a more innocent scenario, it would be publicizing under auspices of our identity an advertisement of the weight loss medication (less embarrassing) or increasing sexual potency (more reprehensible). Despite everything being said, we have no choice: we are sentenced for using the net at work, and in contacts with our family and friends. It is really sad that instead of interacting with a real person we look at the cold light of the computer screen. Let us quote a fragment of the book by Wrobel [4]:

> Faceless and eyeless others offer unimaginable chances for exchange of information, but award no opportunity for contact. Looking at computer/telephone screens, "talking" to virtual electronic partners, texting or tweeting them, taking an ephemeral break only to listen to a voice mail and to read a routine, incoming fax, slowly but surely, we may transform ourselves into communicative robots. (p.34)

2.4.4 Communication Without Context

Unfortunately, more troublesome questions appear: we are not only uncertain who we communicate with, but now, more frequently we experience the fear of being used by the others. Is this request for a financial support for the treatment of cancer a scam? Did we become a victim of identity theft when providing our Social Security number (and we have experienced it because somebody used one of our numbers filling his/her tax return)? Is this demand for verification of the password an attempt to wangle it from us? Virtuality is expanding at the cost of reality and the side effect is the raise of uncertainty, suspiciousness, and lack of security. The result is that the "mechanics of trust" undergoes a dramatic change because anonymity, unfortunately, promotes deceit. On the other hand, a personal communication, face-to-face type, builds trust faster and more effectively.

2.4.5   Technology "Changes" the "What" and "How"

As we have already mentioned, e-Mental Health creates new opportunities for providing the needed assistance to the patients and clients, but certain worries related to telepsychiatry were expressed as well. McLaren et al. [5] pointed out that important non-verbal cues are often missed during videoconferences. Hilty et al. [1] indicated that signal delays typical of equipment which is not of state-of-the-art quality causes a turn-taking conversation problem. Overall, the psychiatrists concerns with e-Mental Health were summarized by Hilty et al. [1] in the following way:

> Concerns surfaced about: technical problems (e.g. unclear picture, video freeze); decreased ease with the process; decreased ability to express oneself; and poorer quality of the interpersonal relationship.

The following is another, quite disturbing question related to so common use of the Internet: what happened to our privacy? It happens that the writers had unfortunate, personal experiences with the time when the part of Europe was under the Soviet thumb and remember well the fear of surveillance orchestrated by the secret police or the anxiety caused by the possibility that the neighbor is an informer and reports on our activities. Thirty years later, we would still sometimes speculate that there was not a Mark Zuckerberg behind the *Facebook* invention, but a "big brother" or secret agents because they do not have to spy, monitor, and eavesdrop anymore, etc. Our willingness of informing the whole world about our whereabouts, with whom, what, when, and how many times we are doing certain things, makes government's spying unnecessary. We live in a world of socially accepted and widespread exhibitionism – everybody may become a celebrity under condition of having a habit of making public announcements of whom one dates, how often, and how seriously she argues/breaks up/reunite with her partner. The paradox of this phenomenon comes from the fact that matters which we would not be willing to discuss in a group of six people, are announced to hundreds of "friends" on *Facebook* in hope of getting the widest possible approval. In this way, we became the Fausts of the twenty-first century who traded with the devil the intimacy for "I like" marks.

The fact of having dozens, if not hundreds, of friends has to lead to a superficial, hackneyed communication which is focused on spectacular effect that is to lead to the wide acceptance and appreciation. We have created the informative bazaar where everything is for sale and all sale gimmicks are allowed. Authenticity is a major victim here, and the biggest winner is the appearance.

2.4.6   "Orwell's 1984" Revisited

Our use of cellular phone and satellite navigation allow the governmental agencies not only to track our location, but as the recent scandal surveillance scandal revealed by Snowden [6], to record our telephone conversation. Because today's smart phones store an impressive amount of information about us, it is very important that our privacy related to their use is protected. Fortunately, it was recognized by the recent U.S. Supreme Court decision.

> The Wednesday [June 26, 2014 - J.W.] Supreme Court decision of Riley v. California isn't just a landmark ruling on cell phone privacy. It also represents a dramatic shift in the high court's attitude toward technology and privacy. The Supreme Court's new attitude is best summarized by a single sentence in the opinion. The government had argued that searching a cell phone is no different from searching other items in a suspect's pocket. That, the court wrote, "is like saying a ride on horseback is materially indistinguishable from a flight to the moon." [7]

2.5   Discussion

It is true that the Internet makes it possible to get many things done without leaving home, but when we are visiting the post office we have an interaction with a person, not a machine. Going to the bank creates an opportunity to exchange some words with a man who assists us, buying a plane ticket in a tourist agency is connected with having a conversation on our vacation plans. By choosing the faster and easier way, we shut the prospect of the interactions with people who were taking care of us. Of course, the computer type way will be "faster and easier," but only under condition that we own an alphabetical notebook of all passwords where, among dozens of sophisticated codes we can identify the one for the postal services, the one for the bank, that one we should use when buying a discount ticket, etc. A similar situation happens when it comes to pictures. In the past, we had significantly less of them, but at least we possessed them in a physical way. Today, we are alleged owners of thousands of pictures (we do not have to worry about the costs of the film and developing of it) but in most cases they are somewhere in the computer's memory instead of sitting in a photo album that at least from time to time is watched.

Practically unlimited possibility of publishing everything by everybody leads sometimes to violation of privacy, to posting comments which are offensive, rude, or falsified, but accessible to all web users. In extreme situations, like posting telephone made videos that document sexual harassment of underage girls by their male colleagues, we have to deal with suicidal deaths of the victims who were not able to carry the stigma of shame.

It is true that the Internet is the well of knowledge, but is it always the objective one? Many, among popular news sites, post information that is carefully selected in the way that is to direct opinion of the readers. They are either removed from the context or presented in a selective way, and despite the fact that they are true, because the other news events are ignored, they say only a part of the truth and in this way manipulate the reader's way of thinking.

We have already mentioned how computerization expanded abilities and range of the influence of science, including medicine. Are we, however, fully aware of what may happen when there will be a serious shortage of power or when terrorists will get an access to most vital centers of the computer management? The cover of the American magazine *The Week* [8] issued on May 30, 2014, announces: *World War 3.0. The U.S.'s new offensive against China's cyberthieves*, suggesting that all of us face dangers that are difficult to imagine.

2.5.1 Hazards That Affect Mental Well-Being

The danger does not come only from outside. When we rely too much on technological shortcuts, that is, in simple arithmetic, when instead of multiplying from memory or by the means of paper and pencil, we escape to the telephone calculator – in a longer range it leads to alarming phenomenon of biological atrophy about which the already mentioned Tim Wu writes. For our disadvantage, not only our mind becomes ponderous but our body as well; and mainly seating lifestyle promotes obesity, cardiovascular diseases, and type II diabetes.

Finally, how do we recognize that when it comes to the use of the Internet, we have already left the safe territory and entered into domain of addiction (see Chap. 14 which discusses pathological use of this technology)? Let us briefly formulate what creates the main criterion of addiction, based *DSM-5* [9] criteria (pp. 282–283) for gambling disorder (there is still no Internet related addiction officially defined). We are dealing with it when our activities negatively affect our functioning in society, at work, with family, and in contacts with others. If, for example, the amount of time which is spent by a young person on social network causes that there is a shortage of time when it comes to homework, test preparation, or leads to sleep deprivation and taking naps during classes, then we have a problem. If a child avoids going outside, meetings with friends, being active in sports because of the computer then we may suspect that it is the result of compulsion. If we plan to spend just one hour in front of the monitor, because it is the amount of time that we can afford, whereas three hours later we are still not where we should be, it means that it is not us anymore who decide about our activities. If watching pornography and masturbating in front of the computer screen translates first to negligence of intimacy with one's wife and later lack of either strength or will to have one, it means that the time has come to see a therapist. If thinking about using a computer prevents us from drawing pleasure from what we are doing at a given moment, if it does not allow to focus on conversation or the task we are conducting, it means that we have lost control over the Internet domain of our life. If, when in office, we cannot resist temptation of looking at the web-page that excites us despite knowing that somebody can notice it and, as result, we can lose our job, if we are not able not to read and answer the text while driving and being fully aware of the danger of collision, then it means that we allowed technology that was to make our life easier to enslave us.

Conclusions

Inventions, including the Internet, create many opportunities for the human race but at the same time they bring a lot of dangers. However, we should realize that the effects of the scientific progress themselves, without the prime mover of their creator, and later customer, who starts using them for his/her beneficial or destructive purposes, are mostly neutral. It is us who give meaning to our lives and their instruments. Arsenic is very useful in production of glass, conservation of wood or in dentistry, but it is also a deadly poison. At the beginning of the twentieth century, the workers in despair were destroying machines because they had believed that they were taking jobs away from them. Today, thanks to robots and automatization, a "physical laborer" description less and less frequently reflects a situation in which a worker has to indeed use the strength of his muscles. Thanks to inventions, our daily tasks are less difficult and accomplishing them requires less time than in the past. Theoretically, we can have it more, under the condition that in front of temptation of more and more technologically sophisticated and spectacular but at the same time very possessive toys, we will have enough common sense not to allow them to enslave us.

2.6   Summary

The invention of the Internet creates enormous opportunities, and, at the same time, serious dangers. The paradox is that the similar qualities, depending on who is using them and for what purpose, could be turned either for our advantage or disadvantage. This chapter discusses the opposing views of several aspects of the use of the Internet focusing on ways in which it positively and negatively affects the life of those who depend on it.

The reasonable, balanced, and careful deployment of this technology led to revolutionary increase in opportunities to disseminate, share, obtain, accumulate, and store information and interpersonal contacts.

The abuse and malicious misuse of the Internet -and the instruments that operate thanks to it-result in many unfortunate phenomena: "tyranny of tiny tasks" related to the use of the e-mail technology, the Internet deception, which includes scams, cyber crimes, and smearing, that negatively affects the mechanics of trust, voluntary compromise of our privacy by the wide use of the social networking, the atrophy of certain brain activities because of choosing the technological shortcuts, manipulation of the public opinion, the phenomenon of the Internet addiction, and gradual decrease in face to face interpersonal communication which is being replaced by communing with the cyber gadgets.

References

1. Hilty DM, et al. Effects of telepsychiatry on the doctor-patient relationship: communication, satisfaction, and relevant issues. Primary Psychiatry. 2002;9:29–34.
2. Hilty DM, Yellowlees PM, Nesbitt TS. Evolution of telepsychiatry to rural sites: change over time in types of referral and PCP knowledge, skill, and satisfaction. Gen Hosp Psychiatry 2006;28(5):367–73.
3. Wu T. The problem with easy technology. Posted on The New Yorker blog "Elements" on February 25, 2014. http://www.newyorker.com/online/blogs/elements/2014/02/the-problem-with-easy-technology.html.
4. Wrobel J. Contact. The tale of human longing for fulfilling communication. San Diego: Wisdom Moon Publishing; 2013.
5. McLaren P, et al. An evaluation of the use of interactive television in an acute psychiatric service. J Telemed Telecare. 1995;1:79–85.
6. Snowden E. Here's how we take back the Internet. Posted on TED website on March 2014. http://www.ted.com/talks/edward_snowden_here_s_how_we_take_back_the_internet.
7. Lee TB. The most important sentence in the Supreme Court's cell phone privacy ruling. Posted on VOX.com website, on 26 June 2014. http://www.vox.com/2014/6/26/5843586/the-most-important-sentence-in-wednesdays-cell-phone-privacy-ruling.
8. Chinese hackers indicted for cybertheft. The editorial page (The main stories…). The Week. 2014;14(670):2.
9. Desk reference to the diagnostic criteria from DSM-5. Washington, DC: American Psychiatric Association; 2013.

Part II

Prevention, Early Detection and Health Promotion

Donald M. Hilty

e-Mental Health Improves Access to Care, Facilitates Early Intervention, and Provides Evidence-Based Treatments at a Distance

3

Erica Z. Shoemaker and Donald M. Hilty

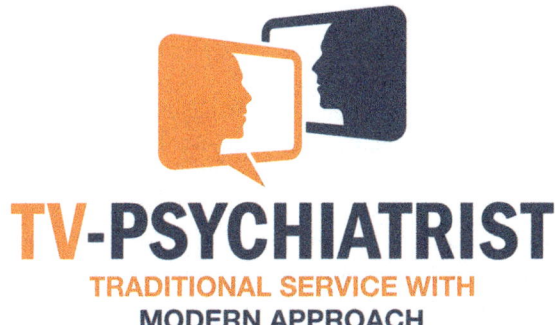

Contents

3.1	Introduction	44
3.2	Access and Service Delivery	45
	3.2.1 eMH Application: Services and Models	45
	3.2.2 eMH and Populations Based on Age and Setting	46
3.3	Access to Cadillac Care	47
3.4	eMH May Be Superior to In-person care for Some Populations	50
3.5	Discussion	53
	Conclusions	54
	References	54

E.Z. Shoemaker, MD
Department of Psychiatry and Behavioral Sciences, Keck School of Medicine at USC
and LAC+USC Medical Center, 2250 Alcazar Street, CSC, Suite 2200,
Los Angeles, CA 90033, USA

D.M. Hilty, MD (✉)
Keck School of Medicine, University of Southern California, Los Angeles, CA, USA
e-mail: donh031226@gmail.com

© Springer International Publishing Switzerland 2016
D. Mucic, D.M. Hilty (eds.), *e-Mental Health*,
DOI 10.1007/978-3-319-20852-7_3

Abstract

Our current healthcare system in the United States is characterized by problems with access to timely and evidence-based care, particularly for mental disorders. e-Mental Health (eMH) improves access to care regardless of the point-of-service or barriers involved. Its effectiveness across age, population, and disorders is as good as in-person care, though adjustments for some populations in the approach are necessary. Early intervention is an example of "Cadillac" care or a best evidence-based approach that is easier to distribute via telemedicine. Cadillac care delivered via eMH has the potential to bring evidence-based early-intervention modalities to very young children and their families. However, early access to care is also critical for all populations, particularly those with cultural or medical disadvantages. It appears that eMH may be preferable or better than in-person care in some instances.

3.1 Introduction

Our current healthcare system in the United States is characterized by problems with access to timely care, especially timely care for mental disorders. For example, examination of data from the National Comorbidity Survey Replication in 2005 found that only 41 % of Americans with a mental disorder over the previous 12 months received any treatment for their condition in the prior year [1]. Only 28 % of Americans with a mental disorder in the past year received treatment from a psychiatrist or non-psychiatrist mental health professional [1]. Further examination of this same survey showed very worrisome data about timely care: among those who do receive care, the median delay in treatment initiation after initial disorder onset ranges from 6 to 23 years across disorders [2]. Even among those with common disorders – mood disorders, generalized anxiety disorder, panic disorder, or drug dependence – only 25–40 % of make initial treatment contact in the first year of disorder onset [2]. Thus critical time is lost in the identification and early intervention with mental illness.

A 2012 Institute of Medicine report, Crossing the Quality Chasm, brought into focus that the American healthcare system has challenges not only with access to *any* care, but access to quality, evidence-based care [3]. This report called on healthcare providers and organizations in the United States to close the gap between care that we know is effective (i.e., evidence-based care) and care that we actually deliver (often fragmented care with interventions that are convenient but not necessarily evidence-based). Nowhere is this chasm wider than in our healthcare system's treatment of mental disorders in patients. This is despite remarkable proliferation of somatic and psychosocial treatments that are well tolerated and research supported in recent decades [4].

The Institute for Healthcare Improvement (IHI) is an agency that has sprung up to assist healthcare systems in their transformation to higher-quality systems

[5]. One IHI initiative, the Triple Aim, consists of: (1) better population health, (2) better patient experience of care and better quality and safety of care, and (3) reduced cost. In order to achieve better population health – the population here being a medical center's patients or an insurance company's subscriber – a healthcare system can improve the mental health of its patient population by investing in interventions to promptly treat minor and major mental illness. eMH has demonstrated efficacy in providing treatments for mental disorders that are more accessible and acceptable to patients; as such, it has the potential to help healthcare systems reduce the burden of psychiatric illness in a population.

eMH's effectiveness has gone through three phases [6]. First, it was judged effective in terms of increasing access to care, being well accepted, and having good educational outcomes [6]. Second, the validity and reliability of eMH compared to in-person care showed no differences [7, 8]. This assessment moved forward into formal "as good as" or non-inferiority studies [9], which have also had positive results. Lastly, its current evaluation is in the muddy areas of costs/economic assessments, but even there, we have excellent approaches and frameworks [7, 10, 11]. A Practice Parameter exists from the American Association of Child and Adolescent Psychiatry [12].

This chapter will help the reader to:

1. Highlight eMH's role in improving access to care for people with access, medical, cultural, geographic, and other barriers
2. Highlight eMH's role in bringing evidence-based child and adolescent care to children and families, especially intensive psychosocial care
3. Highlight situations in which eMH may, in fact, provide superior care to in-person psychiatric services
4. Demonstrate how 1, 2, and 3 may serve to reduce the incidence of mental disorders and reduce the suffering and disability caused by these disorders

3.2   Access and Service Delivery

3.2.1   eMH Application: Services and Models

The service points at which eMH can be used to enhance care are theoretically limitless: clinics, emergency rooms, patients' homes, nursing homes, homeless shelters, hospices, schools, forensic facilities, and at the battlefront. A full range of evaluation, consultation, and treatment services has been carried out by telemedicine. Especially surprising is the breadth of psychotherapeutic interventions that have been provided using eMH. Initial studies focused on satisfaction, working alliance between the patient-provider, and communication changes [6, 13], and it appeared that no significant problems were arising once the technology bandwidth had increased [8]. Reports on therapy and even more broadly defined "e-therapy" have been done [14].

Studies in adults generally involve patients with depression and anxiety – often military populations with PTSD – and these studies show comparative efficacy of eMH to in-person services. Incidentally, eMH sometimes is better (as mentioned above), though a preliminary anger management group study on therapeutic alliance and attrition showed a lower alliance with the telegroup leader than with the in-person leader [15]. The core issues are the impact of technology, patient education, exploring the virtual connection [16], and adjusting some behaviors (e.g., handing a tissue box, sighing, pat on the shoulder, handshake) to verbal statements conveying the same thing (e.g., empathy) [17]. Guidelines for therapy by videoconferencing have been explored [18].

3.2.2 eMH and Populations Based on Age and Setting

3.2.2.1 Child and Adolescent Populations

Child telepsychiatry research has moved beyond feasibility, acceptability, and good initial outcomes [19, 20]. Though studies are preliminary, it appears that interviews for collecting the history, mental status/physical examination, and family data go well. Some child populations (see below) may do better with eMH than in-person care [21].

It is true that providing quality child and adolescent psychiatry care will require a higher level of organization and more planning before a patient visit [22]. When useful and permitted by the patient and family, Web- or phone-based questionnaires may pre-diagnose patients before a visit [23], and the mental health clinician may be able to gather useful collateral from the referring team prior to a visit [24]. The patient-side interview room will need to be large enough to accommodate the child, their family, and often a patient-side staff member [22]. The camera and microphone setup should be flexible to allow a wide view of the room (to catch patient-family interactions), and the room should be equipped with child-size furniture and toys. Ideally, should the consultant need to observe the child's play in order to inform their assessment, they could ask patient-side staff to play with/draw with the child [25]. Lastly, as with all child and adolescent psychiatry, the clinician should be very transparent as to who else is viewing the encounter on the provider's side, and whether the encounter is being videotaped.

3.2.2.2 Other Populations and Settings

Reports in adult patients show eMH results in improvement in depression [26–28], reductions in length of hospitalization [29, 30], more appropriate medication use [27, 30], symptom reduction of disorders [27, 29, 30], and improvements in portion of psychotherapy judged to be evidence-based for PTSD [31, 32].

Geriatric data are emerging, but more studies are needed in medicine and eMH [33]. Obstacles include access to service, functional challenges, primary care provider attitudes, and lack of psychiatrists [34] and perhaps what could be called a lack of nursing home "ownership" by any one provider to formalize a clinical approach. Nursing home eMH studies have been effective in terms of informal measures [35], mainly focusing on depression or dementia, with evaluation more facile and more efficient use of consultant time. Assessment, cognitive intervention, and outcomes have been similar to in-person [35] and a new development is telemonitoring of depression in the home, which facilitates connectedness [36]. Extra attention to helping older adults access the technology, especially if they have difficulties with their hearing or vision, is required, but acceptance of eMH appears fine, and it was better than adults in one study [17].

eMH models of clinical care and education have pros and cons [8, 37], including their level of overall intensity, cost, feasibility, and depth of the relationship between the eMH provider, the private care practitioner, and patient. Low intensity models include tele-education, formal case review [38] and in-person, telephone, or e-mail doctor-to-doctor "curbside" consultations. Moderate intensity models include disease management for depression [17] or an integrated program of mental health screening, therapy on site, and telepsychiatric consultation (phone, e-mail, or video) [39] or asynchronous telepsychiatry (ATP) to primary care in English and Spanish-speaking patients in primary care [40]. High intensity models are typically the ones previously mentioned involving collaborative care [41–43].

Special settings and populations also include involuntary, inpatient, and incarcerated – and those in emergency rooms – and related to the PCMH.

3.3 Access to Cadillac Care

eMH increases access, in general, and can be used to provide what we will colloquially call "Cadillac care," meaning evidence-based treatment delivered by expert clinicians. One tool that many healthcare systems are using to meet the Triple Aim is the Patient-Centered Medical Home [44]. The PCMH model emphasizes the primary care clinicians providing the majority of care. Many medical homes work to integrate behavioral health or care for mental disorders into their panel of services that can be provided in the medical home. One way to do this is to embed generalist mental health clinicians in primary care clinics. However, if we are interested in quality care, not just access to care, we need to acknowledge that, "Some evidence-based practices may prove too complex for universal dissemination [to generalists], and the time and expense required for quality dissemination and implementation preclude large-scale training in the treatment of low base rate disorders" [4]. By supplementing the care that can be reasonably provided by generalists in integrated care settings with expert, evidence-based interventions delivered by eMH, our healthcare systems can truly move to prevent and reduce the severity of mental illness.

Example 1: Providing Linguistically and Culturally Expert Care The utility of tele-translation services is obvious. While most healthcare providers aim to use in-person providers, these interpreters are often staff members serving a double function, and they have received little formal training. The use of family members for interpreting is fraught with pitfalls, both practical and ethical. Staff members – even nurses – and family members are prone to miscommunicate patient complaints or de-emphasize critical pieces of the patient report [45–47]. Use of interpreters via videoconferencing therapy technology may be especially useful for languages that are relatively rare, such as sign language [48].

Beyond language expertise, eMH has been shown to be useful in bringing culturally expert services to populations who have specialized cultural needs [7, 8, 11]. Culture is known to influence a number of aspects of an individual's healthcare, including attitudes toward different treatments, the provider-patient relationship [39, 49], and an individual's willingness to engage in the use of technology. One study has shown that Asians, especially Koreans, were more likely to form online relationships than Caucasians [50]. While culture may affect outcomes, poverty and education – common disparities across culture – may also have impact; poverty for African Americans was a greater influence than ethnicity/culture in one study [51]. Just like with in-person psychiatry, when cultural issues seem especially relevant, a clinician can use the Outline for Cultural Formulation and Cultural Formulation Interview from the Diagnostic and Statistical Manual of Mental Disorders, Fifth Edition [52], to clarify their formulation of a patient.

The University of Colorado School of Medicine's Center for Native American TeleHealth and TeleEducation (CNATT) has done several studies looking at acceptability of mental health services delivered by interactive videoconferencing with patients from Native American populations. They have conducted studies with children and adolescent patients in Rapid City, South Dakota [53] and with adult male veterans from a Northern Plains tribe [54]. In both studies the authors were concerned that videoconferencing technology itself might be off-putting to this population and result in low patient satisfaction. They likewise theorized, however, that both the patient-side and teleprovider-side clinicians were expert and experienced in the treatment of people from local Native American populations, and this expertise might offset patient discomfort about the videoconference technology. Both with child and adult patients, the patient and provider satisfaction with eMH was high. This same research group has now extended itself even further out of its usual form of practice, using eMH to help train psychiatrists in Cambodia [53].

Example 2: Providing Expert Care for Disorders Requiring Combination Inpatient Hospitalization and Family Psychotherapy Anorexia nervosa is a severe and life-threatening mental illness. Treatment for this disorder may require inpatient stabilization, nutritional rehabilitation, and multidimensional psychotherapeutic care [55]. In adolescents, the addition of family therapy has been found to help patients gain weight, reduce depression, and reduce family conflict (APA Guideline). In keeping with these guidelines, Goldfield and Boachie reported on a case in which they used eight sessions of family therapy delivered via eMH to a girl with anorexia in an inpatient psychiatric unit in Ottawa while her family was at home in a small town in Northern Ontario [56]. This girl's eating disorder was severe enough that she required a specialized inpatient hospitalization, but it was not feasible for family to travel from rural Ontario to Ottawa to participate in family therapy. eMH allowed them to add family therapy – an evidence-based intervention – to their usual inpatient care. They reported that by the end of her hospitalization, the patient felt emotionally closer to her father, had accepted that she had an eating disorder, and was taking responsibility for her recovery. She was discharged with a BMI of 19.5. The staff of the inpatient unit felt that provision of this family therapy was integral to this girl's recovery on their unit [56].

Example 3: Providing Expert Care for Low-Frequency Disorders in Very Young Children James Comer's seminal work in the use of videoconferencing for treatment of very young children with psychiatric disorders shows that effective treatment requires very active involvement of both parents and child (Internet-based) [57]. A pilot study of cognitive behavioral therapy for obsessive-compulsive disorder (OCD) delivered to the family's home, for five children between 4 and 8 years old, used Freeman and Garcia's 2009 treatment manual [58] supplemented with Internet-based computer games designed to help young children understand CBT concepts [59]. The CBT protocol states, "Throughout treatment, parents are included in structured ways to address issues of family functioning and parenting: (1) parents are trained as coaches for their children and play key roles in shaping treatment and ensuring out-of-session adherence and motivation; (2) treatment addresses parental accommodation of child symptoms; and (3) treatment has an "exposure" function for parents as well, as they are asked to tolerate their own distress while assisting their children with difficult exposure exercises and homework tasks. Parents learn to use differential attention, modeling, and scaffolding techniques to manage child symptoms." Computer games supplemented the curriculum to help the young child understand CBT concepts. All five children had some response, and three children no longer met criteria for OCD at the end of the trial [59]. While one would be tempted to dismiss the pilot's findings, anxiety disorders and OCD in children tend to be chronic, episodic illnesses. Effective intervention with preschoolers with OCD has the potential to reduce the severity and chronicity of this debilitating illness (Table 3.1) [59].

Table 3.1 Summary of advantages of eMH

Geographic access	Bring care to where the patients are	Rural areas Underserved urban areas Primary care clinics School Juvenile justice settings Nursing homes
Access to evidence-based practices, administered by highly trained providers	Cadillac care	Linguistically or culturally specialized care Children's ADHD eMH treatment study CBT for OCD Parent-child interaction therapy for disruptive behavior disorders Family Therapy for Anorexia Nervosa

May be superior to in-person care	Patients may prefer it
	Providers may prefer it
	Ecological Validity
		Anxious and autistic patients may be relieved by the added distance and less confrontation
		Patients who feel stigmatized by having to seek treatment may be more likely to participate (military veterans)
		Teenagers may be attracted to the technology
		When done in-home, very private
		Better continuity:
		    Allows providers safety in situations perceived as dangerous (correctional)
		    Provider can continue to treat patient even if the provider moves
		Allows specialization
		    Providers can specialize in certain EBP and provide enough volume of services to be financially viable
		    Providers can provide specialized linguistic and cultural services
		Child and adult behavior can be observed in the home
		Child behavior observed in the classroom
		Family-based treatments can be provided in the home

3.4   eMH May Be Superior to In-person Care for Some Populations

Though inconceivable to all of us in the 1990s, when systematic application and evaluation of eMH began, the literature indicates there may be instances in which eMH is a preferred option over in-person care (Table 3.2) [8].

Example 4: eMH May Be More Acceptable for Veterans with PTSD Patients than In-Person Care Patients with anxiety disorders and PTSD often experience worry, fear, phobic avoidance, panic attacks, and other anxiety experiences that prohibit seeking help. Ironically, symptoms of their mental illness prevent them from

Table 3.2 Common factors in situations in which eMH may be superior to in-person care: common denominators of this success

Anxiety/avoidance	Anxious patients may prefer eMH as feeling less confrontational, less intimate (and therefore more tolerable)
Novelty	Teenagers may find eMH fun or "more like a videogame"
Direction or cueing	Patients with Autism or ADHD may be better able to attend technological interface better than an in-person interview
Distance and privacy	Patients who live in small communities (tribal reservations) or who feel a high degree of stigma (military veterans, patients with substance abuse problems) may especially appreciate more physical and psychological distance
Authenticity of the interaction	Patients may "let their guard down" and demonstrate more ecologically valid behavior over eMH than in-person

seeking treatment for their mental illness. Military veterans may be burdened with attitudes that make them feel even more stigmatized by mental illness than their civilian peers, and this feeling of stigmatization raises the psychological obstacles to local treatment even higher. Many studies are in progress to reach veterans by phone, e-mail, chat rooms, and other technologies – for individual and group contact – to overcome some of these obstacles and to reduce isolation [27, 60]. In order to address the needs of veterans, investigators have studied eMH for the treatment of veterans with PTSD, panic, and depression. Telephone and eMH studies employing CBT for PTSD have been found effective [61]. In the Bouchard study, patients and providers reported that a strong therapeutic alliance was noted in all three dimensions of the treatment alliance. Both provider and patients reported that the technology did not interfere with feeling immersed in the treatment, and patients made comments like, "I'm glad you are here, it helps me so much."

Example 5: Autistic Children and Adults May Prefer eMH to In-Person Care Pakuyrek described the case of a 5-year-old boy who referred for developmental concerns, including stereotypical behaviors, preoccupations, and social difficulties, in addition to poor attention and task completion [21]. Prior to the session, the mother and local providers told the eMH provider that the boy did much better with visual strategies. At times, he was standing only about a foot away from the monitor's camera, staring directly into it the entire time. This was despite his long and well-known history of poor eye contact and a tendency to avoid social interactions. The mother later reported that she had never seen her son so comfortable with any new situation, let alone with a total stranger. To his mother's surprise, the boy not only finished an hour-long session, but also managed to answer all of the examiner's questions.

Example 6: Teenagers' Affinity for Technology Leads to High Acceptability of eMH Another population that may prefer eMH to in-person services is teenagers. Teenagers are notorious for two characteristics that can be leveraged to one's advantage: (1) their affinity for technology and (2) their preoccupation with privacy and confidentiality. Multiple authors have described teenagers' affinity for eMH. Kaliebe, in his review of the use eMH in juvenile justice settings noted, "youths seem to be more open in disclosing personal information, and the interactions are more relaxed than in a traditional face-to-face encounter with this population," and that, in general, "the kids really like it" [62]. Savin described a case of treating a 13-year-old boy with poor performance in school. One of this boy's strengths was his interest in and proficiency using technology; the eMH psychiatrist used discussing the video-conferencing therapy as a means to engage this reluctant teenager [25]. Furthermore, using the Internet to engage teenagers around their favorite music or movies is quite natural when provider and patient are already communicating via computer screens [25]. While not explicitly tested yet, we should keep in mind that teenagers are likely to appreciate the greater degree of privacy that eMH delivered in the home can provide; as eMH reduces barriers to treatment for anxious patients, it may also reduce barriers to treatment for self-conscious teenagers.

Example 7: eMH Can Provide Improved Ecological Validity of Treatment Expert services delivered in the family's home may, in fact, have an advantage over expert services delivered in a clinic in that they provide access to see baseline parent and child behavior in the home (for young children, the principal site of the behaviors) and access to observe if changes in behavior have truly occurred in the home. This gets to the issue of ecological validity; children (and their parents) often behave better in a clinician's office than in the "real world," and eMH gives the clinician access to that family's "real world."

Dr. Comer's group has used videoconferencing therapy in implementing Parent Child Interactive Therapy (PCIT) in the home context. In-person PCIT is a parent-training modality in which a therapist coaches a parent in real-time through the use of a 2-way mirror and a bug-in-the ear technology. PCIT is generally split into two parts; the first half focuses the parent on developing a warm and responsive parenting style by training the parent to be an enthusiastic and responsive play partner, and the second half focuses on coaching the parent to train the child on being compliant with parent commands. PCIT is a highly evidence-based treatment; it is listed in the National Registry of Evidence-based Programs and Practices in 2009 [57]. PCIT delivered via videoconferencing therapy replaces the office technology of the two-way mirror with a webcam, an in-room omnidirectional microphone, and a Bluetooth-based bug in the parent's ear [57]. Dr. Comer reports that some parents report experiencing the Bluetooth earpiece as having a "fairy godmother" help them through difficult parenting moments, a comment that speaks directly to this treatment's acceptability to parents of young children (private communication, James Comer).

In child psychiatry, the second "native" environment in which a clinician would like to observe the child is in their school. There are several programs that have overcome geographic barriers to care using eMH [63]. As yet, few clinicians are observing children in the class or schoolyard via webcam, likely because of concerns over patients' peers' privacy. Barretto, however, reported a case of using eMH to provide functional behavioral analysis for a child's Applied Behavioral Analysis

Treatment. In this case, the ABA therapist directed the teacher how to implement the ABA plan while observing the teacher and child via a webcam [64]. The author credited access to this in-school, "in vivo" data as an element in the success of this child's plan [64].

Example 8: Culture, Diversity, and Language A 52-year-old Mexican American woman in treatment with her primary care provider for depression, suffered from low mood, tearfulness, and a host of somatic complaints [65]. Escitalopram was started at 10 mg, and after 4 months of treatment, her depression had persisted. The patient was referred to the telepsychiatry, and instead of the usual male Caucasian provider, the 60-min evaluation was done by a 30-year-old "pinch-hitter," a Mexican-American female psychiatrist who spoke Spanish. The patient spoke of many medications by color, stating that they "all helped very much," but she did not know which one was for depression. When asked about adherence with the medication, she complimented her provider, but then asked with trepidation "Is there any problem taking so many medications together, especially when you increase the doses?" The provider joined in the last 10 min with an interpreter to discuss the patient's concerns, questions, the treatment plan, and safety of the plan. Adherence was intact with the medication at follow-up at 2 months later (now overall, month 6) weeks with a partial response, then again at 4 months (now overall, 8 months) with full mood response and hardly any somatic complaints at a dose increase to 20 mg.

3.5   Discussion

We began this chapter discussing the directive for healthcare systems to provide mental health services that are not limited by geographical proximity to urban areas with large numbers of mental health professionals. We have shown that eMH can provide access to mental healthcare for diverse populations in a variety of settings. This would include care within the Patient-Centered Medical Home (primary care clinic), as well as care delivered in the home or school setting.

However, for the large number of patients who require specialized care delivered by a highly trained and expert clinician, eMH also provides a way to provide the so-called Cadillac care. This Cadillac care may be highly acceptable to patients, as the patient can stay in a comfortable environment of their home or school. eMH has tremendous potential advantages for providers as well. Comer and Barlow posit that future specialty mental health clinics may be located, not in a brick-and-mortal setting, but online. This arrangement would liberate providers to specialize in a narrow band of populations, disorders, and treatments in which they could become truly expert. It would also liberate patients with specialty conditions from having to receive their expert treatment in large metropolitan areas or at large teaching hospitals [4].

As we better learn how to integrate synchronous and asynchronous use of eMH throughout our system, we will likely evolve to using hybrid care, providing a spectrum of generalist in-person care to eMH used for expert consultation to expert treatment via videoconferencing therapy [66, 67]. This hybrid care has the potential to provide care that is superior for many patients and many mental health conditions.

Conclusions

The potential for eMH to broaden access to care and access to high-quality specialized care is starting to be recognized widely. This development is exciting not only because it has the potential to relieve the suffering caused by mental disorders in the population currently, but also because the early intervention (especially with young children) that is feasible through eMH has the potential to prevent suffering and disability in future populations. Even the World Health Organization is surveying telemedicine opportunities and developments in member states [68].

References

1. Wang PS, Lane M, Olfson M, et al. Twelve-month use of mental health services in the United States results from the National Comorbidity Survey Replication. Arch Gen Psychiatry. 2005;62:629–40.
2. Wang PS, Berglund P, Olfson M, et al. failure and delay in initial treatment contact after first onset of mental disorders in the National Comorbidity Survey Replication. Arch Gen Psychiatry. 2005;62:603–13.
3. Institute of Medicine (US) Committee on Quality of Health Care in America: crossing the quality chasm: a new health system for the 21st century. Washington, DC: National Academies Press (US); 2001. 28 Feb 2015. At: https://www.iom.edu/Reports/2001/Crossing-the-Quality-Chasm-A-New-Health-System-for-the-21st-Century.aspx.
4. Comer JS, Barlow DH. The occasional case against broad dissemination and implementation: retaining a role for specialty care in the delivery of psychological treatments. Am Psychol. 2014;69:1–18.
5. Institute for Healthcare Improvement: The Triple Aim. Optimizing health, care and cost. Heatlhc Exec. 2009;24:64–6.
6. Hilty DM, Liu W, Marks SL, et al. Effectiveness of telepsychiatry: a brief review. Can Psychiat Asso Bull. 2003;35(5):10–17.
7. Yellowlees PM, Shore JH, Roberts L, et al. Practice guidelines for videoconferencing-based telemental health. Tel E Health. 2010;16:1074–89.
8. Hilty DM, Ferrer D, Callahan EJ, et al. The effectiveness of telemental health: a 2013 review. Tel J e-Health. 2013;19(6):444–54.
9. Richardson LK, Frueh BC, Grubaugh AL, et al. Current directions in videoconferencing telemental health research. Clin Psychol. 2009;16(3):323–8.
10. Shore JH, Mishkind MC, Bernard J, et al. A lexicon of assessment and outcome measures for telemental health. Tel e-Health. 2013;3:282–92.
11. Hilty DM, Yellowlees PM, Nasatir SEH, et al. Program evaluation and practical, step-by-step program modification in telemental health. Behavioral telehealth series volume 1- clinical video conferencing: program development and practice. Springer Press, New York, NY. 2014. pp. 105–134.
12. Myers K, Cain S, Work Group on Quality Issues. American academy of practice parameter for telepsychiatry with children and adolescents. J Am Acad Child Adol Psychiatry. 2008;47(12):1468–83.
13. Hilty DM, Nesbitt TS, Marks SL, et al. How telepsychiatry affects the doctor-patient relationship: communication, satisfaction, and additional clinically relevant issues. Primary Psychiatry. 2002;9(9):29–34.

14. Postel MG, de Haan HA, de Jong CA. E-therapy for mental health problems: a systematic review. Tel e-Health. 2008;14:707–14.
15. Greene CJ, Morland LA, Macdonald A, et al. How does tele-mental health affect group therapy process? Secondary analysis of a noninferiority trial. Consult Clin Psychol. 2010;78:746–50.
16. Glueck D. Establishing therapeutic rapport in telemental health. In: Turvey CL, Myers K, editors. Telemental health. New York, NY: Elsevier; 2013. p. 29–46.
17. Hilty DM, Marks SL, Wegeland JE, et al. A randomized controlled trial of disease management modules, including telepsychiatric care, for depression in rural primary care. Psychiatry. 2007;4(2):58–65.
18. Nelson EL, Duncan AB, Lillis T. Special considerations for conducting psychotherapy via videoconferencing. In: Myers K, Turvey CL, editors. Telemental health: clinical, technical and administrative foundations for evidenced-based practice. San Francisco: Elsevier; 2013. p. 295–314.
19. Pesamaa L, Ebeling H, Kuusimaki ML, et al. Videoconferencing in child and adolescent telepsychiatry: a systematic review of the literature. J Tel Telecare. 2004;10:187–92.
20. Myers KM, Vander Stoep A, McCarty CA, et al. Child and adolescent telepsychiatry: variations in utilization, referral patterns and practice trends. J Tel Telecare. 2010;16:128–33.
21. Pakyurek M, Yellowlees PM, Hilty DM. The child and adolescent telepsychiatry consultation: can it be a more effective clinical process for certain patients than conventional practice? Tel J e-Health. 2010;16:289–92.
22. Hilty DM, Shoemaker EZ, Myers K., et al. Issues and steps toward a clinical guideline for telemental health for care of children and adolescents. J Child Adol Psychopharm (in press).
23. Brondbo H, Mathiassen B, Martinussen M, et al. Agreement on web-based diagnoses and severity of mental health problems in a Norwegian child and adolescent mental health Service. Clin Pract Epidemiol Ment Health. 2012;8:16–21.
24. Glueck DA. Telepsychiatry in private practice. Child Adol Psychiat Clinics N Amer. 2011;20(1):1–11.
25. Savin D, Glueck DA, Chardavoyne J, et al. Bridging cultures: child psychiatry via videoconferencing. Child Adoles Psyhiatr Clin N Am. 2011;20:125–34.
26. Ruskin PE, Silver-Aylaian M, Kling MA, et al. Treatment outcomes in depression: comparison of remote treatment through telepsychiatry to in in-person treatment. Am J Psychiat. 2004;161:1471–6.
27. Fortney JC, Pyne JM, Kembrell TA, et al. Telemedicine-based collaborative care for posttraumatic stress disorder: a randomized clinical trial. JAMA Psychiatry. 2015;72:58–67.
28. Moreno FA, Chong J, Dumbauld J, et al. Use of standard webcam and internet equipment for telepsychiatry treatment of depression among underserved Hispanics. Psychiatric Serv. 2012;63:1213–7.
29. O'Reilly R, Bishop J, Maddox K, et al. Is telepsychiatry equivalent to face to face psychiatry: results from a randomized controlled equivalence trial. Psych Serv. 2007;258:836–43.
30. de las Cuevas C, Arrendondo MT, Cabrera MF, et al. Randomized controlled trial of telepsychiatry through videoconference versus face-to-face conventional psychiatric treatment. Tel J E Health. 2006;12:341–50.
31. Morland LA, Greene CJ, Rosen CS, et al. Telemedicine for anger management therapy in a rural population of combat veterans with posttraumatic stress disorder: a randomized noninferiority trial. J Clin Psychiat. 2010;71:855–63.
32. Frueh BC, Monnier J, Yim E. Randomized trial for post-traumatic stress disorder. J Tel Telecare. 2007;13:142–7.
33. Botsis T, Demiris G, Peterson S, et al. Home telecare technologies for the elderly. J Tel Telecare. 2008;14:333–7.
34. Sheeran T, Dealy J, Rabinowitz T. Geriatric telemental health. In: Myers K, Turvey CL, editors. Telemental health. New York: Elsevier; 2013. p. 171–95.
35. Rabinowitz T, Murphy K, Amour JL, et al. Benefits of a telepsychiatry consultation service for rural nursing home residents. Tel J E Health. 2010;16:34–40.

36. Sheeran T, Rabinowitz T, Lotterman J, et al. Feasibility and impact of telemonitor-based depression care management for geriatric homecare patients. Tel J e-Health. 2011;17:620–6.
37. Hilty DM, Yellowlees PM, Cobb HC, et al. Models of telepsychiatric consultation-liaison service to rural primary care. Psychosomatics. 2006;47(2):152–7.
38. Dobbins ML, Roberts N, Vicari SK, et al. The consulting conference: a new model of collaboration for child psychiatry and primary care. Acad Psychiatry. 2011;35:260–2.
39. Yellowlees PM, Marks SL, Hilty DM, et al. Using e-health to enable culturally appropriate mental health care in rural areas. J Tel e-Health. 2008;14(5):486–92.
40. Yellowlees PM, Odor A, Patrice K, et al. Transcultural psychiatry made simple: asynchronous telepsychiatry as an approach to providing culturally relevant care. Tel e-Health. 2013;19(4):1–6.
41. Fortney JC, Pyne JM, Mouden SP, et al. Practice-based versus telemedicine-based collaborative care for depression in rural federally qualified health centers: a pragmatic randomized comparative effectiveness trial. Amer J Psychiatry. 2013;170(4):414–25.
42. Richardson L, McCauley E, Katon W. Collaborative care for adolescent depression: a pilot study. Gen Hosp Psychiat. 2009;31:36–45.
43. Myers KM, Vander Stoep A, Zhou C, et al. Effectiveness of a telehealth service delivery model for treating attention-deficit hyperactivity disorder: results of a community-based randomized controlled trial. J Amer Asso Child Adol Psych. 2015;54(4):263–74.
44. Crabtree BF, Nutting PA, Miller WL, et al. Summary of the National Demonstration Project and recommendations for the patient-centered medical home. Ann Fam Med. 2010;54(4) 8 Suppl 1:S80–90.
45. Brooks TR. Pitfalls in communication with Hispanic and African-American patients: do translators help or harm? J Nat Med Asso. 1992;84:941.
46. Brua C. Role-blurring and ethical grey zones associated with lay interpreters: three case studies. Communication Med. 2008;5:73.
47. Elderkin-Thompson V, Silver RC, Waitzkin H. When nurses double as interpreters: a study of Spanish-speaking patients in a US primary care setting. Soc Sci Med. 2001;52:1343–58.
48. Lopez AM, Cruz M, Lazarus S, et al. Use of American Sign Language in telepsychiatry consultation. Telemed J E Health. 2004 Fall;10:389–91.
49. Berger JT. Culture and ethnicity in clinical care. Arch Int Med. 1998;158:2085–90.
50. Matei S, Ball-Rokeach SJ. Real and virtual social ties: connections in the everyday lives of seven ethnic neighborhoods. American Behavioral Scientist. 2001;45:550–64.
51. Mossberger K, Tolbert CJ, Gilbert M. Race, place, and information technology. Urban Affairs Review. 2006;41:583–620.
52. American Psychiatric Association. Diagnostic criteria from DSM-5. Washington, DC: American Psychiatric Publishing; 2013.
53. Savin DM, Legha RK, Cordaro AR, et al. Spanning distance and culture in psychiatric education: a teleconferencing collaboration between Cambodia and the United States. Acad Psychiatry. 2013;37(5):355–9.
54. Shore JH, Brooks E, Savin D, et al. Acceptability of telepsychiatry in American Indians. Tel e-Health. 2008;14(5):461–6.
55. American Psychiatric Association Practice Guidelines, Eating Disorders (Anorexia Nervosa). 28 Feb 2015. http://www.psychiatry.org/practice/clinical-practice-guidelines.
56. Goldfield GS, Boachie A. Delivery of family therapy in the treatment of anorexia nervosa using telehealth. Telemed J E Health. 2003 Spring;9(1):111–4.
57. Elkins AL, Comer JS. Parent–child interactive therapy (PCIT). 28 Feb 2015. http://findyouthinfo.gov/node/49884.
58. Freeman JB, Garcia AM. Family-based treatment for young children with OCD: therapist guide. New York, NY: Oxford University Press; 2009.
59. Comer JS, Furr JM, Cooper-Vince C, et al. Rationale and considerations for the internet-based delivery of parent–child interaction therapy. Cogn Behav Pract. 2015;22(3):302–16.

60. Price M, Gros DF. Examination of prior experience with telehealth and comfort with telehealth technology as a moderator of treatment response for PTSD and depression in veterans. Int J Psychiatry Med. 2014;48(1):57–67.
61. Bouchard S, Paquin B, Payeur R, et al. Delivering cognitive-behavior therapy for panic disorder with agoraphobia in videoconference. Telemed J E Health. 2004 Spring;10(1):13–25.
62. Kaliebe K, Heneghan J, Kim TJ. Telepsychiatry in juvenile justice settings. Child Adol Psychiat Clin. 2011;20(1):113–23.
63. Cunningham DL, Connors EH, Lever N, et al. Providers' perspectives: utilizing telepsychiatry in schools. Telemed J E Health. 2013;19(10):794–99.
64. Barretto A, Wacker DP, Harding J, et al. Using telemedicine to conduct behavioral assessments. J Appl Behav Anal. 2006 Fall;39(3):333–40.
65. Cerda GM, Hilty DM, Hales RE, et al. Use of telemedicine with ethnic groups. Psychiatr Serv. 1999;50(10):1364.
66. Yellowlees PM, Nafiz N. The psychiatrist-patient relationship of the future: anytime, anywhere? Review of Psychiatry. 2010;18(2):96–102.
67. Hilty DM, Yellowlees PM. Collaborative mental health services using multiple technologies – the new way to practice and a new standard of practice? J Amer Acad Child Adol Psychiatry. 2015;54:245–46.
68. World Health Organization. Telemedicine opportunities and developments in member states. Results of the second global survey on eHealth. Geneva: WHO Press; 2011.

How to Build, Evaluate, and Increase Your e-Mental Health Program Efficiency

4

Donald M. Hilty, Erica Z. Shoemaker, and Jay Shore

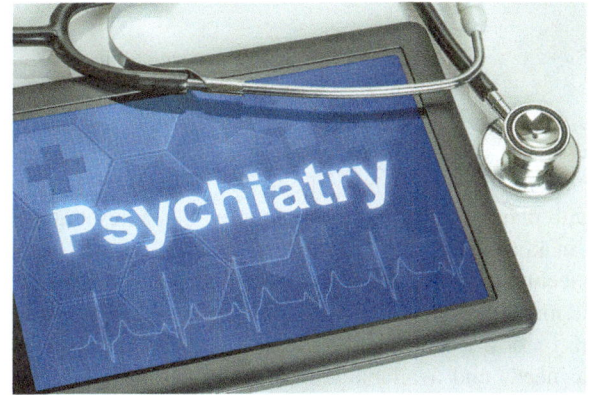

D.M. Hilty, MD (✉)
Keck School of Medicine, University of Southern California,
Los Angeles, CA, USA
e-mail: donh031226@gmail.com

E.Z. Shoemaker, MD
Department of Psychiatry and Behavioral Sciences, Keck School of Medicine at USC and
LAC+USC Medical Center, Los Angeles, CA, USA

J. Shore, MD, MPH
University of Colorado Depression Center, Aurora, CO, USA

Centers for American Indian and Alaska Native Health University of Colorado,
Aurora, CO, USA

© Springer International Publishing Switzerland 2016
D. Mucic, D.M. Hilty (eds.), *e-Mental Health*,
DOI 10.1007/978-3-319-20852-7_4

Contents

4.1   Introduction 60
4.2   Program Evaluation: The Basics, Formal Steps,
      and Input from Business 61
      4.2.1   Effectiveness Defined: New and Old Ideas 61
      4.2.2   Overview of "Good" Program Evaluation 62
      4.2.3   Organizational, Leadership, and Team Fitness 63
      4.2.4   Questions to Reflect on for Setting Appropriate Goals 64
4.3   Measuring Outcomes: An Overview on the Approach and Setting Targets 66
      4.3.1   Overview 66
      4.3.2   Evaluation Parameters 67
      4.3.3   Models of Care: How to Select Them and Impact on Evaluation 68
4.4   The Evidence Base for Clinical Outcomes 69
      4.4.1   Cost/Economic Outcomes 69
      4.4.2   Clinical Outcomes 71
4.5   Discussion and Conclusion 72
References 73

Abstract

Objective: This chapter discusses the prioritization of outcomes and evaluation in the provision of synchronous telemedicine (i.e., videoconferencing, STM) services. *Methods:* This organizational approach may be a shift from seeing what happens with planned services to planning the outcomes and then designing the services—in advance. *Results:* Basic and advanced areas of evaluation (e.g., satisfaction, technology, cost, clinical and other outcomes) are suggested and involve the many participants in STM in a systematic framework. It also offers suggestions on how to do a needs assessment and how to adjust priorities based on specific needs and available resources in a program. Examples of project improvement apply ideas from theory to clinical and other associated outcomes. References and resources of information are provided for further review. *Conclusion:* The readers acquire knowledge, skill, and a framework to improve existing programs and help their many participants.

4.1   Introduction

Changes in global healthcare evolve slowly or rapidly, based on existing clinical and economic models of care. In the USA, patient-centered care, the affordable care act, and other forces are reshaping services significantly. More accountability is expected of clinicians, clinics, and health systems—by both consumers and payers. Focus is being placed on accessible, safe, and quality care. New models move quality improvement from a "good" peripheral idea to a central role in the care process. Integrative methods for care (e.g., medicine and psychiatry), health systems (e.g., stepped care), and an emphasis on teamwork shift us from solitary interest in medicine to a combined interest in medicine, economics, and evaluation.

Versatile approaches like STM facilitate efficiency and flexibility in approach for thoughtful program evaluation. e-Mental health, e.g., synchronous telepsychiatry (STP), has shifted the focus from efficacy of interventions to effectiveness, with an emphasis on comparing it to in-person care [1]. eMH's almost immediate adaptation into primary care services led to new implementation of collaborative care models [1–3] in addition to standard phone/e-mail "curbside" consultations between physicians and regular consultation models. Additionally, web-based data management, electronic health records (EHRs), stepped models of care, and other innovations are facilitating increased reliance on STP methods [4–6], but asynchronous TP (ATP) [7] and other technologies are fast moving due to regular life (e.g., smartphones for reflection, self-assessment, and communication to providers) [8].

Program evaluation has become increasingly important to meet program, patient, provider, and externally driven (Joint Commission, reimbursement) needs—and more accountability is expected by both consumers and payers. A contemporary view is that we want to do "good" care, make a difference, and self-improve rather than being attached to the slow evolution of changes in care (i.e., "doing things the same old way")—a partially true criticism of medicine's attempts to preserve healing through the doctor-patient relationship, standards of care, and best practices. Contemporary program evaluation and outcome work is *a substantial shift* in philosophical approach for some, from seeing what happens with planned services to planning the outcomes and then designing the services—in advance. Now, it is patient, learner, and outcome centered, whereby the end product determines what is built or put in place—hence assessment includes satisfaction, technology, cost, clinical, process of care, and other outcomes. Accordingly, the contemporary program evaluation incorporates programmatic changes based on iterative evaluations and trials.

This chapter will help the reader to: (1) grasp the philosophical approach and methods of clinical, program, and system evaluation; (2) assess the program from clinical care coordinators to specialists, team/interdisciplinary roles, administration and leadership through use of a needs assessments, and accountability; and (3) focus on clinical evaluation to set "appropriate" goals and make meaningful changes using regular standards of care, built-in "required" payer/accreditation measures, and advanced (i.e., screening, self-report questionnaires, clinician administered) options for quality improvement. Examples of project improvement apply ideas from theory to clinical and other associated outcomes. References and resources of information are provided for further review.

4.2   Program Evaluation: The Basics, Formal Steps, and Input from Business

4.2.1   Effectiveness Defined: New and Old Ideas

Evaluation of eMH and now other modalities has gone through three phases. First, a review of eMH's effectiveness considered it effective in terms of providing access to care, as being well accepted, and as having good educational outcomes [9].

Second, a transition moved into satisfaction beyond patients, costs/economics, and validity and reliability of clinical care compared to in-person services [10]. Third, a recent publication focused on clinical effectiveness as a bottom-line way to evaluate eMH [1], and the current evidence base generally supports the assumption that a broad array of in-person services can be replicated effectively via eMH. Yet we must remain cognizant of this assumption and therefore not gear program evaluation to answer the question "are eMH services effective?" but, rather, to answer "are eMH services effective to do "what" for "whom," "when" and "at what financial, administrative, and clinical, costs?"

4.2.2 Overview of "Good" Program Evaluation

The depth and breadth of eMH program evaluation depend on a program's goals, resources, and limitations. Informal, semiformal, and formal assessment procedures can be chosen or mixed and matched to meet a specific program's needs. Well-planned informal procedures (such as conversations with staff, group-based identification of weekly struggles and successes) can be powerful tools to help guide ongoing implementation. Semiformal assessment could be limited to well-timed 4-question survey at the start of care and on follow-up. Formal inclusion of clinician-administered instruments is highly valid and reliable but time consuming, and sometimes the data are unused or unanalyzed.

Feasibility is a good starting (and ending) place for program evaluation. It is usually defined in terms of operational, economic, technical, market, resource, and cultural or financial feasibility. Demonstrating the feasibility of a program would come before demonstrating the clinical effectiveness of a program—this is simply tested in research (pilot study), business (test market), and politics (straw poll). Quantitative aspects of feasibility are often based on needs identified in historical data, financial or service utilization projections, or measures of how desirable the planned services are to patients, providers, managers, and stakeholders. Qualitative aspects may include a description of the product or service and descriptions of how well a proposed system solves current problems and takes advantage of opportunities or fits in with existing business environments, policies, and overarching goals. Lastly, the concept of feasibility remains important at every new phase of program development and evaluation—it informs the next step(s) by iterative process.

Finally, program evaluation helps to plan most, but not all, outcomes, so there are some basic rules. First, an early as possible is key. If we are committed to the principles of ongoing program evaluation for the improvement of services, it makes little sense to do the hard part (i.e., building those services) without the benefit of thoughtful stepwise evaluation. The challenge is to operationalize and merge the evaluative process with external, defined, and measurable set of hypotheses and goals. Second, incremental planning is suggested as time is limited, and ultimately it is safer to be responsible and conservative in implementation. A basic plan with an option or two for expansion can work well. Third, there will be problems and conflicts—how you handle them is key, particularly for the working culture and moving ahead. For eMH, there are at least two or more sites of care, scheduling, technology, shared clinical space, and other issues.

4.2.3   Organizational, Leadership, and Team Fitness

Good evaluation of outcomes related to eMH begins with a program and its fitness: organization, function, leadership, team members, experience, and many other parameters. When designing a program, thought should be given to team members, affiliations, personnel competencies, level of on-site and remote-site buy-in, and resources all in relation to specific and measurable program goals. A brief analysis of setting up a team well suited for ongoing program evaluation will be helpful. Each component of a high-functioning eMH team should have a plan for evaluation, and plans can be as simple, involved, formal, or informal as you think necessary. A "good" or responsive team adapts to and creates change. An under-identified area of program evaluation is in attending to team characteristics and mores that promote responsiveness and effectiveness. Assessing shared team processes promotes efficiency in leadership and course correction. Team-based resources and the qualities of a high-functioning team are in Table 4.1.

Table 4.1 Team-based resources and the qualities of a high-functioning team

Team resources:
Leadership staff
Clinical staff
Patient-side clinical support staff: walk patients to eMH rooms, administer measures
Patient- and provider-side referral sources: clinical staff to provide referrals for eMH
Patient- and provider-side technical support: hands-on responsive personnel
Administrative support: business manager, scheduling staff, clerks
Data entry support: for program evaluation
Statistician/analyst: to investigate data
Protected team time: meetings to celebrate success, review, and problem-solve
Protected clinician time: adequate time for clinicians to manage eMH encounters
Time for resource protection: to effectively convey evaluation results to stakeholders
Evaluation resources: assessment plans, clinical measures, process-oriented measures
Qualities of a high-functioning eMH program:
Unified goals
Vitality, purpose, and sense of professional well-being
Interdisciplinary collaboration: ability to share knowledge and respect varied experiences and skill sets
Role definition with overlapping/interchangeable responsibilities
Clear nondefensive communication
Personal support
Stability
Productive conflict resolution

4.2.4 Questions to Reflect on for Setting Appropriate Goals

Question 1 How formal does a team member's training or a program plan have to be, in order to do "good" evaluation of outcomes and improve our program?

Ultimately, there is a range of how ambitious a program's goals are, its funding, skills of team members (e.g., rural groups may not have all parts), and the level of support from administration. Deciding on the depth and breadth of eMH evaluation and outcomes is comparable to someone considering additional degrees or training. Let's assume a person who has a role in an eMH program and who has an undergraduate degree, 5 years of experience, and some professional training wants to learn more about business to learn an approach to grants, managing a team, financial stability, and outcomes/evaluation. What are his/her options?

- *Informal approach*: This might be a clinician who wants to better evaluate his/her impact or whose medical/hospital director wants to demonstrate quality improvement related to the clinical care. He/she might learn from another colleague with a model or project, take a course on quality improvement, or become familiar with some scale (completed by the patient, spouse, or him-/herself) to add to the services. He/she spends limited time, has a tangible outcome, and improves.
- *Semiformal approach*: This team member, a clinic manager, may be doing well and be promoted to a managerial position in a program, but lacks the "next" skill or knowledge set (or the approach to reframe his/her new role within the organization). Mentoring will help but takes time. An executive Masters in Business Administration (MBA) full time for about 1 year or spread half time over 2 years might provide knowledge and some skills of business administration and teach him/her how to hire or supervise additional team members with skill sets needed. (Another example of this level of approach may be a clinician who takes a course on research design and outcomes for clinical trials.)
- *Formal approach*: This team member, a skilled clinician and novice researcher, wants to take a leadership role and improve evaluation. He/she may be unsure of the way to move forward or there may be more than one viable option, but the requisite goal is more expertise, independent function and leadership. A Masters in Public Health (MPH) with a focus in health services or a 2-year MBA (both business and team evaluation skills) or a Masters in Clinical Research (design, outcomes, quantitative/qualitative skills, logic models/approach, clinical measures, statistical analyses) may be good.

Question 2 Is the program aligned with the overall organization's goals?

Alignment of missions involves multiple levels. First, consider the missions of the program and its organization. Second, consider the missions of collaborating programs/sites/organizations. Lastly, consider the overall mission. Key demonstrations of alignment are in contract agreements and negotiated time of consultants (if applicable) and of its setting up the program team: is there alignment of clinical, administrative, technical, and financial aspects?

Funding and payment usually set up the framework for the infrastructure, and all of this affects the ease and scope of evaluation. Health system design and ability to adapt vary widely. Private practice, academic health center, public sector, and other settings adapt their practices, staffing, and organization of information, e.g., electronic health record (EHR), to meet many goals. Caution is warranted before automatically assuming that in-place EHR, quality improvement (QI), and other processes can easily be used to save time/money or avoid duplication. Key issues are who controls access, the primary mission of a committee vs. the evaluation mission, and flexibility of all the parties.

Question 3 What are the do's and don'ts of program evaluation?

There are some very effective do's and don'ts of program evaluation (Table 4.2). Consensus of breadth and depth is a starting place. Reevaluation occurs a time or two as things move forward and questions arise about priorities, options, scope, and practical issues (e.g., how much data to collect).

Question 4 Evaluating costs outcomes: what scope to choose and how much to spend?

Cost and value assessment overlap [11] and a standard semi-systematic plan would aid programs significantly. Typically, there is a cost for clinicians' time, travel (provider or patient, direct and/or indirect), technology (bandwidth, hard- and software), staff (direct and indirect), administration, and others. This topic is parsed out in the section below.

Table 4.2 Do's and don'ts of evaluation

The "do's" of evaluation almost always include:
Adopt standardized measures already used, in this case in in-person care or in eMH published projects. They typically have undergone multiple iterations, levels of review, and sometimes psychometric testing
Use specific measures unless generalized measures with different parts are efficient. This arises and is demonstrated in the project section (below) for the study on the treatment of depression (and anxiety) in primary care. The Beck Depression Inventory (BDI) [62, 63] could be used to grade severity of depression or a broader net of information could be obtained by using the Symptom Checklist (SCL)-90 (or a shorter version; has anxiety, somatoform, and other screenings) [64]. The compromise was using the BDI because the primary interest of the study was depression
Check for disorders that confound measures. Checklist screened for anxiety and somatic symptoms that were confounding variables of outcomes (a 20-item version that had been researched to be consistent with findings of the SCL-90-R); no separate anxiety scale was therefore needed. For substance abuse, the Alcohol Use Disorders Identification Test was recommended (AUDIT) [65]
Have self-report/patient completion if it is accurate. This comes down to time and money. The clinician-administered alcohol 4-item CAGE [66] alternative was better than the AUDIT, but patients could fill out the latter one. The BDI is patient completed. So was the SCL-20. How much can a patient do, particularly one that is depressed? The BDI-30 original is the best, but the BDI-13 was chosen due to little drop off statistically; the drop off was judged as too much for the BDI-7 [67]. Many now use the BDI-II [68]. If this is a mania study, using a screening scale that is patient self-report is notoriously poor, though, and is best avoided altogether

(continued)

Table 4.2 (continued)

Collect data and do the evaluation prospectively rather than retrospectively. Why? If you look back and analyze data, it will double or triple your administration/staff time and there will be "holes" in what was collected compared to what you really "want" or need
Make sure you know (or someone knows) what you are doing. If you don't, does a team member know about these things? Do you need an academic type, a statistician or a person who does evaluation for a living to help? Get them involved earlier, not later. The time is worth the money every time
For a grant or contract, on the "good" end shoot for 30 % of the budget for evaluation, at a minimum 20 %; less than that will probably haunt you, unless the research/evaluation is so engrained in a clinical EHR that things are truly automatically collected and can be extracted and analyzed with ease, in other words, one you literally set up and control
Evolve from nascent to specific targets
From aim 1: To determine the efficacy of telemedicine for the provision of mental health services in rural primary care settings. *Hypothesis 1:* The intervention group, when compared to the control group, will demonstrate significantly decreased depressive symptoms per structured psychiatric interview and better outcomes
To aim 2: To determine the effectiveness of collaborative care facilitated by telemedicine for the provision of mental health services in rural primary care settings. *Hypothesis 2:* The intervention group, when compared to the control group, will demonstrate significantly decreased depressive symptoms as determined by BDI self-report questionnaires and a structured psychiatric interview at 3, 6, and 12 months after study entry
General "don'ts" are many and these may be considered in two groups. First, one set of don'ts is inferred from reading the do's. Another set of don'ts includes but is not limited to:
Collect "extra" data. If it is not immediately relevant, do not spend time on it. Folks put too much in front of patients to self-report, have clinicians fill out too many needless surveys, and have more data—so much—they will never get to it
Measure obvious things unless you have to. Satisfaction studies never got off the ground as telemedicine was so well received (i.e., 95 + % of patients and providers had high satisfaction). If a grant agency wants it measured, then you have no choice
Ignore even minor expectations the grant agency
Ignore the changes or upgrades in the literature; don't try to update everything with the latest and the best—not always necessary
Automatically assume that in-place EHR, quality improvement (QI), and other processes can easily be used to save time/money

4.3 Measuring Outcomes: An Overview on the Approach and Setting Targets

4.3.1 Overview

The drive to provide quality care is the primary stimulus for evaluation and research into outcomes. These are probably best summarized by three resources:

1. The eMH Group of the American Telemedicine Association (ATA) has thoroughly evaluated specific dimensions [11]: an expert consensus process which resulted in a lexicon for outcomes in the areas of patient satisfaction (i.e., access,

distance to service, use of), provider satisfaction, process of care (e.g., no-shows, coordination, completion of treatment), communication (e.g., rapport), reliability/validity (e.g., assessment, treatment vs. in-person), specific disorder measures (e.g., symptoms), cost (i.e., length of service, travel, hard- and software), and other administrative factors (e.g., facility management, team staffing). Limitations were that the group had a difficult time prioritizing which factors were the "most" important and thus could not prioritize recommendations. The suggested approach above is shaped significantly by a customized plan for each program.

2. A review on effectiveness specific to models, populations, settings, and other topics [1]: highly organized and comparative tables of clinical, cost, ethnic populations, and other outcomes for adult populations, along with prose descriptions of the rest. It was limited in scope such that tables for child and adolescent patients and many settings were not included.

3. An extensive chapter on program evaluation that has sections on clinical, cost, and other areas of eMH care [12]: even great depth than this chapter, but not including examples of project improvement nor (now) the latest outcomes, including the child and adolescent studies in depth.

4.3.2   Evaluation Parameters

4.3.2.1 Feasibility
Feasibility may be described in terms of operational, economic, technical, market, resource, or financial feasibility. Feasibility parameters include a description of the product or service, accounting statements, details of the operations and management, and policies, financial data, and legal requirements. Generally, feasibility studies precede technical development and project implementation.

4.3.2.2 Validity
For eMH and medicine, the most important issue is whether eMH works similar to the way we know in-person care works for a variety of disorders and treatments. Good satisfaction, ability to establish a therapeutic relationship to "experience" the provider, and a user-friendly perception are all good indicators of validity. eMH does most if not all things done in person (e.g., smell alcohol on a patient, check for extrapyramidal side effects or tremor, see all movements); proxies at the remote site may be trained and used.

4.3.2.3 Reliability
In the psychometrics, reliability is used to describe the overall consistency of a measure. Measurements of people's height and weight are often extremely reliable. One early study of telepsychiatry had patients treated in in-person and telemedicine "arms" mixed together, and no differences were noted [13]. A recent study of ADHD at a distance used synchronous telepsychiatry (STP) and asynchronous telepsychiatry (ATP, i.e., web-based) approaches for further training, data collection, and

monitoring with positive clinical outcomes [14]. Other eMH evidence bases show high reliability and validity started at 384+ KBPS and asynchronous [7] and other telephonic options [15, 16]. No major problems have been noted, but preliminary results are all that is available for some populations (e.g., geriatric psychiatry).

4.3.2.4 Satisfaction

Satisfaction is colloquially used in relation to life, purchases, work, relationships, and other common experiences. It is affected by culture, personality, state (e.g., depression), trait (i.e., personality), values, past experiences, expectations, and other factors. The eMH evidence base for satisfaction is soundly superior (STP more so than Skype-level technologies) with patients and providers willing to use it in order to connect despite state (e.g., depression), trait (i.e., personality), culture, and language dimensions. Patient satisfaction is a proxy for quality, access, affordability, and ability to connect, while provider satisfaction has additional dimensions of the ease of technology integration into clinical workflow, perceived value of better service, or access to specialists.

eMH appears better in overcoming obstacles related to geography, time zones, and delays of time for treatment. Cultural issues highlight how technology might better connect folks (e.g., providing access to the patient's primary language, same culture providers, communication with a provider outside of one's in-group). Ironically, the medical home's focus of care on the primary care clinic may work or not, as some prefer other settings (e.g., religion or spiritual centers) or other practitioners (e.g., shaman, priest, other). eMH has cued patients to think about things they should have (or had) already in their doctor's visit or in using technology. There are subtle differences like not handshaking or using empathic comments rather than passing a tissue.

4.3.2.5 Cost/Economics

Next section, please.

4.3.2.6 Clinical Outcomes

Next section, please.

4.3.3 Models of Care: How to Select Them and Impact on Evaluation

A summary of eMH models of care reviewed the pros and cons of each model [1, 17], and other models have been thoroughly studied and well articulated [18].

4.3.3.1 Low Intensity

- Case review of diagnosis and discussion may change the diagnosis and treatment plan significantly [19, 20]. Provider knowledge, skills, and complexity of questions improve over time [21], particularly in rural private care practitioners (PCP) [22].
- In-person, telephone, or e-mail doctor-to-doctor "curbside" consultations are a central feature of clinical practice [17, 23], meeting 33 % of PCPs' informational needs [24–27]. Overall, these consultations do not include patient evaluations,

but they are inexpensive, rapid, brief, and often readily available [28]. A more in-depth system was a 24-h warm-line, multispecialty phone and e-mail physician-to-provider consultation system for adults and children with developmental disabilities [29].

- Cultural consultation to rural primary care using telemedicine [30, 31].
- Disaster response to a bioterrorism attack was evaluated as feasible in terms of training and consultations [32].

4.3.3.2 Moderate Intensity
- An integrated program of mental health screening, therapy on site, and telepsychiatric consultation (phone, email, or video), with continuing medical education (CME) and training on screening questionnaires [33, 34], has improved outcomes and site-based staff skills.
- A randomized controlled trial (RCT) for depression in adults, using disease management and telepsychiatric consultation vs. usual care over 12 months, improved the care of both groups, as the "usual care" group benefited from the Hawthorne effect and skill development of the providers, in addition to curbside consultations [35].
- Asynchronous telepsychiatry (ATP) to primary care are feasible, valid, and reliable in English- and Spanish-speaking patients in primary care [31, 36] (similar methods are used in radiology, dermatology, ophthalmology, cardiology, and pathology). One ATP model uses a basic questionnaire for screening by the provider of the patient, video capture of that interview, and uploading of patient histories for a remote psychiatrist for review in an HIPAA-adherent manner [37]. Diagnosis and treatment recommendations are made and PCPs implement care successfully about 80 % of the time and the model is cost-effective [38].

4.3.3.3 High Intensity
- Collaborative care, which has now been more formally applied to telemedicine [2, 39, 40], has encouraging results. The virtual collaborative care team was able to produce better outcomes than the traditional "gold standard" methodology of primary care psychiatry [2].
- Child collaborative care for children with ADHD at a distance used STP and ATP (i.e., web-based) approaches for further training, data collection, and monitoring and showed positive clinical outcomes [14].

4.4 The Evidence Base for Clinical Outcomes

4.4.1 Cost/Economic Outcomes

With regard to cost, there is benefit to delineate between differing types of cost analyses [12, 41]. The cost-offset model, which implies treating mental conditions may reduce other health costs, is widely used. Cost-minimization analysis implies the same effectiveness model but different (lower) costs. Cost-effectiveness assesses intervention costs vs. alternative expenditures; a subtype is cost-utility analysis, which includes data on health-related quality of life measures (i.e., quality-adjusted life years). Cost-benefit analysis values all outcomes by translating them into economic terms to the degree possible and is particularly important when an intervention appears far too expensive at face value (or cross section) but not longitudinally (e.g., a transplant helps someone live and work an additional 50 years; this calculation gets into quality of life years analysis).

The eMH group of the ATA has thoroughly evaluated specific dimensions [11]. Economic evaluation that incorporates standard eco-general, clear definitions does not exist for many of the cost structures. This may be appropriate as costs are derived and perceived differently. There are several cost factors that were identified as important to measure objectively. Until final definitions are set, each cost factor should be operationalized and reported. Consideration should also be given to what is sunk or similar cost of care as usual (provider time). In general, clear definitions do not exist for many of the cost structures. The eMH evidence base related to cost is best presented elsewhere [12].

Generally, programs vary in calculations in terms of cost, but these may be potentially, arbitrarily, stratified into tiers of quality of assessment, though technically these should be formally stratified by research and data.

4.4.1.1 Regular Tier Quality
- Patient only
- Technology direct but limited (e.g., rent of lines)
- One-time (i.e., one service) cost, the cost if a certain number of consultations are done or the cost per additional service (i.e., using eMH sometimes we provide services not previously available)

4.4.1.2 Above-Average Quality
- Patient, provider, and clinic, limited direct and indirect (e.g., cost of travel, missed work, avoiding higher-care option, cost offset by reduced visits to PCP by treatment of depression)
- Technology, direct and indirect, but limited (e.g., above, hardware, software)
- A "break-even" model cost based on number of consultations or use over time, some cost-benefit calculation

4.4.1.3 Very High Quality
- Patient, provider, staff, clinic, community (e.g., cost of flow of services and associated spending on gas, shopping, and hotels for travel to urban center), and administrative

- Technology, direct and indirect, comprehensive (above, depreciation, upgrades), and including "live" technical participation (e.g., remote control or live Q&A to problem-solve one or both ends of video)
- Sophisticated analyses including impact on utilization of services, calculation of quality of life years, cost-effectiveness; need for economist or other expert

4.4.2 Clinical Outcomes

4.4.2.1 Overview and Adults

Results regarding age, disorder, and ethnic population are encouraging, overall [1, 12, 42]. Videoconferencing appears to be as effective as in-person care for most parameters, such as feasibility, outcomes, age, and satisfaction with a single assessment and consultation or follow-up use. Illnesses studied have been depression [2, 39, 43], PTSD [44–48], substance use [49], and developmental disabilities [50]. Comparison of treatment may be based on samples of the same disease state and in-person care.

The majority of research has focused on practical, straightforward assessments like symptoms, satisfaction, and basic costs. Pre- and posttreatment measurements, with a screening questionnaire or a general index like global assessment of function [51], are simple yet meaningful, usually with the hope of showing response (50 % reduction of symptoms) or remission. Other things worthy of more attention are quality of life, work attendance/absenteeism, compliance/adherence, or psychosocial measures (unit cohesiveness, social isolation). Patient adherence to treatment plans is limited in medicine, but number of visits, duration of treatment, and number or % of modules completed are helpful. Care performance, e.g., HEDIS (Healthcare Effectiveness Data and Information Set), and treatment utilization (i.e., visits, visit duration/frequency/problem addressed, resources like labs, medications, system-funded travel, devices, consultation, number of referrals made and utilized) measures are useful.

4.4.2.2 Children and Adolescents

The feasibility, acceptability, and sustainability of eMH for children and adolescents have now been shown [52], and it has been hypothesized as preferable for autism-spectrum patients [53]. Primary care patients treated showed improvement in terms of depression and subscales on behavioral checklists [33, 34]. A qualitative study of young people's perspectives on receiving telepsychiatric services revealed that the sessions were helpful, they felt a sense of personal choice during the consultation, and they were generally liking the technology [54], and the practice parameter from 2008 [55] is being updated. Collaborative care for depression [40] and the STP/ATP combination or "hybrid" method for ADHD work well [14].

4.4.2.3 Geriatric

The benefits of eMH are emerging from neuropsychiatric studies and a few geriatric clinical studies. Geriatric data are emerging, mostly on depression and cognition, but more studies are needed in medicine and eMH [56]. Obstacles include access to service, functional challenges, primary care provider attitudes, and lack of psychiatrists [57].

4.4.2.4 Ethnicity, Culture, and Language

Studies are blossoming in terms of specific needs of Hispanics/Latinos, Asians, Native Americans, Eastern Europeans, and those using sign language—all using telepsychiatry for service provision [1]. With patients of different cultural backgrounds, using the patients' primary language allows more comfort in expressing genuine feelings and emotions. A plan for assessment and care for patients with ethnic, cultural, and language issues is essential [33, 36]. Scientific and policy questions are: (1) What tools, methods, and measures are needed to assess the patients, providers, and health systems? (2) What are the intersections of culture, sociodemographics, geography, and technology in health? (3) Will patients' disorder, racial or ethnic identity, or other factors determine whether e-mental health or in-person care is more effective? (4) What is the most cost-effective and feasible way to provide language/interpreting support?

4.4.2.5 Other Special Populations

These include but are not limited to involuntary, inpatient, those needing seclusion and restraint, the incarcerated, and emergencies [10, 12]. The ATA evidence-based practice guideline summarizes and defines key things like mental health evaluation, clinical services/care, regular populations, and populations with special management considerations (e.g., incarcerated) [10]. Measures for consideration include quality of care, the process of consent, and other legal requirements. Guidelines on how to be effective in providing emergency telepsychiatry need to be evaluated [1, 58, 59], though there are one study [60] and one of different programs [61].

4.4.2.6 Psychometrically Sound Instruments and Guidelines

Diagnostic assessment and instruments are specifically described elsewhere [1, 12].

4.5   Discussion and Conclusion

This chapter addressed prioritization of outcomes and evaluation in the provision of eMH services. Basic and advanced areas of evaluation (e.g., satisfaction, technology, cost, clinical, and other outcomes) are suggested for the many participants in eMH in a systematic framework. Process, procedures, levels of depth, and do's and don'ts were offered to give the reader options to learn basic or advanced approaches to eMH, program change, and evaluation/outcomes. It also offers suggestions on how to do a needs assessment and how to adjust priorities based on specific needs and available resources in a program. Examples of project improvement apply ideas from theory to clinical and other associated outcomes.

The information is necessary for clinical leaders, managers, and other team members because they approach, and processes that guide "good" evaluation and outcomes may require a foundation of planning for a program to be successful. Overall, the best standard is a simple yet elegant plan and one that is practical, efficient, systematic, and grounded in the evidence base. Standard do's and don'ts of evaluation should be considered. This chapter attempts to show levels of quality of evaluation options, with varying scope and depth, and examples of how to augment whatever place a program is starting—a plan with sufficient "how to" to get to the next better place incrementally. The chapter is limited in size and depth, but additional references and resources of information are provided for further review. The readers may acquire knowledge, skill, and a framework to improve existing programs and help their many participants.

Acknowledgments American Telemedicine Association, and in particular, the Mental Health Interest Group

University of Southern California Department of Psychiatry and Behavioral Sciences

UC Davis Department of Psychiatry and Behavioral Sciences

References

1. Hilty DM, Ferrer D, Callahan EJ, et al. The effectiveness of telemental health: a 2013 review. Telemed J E Health. 2013;19(6):444–54.
2. Fortney JC, Pyne JM, Mouden SP, et al. Practice-based versus telemedicine-based collaborative care for depression in rural federally qualified health centers: a pragmatic randomized comparative effectiveness trial. Am J Psychiatry. 2013;170(4):414–25.
3. Katon W, Von Korff M, Lin E, et al. Collaborative management to achieve depression treatment guidelines. J Clin Psychiatry. 1997;58 Suppl 1:20–4.
4. Moreno FA, Chong J, Dumbauld J, et al. Use of standard webcam and Internet equipment for telepsychiatry treatment of depression among underserved Hispanics. Psychiatr Serv. 2012;63(12):1213–7.
5. Unutzer J, Choi Y, Cook IA, et al. A web-based data management system to improve care for depression in a multicenter clinical trial. Psychiatr Serv. 2002;53:671–8.
6. Geyer J, Myers K, Vander Stoep A, et al. Implementing a low-cost web-based clinical trial management system for community studies: a case study. Clin Trials. 2011;8:634–44.
7. Yellowlees PM, Odor A, Burke MM, et al. A feasibility study of asynchronous telepsychiatry for psychiatric consultations. Psychiatr Serv. 2010;61(8):838–40.
8. Ottawa ON. Personal wireless device use for wound care consultation: a review of safety, clinical benefits and guidelines [Internet]. Canadian Agency for Drugs and Technologies in Health, May, 2014. 28 Feb 2005. At http://www.cadth.ca/en/products/rapid-response.
9. Hilty DM, Liu W, Marks SL, et al. Effectiveness of telepsychiatry: a brief review. Can Psychiat Asso Bull. 2003;35(5):10–17.
10. Yellowlees PM, Shore JH, Roberts L, et al. Practice guidelines for videoconferencing-based telemental health. Telemed J E Health. 2010;16(10):1074–89.
11. Shore JH, Mishkind MC, Bernard J, et al. A lexicon of assessment and outcome measures for telemental health, ATA, 2013. 28 Feb 2015. At http://www.americantelemed.org/practice/standards/ata-standards-guidelines/a-lexicon-of-assessment-and-outcome-measurements-for-telemental-health#.UwF5Dv0_3-Y OR http://www.americantelemed.org/resources/stan-

dards/ata-standards-guidelines/a-lexicon-of-assessment-and-outcome-measurements-for-telemental-health#.U2bG2xYrfdk.

12. Hilty DM, Yellowlees PM, Nasatir SEH, et al. Program evaluation and practical, step-by-step program modification in telemental health. In: Behavioral telehealth series volume 1- clinical video conferencing: program development and practice. Springer Press, New York. 2014. pp. 75–104.
13. Hilty DM, Nesbitt TS, Hales RE, et al. The use of telemedicine by academic psychiatrists for the provision of care in the primary care setting. Medscape Mental Health. 2000;5:1–11.
14. Myers KM. Effectiveness of a telehealth service delivery model for treating attention-deficit hyperactivity disorder: results of a community-based randomized controlled trial. J Am Acad Child Adolesc Psychiatry. 2015;54(4):263–74.
15. Koenig HG, Cohen HJ, Goli V, et al. Major depression and the NIMH Diagnostic Interview Schedule: validation in medically ill hospitalized patients. Int J Psychiatry Med. 1989;19:123–32.
16. Wells KB, Burnam MA, Leake B, et al. Agreement between face-to-face and telephone administered versions of the depression section of the NIMH Diagnostic Interview Schedule. J Psychiatr Res. 1988;22:207–20.
17. Hilty DM, Yellowlees PM, Cobb HC, et al. Models of telepsychiatric consultation-liaison service to rural primary care. Psychosomatics. 2006;47(2):152–7.
18. World Health Organization: telemedicine opportunities and developments in member states. Results of the second global survey on eHealth. Geneva: WHO Press; 2011.
19. Hilty DM, Marks SL, Urness D, et al. Clinical and educational applications of telepsychiatry: a review. Can J Psychiatr. 2004;49(1):12–23.
20. Dobbins ML, Roberts N, Vicari SK, et al. The consulting conference: a new model of collaboration for child psychiatry and primary care. Acad Psychiatry. 2011;35:260–2.
21. Hilty DM, Yellowlees PM, Nesbitt TS. Evolution of telepsychiatry to rural sites: change over time in types of referral and PCP knowledge, skill, and satisfaction. Gen Hosp Psychiatry. 2006;28(5):367–73.
22. Hilty DM, Nesbitt TS, Kuenneth TA, et al. Telepsychiatric consultation to primary care: rural vs. suburban needs, utilization and provider satisfaction. J Rural Health. 2007;23(2):163–5.
23. Manian FA, Janssen DA. Curbside consultations. JAMA. 1996;275:145–6.
24. Gruppen LD, Wolf FM, Van Voorhees CV, et al. Information-seeking strategies and differences among primary care physicians. Mobius. 1987;7:18–26.
25. Ely JW, Burch RJ, Vinson DC. The information needs of family physicians: case specific clinical questions. J Fam Pract. 1992;25:265–9.
26. Gorman PN, Ash J, Wykoff L. Can primary care physicians' questions be answered using the medical journal literature? Bull Med Libr Assoc. 1994;82:140–6.
27. Dee C, Blazek R. Information needs of the rural physician. A descriptive study. Bull Med Libr Assoc. 1993;81:259–64.
28. Bergus GR, Sinift D, Randall CS, et al. Use of an e-mail curbside consultation service by family physicians. J Fam Pract. 1998;47(5):357–60.
29. Hilty DM, Ingraham RL, Yang RP, et al. Multispecialty phone and email consultation to primary care providers for patients with developmental disabilities in rural California. Telemed J E Health. 2004;10:413–21.
30. Cerda GC, Hilty DM, Hales RE, et al. Use of telemedicine with ethnic groups (letter). Psychiatr Serv. 1999;50:1364.
31. Yellowlees PM, Marks SL, Hilty DM, et al. Using e-health to enable culturally appropriate mental health care in rural areas. Telemed J E Health. 2008;14(5):486–92.
32. Ayers K, Yellowlees PM. Mental health considerations during a pandemic influenza outbreak. Int J Rescue Disast Med. 2009;9(1). doi:10.5580/1481.
33. Neufeld JD, Bourgeois JA, Hilty DM, et al. The e-Mental Health Consult Service: providing enhanced primary care mental health services through telemedicine. Psychosomatics. 2007;48:135–41.

34. Yellowlees PM, Hilty DM, Marks SL, et al. A retrospective analysis of child and adolescent e-mental health. J Am Acad Child Adolsc Psychiatry. 2008;47(1):1–5.
35. Hilty DM, Marks SL, Wegeland JE, et al. A randomized controlled trial of disease management modules, including telepsychiatric care, for depression in rural primary care. Psychiatry. 2007;4(2):58–65.
36. Yellowlees PM, Odor A, Patrice K, et al. Transcultural psychiatry made simple: asynchronous telepsychiatry as an approach to providing culturally relevant care. Telemed J E Health. 2013;19(4):1–6.
37. Yellowlees PM, Odor A, Patrice K, et al. PsychVACS: a system for asynchronous telepsychiatry. Telemed J E Health. 2011;17(4):299–303.
38. Butler TN, Yellowlees P. Cost analysis of store-and-forward telepsychiatry as a consultation model for primary care. Telemed J E Health. 2012;18(1):74–7.
39. Fortney JC, Pyne JM, Edlund MJ, et al. A randomized trial of telemedicine-based collaborative care for depression. J Gen Intern Med. 2007;22(8):1086–93.
40. Richardson L, McCauley E, Katon W. Collaborative care for adolescent depression: a pilot study. Gen Hosp Psychiatry. 2009;31:36–45.
41. Weinstein MC, Stason WB. Foundations of cost-effectiveness analysis for health and medical practices. N Engl J Med. 1977;296(13):716–21.
42. Hilty DM, Shoemaker EZ, Myers KM., et al. Issues and steps toward a clinical guideline for telemental health for care of children and adolescents. J Child Adol Psychopharm. In Press.
43. Richardson LK, Frueh BC, Grubaugh AL, et al. Current directions in videoconferencing telemental health research. Clin Psychol. 2009;16(3):323–8.
44. Ruskin PE, Silver-Aylaian M, Kling MA, et al. Treatment outcomes in depression: comparison of remote treatment through telepsychiatry to in in-person treatment. Am J Psychiatry. 2004;161:1471–6.
45. Morland LA, Greene CJ, Rosen C, et al. Issues in the design of a randomized noninferiority clinical trial of telemental health psychotherapy for rural combat veterans with PTSD. Contemp Clin Trials. 2009;30(6):513–52.
46. Morland LA, Greene CJ, Rosen CS, et al. Telemedicine for anger management therapy in a rural population of combat veterans with posttraumatic stress disorder: a randomized noninferiority trial. J Clin Psychiatry. 2010;71:855–63.
47. Morland LA, Hynes AK, Mackintosh MA, et al. Group cognitive processing therapy delivered to veterans via telehealth: a pilot cohort. J Trauma Stress. 2011;24(4):465–9.
48. Frueh BC, Monnier J, Yim E, et al. Randomized trial for post-traumatic stress disorder. J Telemed Telecare. 2007;13:142–7.
49. Frueh BC, Henderson S, Myrick H. Telehealth service delivery for persons with alcoholism. J Telemed Telecare. 2005;11(7):372–5.
50. Szeftel R, Federico C, Hakak R, et al. Improved access to mental health evaluation for patients with developmental disabilities using telepsychiatry. J Telemed Telecare. 2012;18(6):317–21.
51. Hall RC. Global assessment of functioning: a modified scale. Psychosomatics. 1995;36(3):267–75.
52. Myers KM, Palmer NB, Geyer JR. Research in child and adolescent telemental health. Child Adolesc Psychiatr Clin N Am. 2011;20(1):155–71.
53. Pakyurek M, Yellowlees PM, Hilty DM. The child and adolescent telepsychiatry consultation: can it be a more effective clinical process for certain patients than conventional practice? Telemed J E Health. 2010;16(3):289–92.
54. Boydell K, Volpe T, Pignatello A. A qualitative study of young people's perspectives on receiving psychiatric services via televideo. J Can Acad Child Adolesc Psychiatry. 2010;19:5–11.
55. AACAP. Practice parameter for telepsychiatry with children and adolescents. J Am Acad Child Adolesc Psychiatry. 2007;47(12):1468–83.
56. Botsis T, Demiris G, Peterson S, et al. Home telecare technologies for the elderly. J Telemed Telecare. 2008;14:333–7.

57. Sheeran T, Dealy J, Rabinowitz T. Geriatric telemental health. In: Myers K, Turvey CL, editors. Telemental health. New York: Elsevier; 2013. p. 171–95.
58. Shore JH, Hilty DM, Yellowlees PM. Emergency management guidelines for telepsychiatry. Gen Hosp Psychiatry. 2007;29:199–206.
59. Yellowlees PM, Burke MM, Marks SL, et al. Emergency telepsychiatry. J Telemed Telecare. 2008;14:277–81.
60. Sorvaniemi M, Ojanen E, Santamaki O. Telepsychiatry in emergency consultations: a follow-up study of sixty patients. Telemed J E Health. 2005;11(4):439–41.
61. Williams M, Pfeffee M, Boyle, et al. Telepsychiatry in the emergency department: Overview and case studies. California HealthCare Foundation. December, 2010. 28 Feb 2015. At http://www.chcf.org/publications/2009/12/telepsychiatry-in-the-emergency-department-overview-and-case-studies.
62. Beck AT, Ward CH, Mendelson M. An inventory for measuring depression. Arch Gen Psychiatry. 1961;18:561–7.
63. Beck AT, Steer RA, Garbin MG. Psychometric properties of the Beck Depression Inventory: twenty-five years of evaluation. Clin Psychol Rev. 1988;8:77–100.
64. Derogatis LR, Rickels K, Rock AF. The SCL-90 and the MMPI: a step in the validation of a new self-report scale. Br J Psychiatry. 1976;128:280–9.
65. Saunders JB, Aasland OG, Babor TF, et al. Development of the Alcohol Use Disorders Identification Test (AUDIT): WHO collaborative project on identification and treatment of persons with harmful alcohol consumption, phase II. Addiction. 1993;88:791–804.
66. Ewing JA. Detecting alcoholism: the CAGE Questionnaire. J Am Med Assoc. 1984;252:1905–7.
67. Steer RA, Ball R, Ranieri RF, et al. Dimensions of the Beck depression inventory-II in clinically depressed outpatients. J Clin Psychol. 1999;55(1):117–28.
68. Steer RA, Rissmiller DJ, Beck AT. Use of the Beck Depression Inventory with depressed geriatric patients. Behav Res Ther. 2000;38(3):311–8.

e-Mental Health Toward Cross-Cultural Populations Worldwide

5

Davor Mucic, Donald M. Hilty, and Peter M. Yellowlees

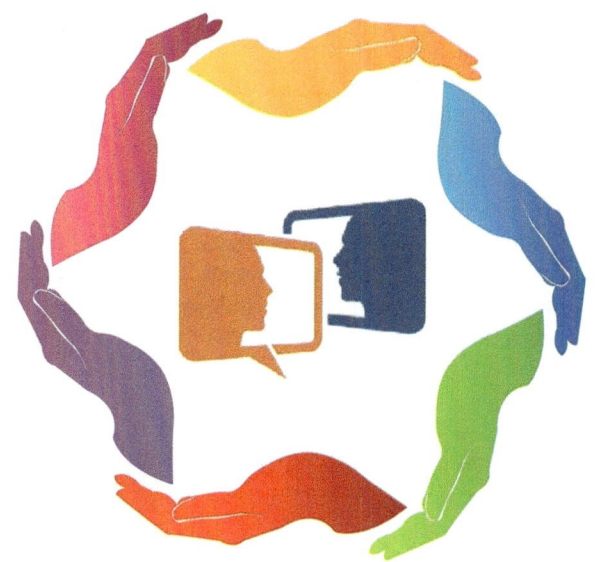

D. Mucic, MD (✉)
The Little Prince Psychiatric Centre, Copenhagen, Denmark
e-mail: info@denlilleprins.org
http://www.denlilleprins.org; http://www.tv-psykiater.dk

D.M. Hilty, MD
Keck School of Medicine, University of Southern California,
Los Angeles, CA, USA
e-mail: donh031226@gmail.com

P.M. Yellowlees, MD, MBBS
Health Informatics Graduate Program, University of California, Davis Health System,
Sacramento, CA, USA

© Springer International Publishing Switzerland 2016
D. Mucic, D.M. Hilty (eds.), *e-Mental Health*,
DOI 10.1007/978-3-319-20852-7_5

Contents

5.1   Introduction   78
5.2   Cross-Cultural Psychiatry and Its Application to EMH..   80
      5.2.1   Cross-Cultural Psychiatry and the Approach to Clinical Care   80
      5.2.2   Cross-Cultural eMH or Telepsychiatry..   81
5.3   Culture, Language, and the Value of eMH..   83
5.4   International Perspectives: Culturally Sensitive Collaborative
      Treatment of Ethnic Minorities Worldwide..   84
      5.4.1   International, Cross-Border Studies...   84
      5.4.2   Development of International eMH Networks?...   85
5.5   Discussion and Conclusions: Change from Within and Without   87
      5.5.1   Changes from "Within" Patients and Providers?...   87
      5.5.2   From "Without"...Societal Perspectives?...   87
Conclusion   88
References..   89

Abstract

Cross-cultural patient mental health-care demands a high standard of communication between the patient and the provider, since linguistic and other differences may influence it and consequently affect quality of care and satisfaction. Geographical distances, culture, religious, and linguistic, make it difficult for some patient populations to access mental health professionals in their desired way. Clinicians with a positive attitude to differences and who advocate for patients may seek out e-Mental Health (eMH) innovations to overcome barriers, increase the quality of mental health care for ethnic minorities, and enhance their own education. Indeed, eMH applications offer new possibilities for reducing disparities in access to relevant mental health care to most vulnerable patient groups, such as refugees, migrants, and asylum seekers worldwide. National and international cross-cultural eMH services may contribute to reduce stigma and improve quality of health care of these groups in their host countries. Equal access to mental health services is a human right, for both domestic and immigrant population in modern communities worldwide.

5.1   Introduction

Physicians and other health-care workers are increasingly being called upon to bridge the cultural differences that may exist between themselves and their patients. This challenge has become ever more urgent due to the rapidly changing demographics. For example, in the United States approximately one-third of the country's population is considered to be minorities now, but by the year 2050 minorities will constitute 54 % of the US population; by 2023, one-half of all children will be minority group members [1, 2]. As the demographic profile of the health-care workforce becomes increasingly diverse, health-care providers must be able to communicate with colleagues in addition to patients [3].

The culture of the patient, clinician and the setting significantly affect health and illness research [4]. Culture refers to a group's shared set of beliefs, norms, and values. Common social groupings (e.g., people who share a religion, youths who participate in the same sport, or adults trained in the same profession) have their own cultures. The culture of the patient includes symptoms, presentation, meaning, causation, family factors, coping styles, treatment seeking, mistrust, stigma, immigration, and overall health status. The culture of the clinician includes communication, primary care, clinician bias, and culture. Culture, society, and mental health service setting issues include financing, evidence-based treatment, culturally competent service, medication, and other factors [5].

Some of the major barriers for ethnic minorities globally to accessing mental healthcare are scarcity of access to care in general, providers they feel comfortable seeking help from, cultural competent interpreters and stigma. Communication between providers (mental health professionals) and patients (ethnic minorities) is therefore more complicated with a third person involved as an interpreter. The Institute of Medicine has recommended that medical school programs "integrate" cross-cultural education into the training of all current and future health professionals and the Liaison Committee on Medical Education changes for 2015 competencies 3.3 (Diversity/Pipeline Programs and Partnerships), 7.5 (Social Problems) and 7.6 (Cultural Competence/Health Care Disparities/Personal Bias)" [6, 3]. Initial reports suggested that residents considered culture as either very important or moderately important in providing care [7], but a recent report contradicts that [3] – it is unknown if this data generalizes internationally.

Fortunately, the use of eMH applications enables opportunities to build the bridges over cultural and linguistic barriers, by connecting patients with professionals that "match" culturally and linguistically [5]. Two convenient "solutions" have been to videoconference an interpreter who knows the same language (e.g., Spanish), but if the interpreter's ethnicity is different (e.g., Asian-American), this may compound the original language problem; the second solution is using interpreters at an academic center for a three-party conference telephone call. Neither of these are the same as in-person service with patient-interpreter cultural, ethnic, and language matching.

This chapter will review the literature, program descriptions, case examples (e.g., innovative programs; the first national and international cross-cultural service), the reader will learn:

1. How eMH can facilitate clinical services to culturally diverse population, which promotes adaptation, values differences, and reduces stigma/discrimination
2. How cross-cultural eMH can facilitate clinical services, which promotes adaptation, values differences, reduces stigma/discrimination, and results in good patient satisfaction
3. International perspectives about culturally sensitive collaborative treatment of ethnic minorities worldwide, when interpreters may not be accessed, and innovative programs to overcome this issue

5.2 Cross-Cultural Psychiatry and Its Application to EMH

5.2.1 Cross-Cultural Psychiatry and the Approach to Clinical Care

Culturally appropriate care has been defined as "the delivery of mental health services that are responsive to the cultural and linguistic concerns of all racial or ethnic minority groups and non-minority groups, including their psychosocial issues, characteristic styles of problem presentation, family and immigration histories, traditions, beliefs and values" [4]. Approaches to clinical care [8] and educational interventions [9, 10] have been described. In California, the primary care providers' (PCP) population is aging and a more diverse set of providers is needed [11] and some medical schools have a specific strategy to recruit Latinos into medical school [12].

More fundamental are concepts that have been defined in the literature that underlie the potential achievement of cultural competence, often referred to as culturally appropriate/sensitive care or individualized personal care [13]. These have been defined as:

- *Stereotyping versus generalization:* Interactions with individuals from a different cultural or ethnic background than one's own have long been characterized by stereotyping. A more appropriate approach would be to make a generalization as to which specific details about the individual can be made, which avoids the derogatory nature of many cultural and ethnic stereotypes.
- *Values of cultural and individual importance:* Different cultural and ethnic groups value the role and perspective of the individual differently. Certain cultural groups are highly individualistic, such as many individuals in the United States and in many western European countries. Other cultural groups, such as many Asian societies, value instead the goals and needs of the group/society as a whole. With regard to mental health care, they may see the problems as individual, family, community, or societal challenges.
- *Worldview:* Individuals, particularly from different cultures, may have great differences in their view of mental health, well-being, treatments, and approaches to care.
- *Ethnocentrism and cultural relativism: This* involves comparing one's own culture's way of doing things with other cultures' approaches. Ethnocentrism refers to the attitude that one's own culture is the "correct" one, while the relativist approach compares other cultures to one's own in a less punitive way.
- *Time orientation:* Adherence to time varies with some cultures predominately present-oriented (i.e., attentive almost exclusively to their immediate needs), while other cultures are traditionally past or future-oriented.
- *Inequity versus egalitarianism:* Cultures are set up in different ways. In theory America has a fairly egalitarian structure where everyone is intended to be equal, with success and power dependent on an individual's personal qualities and accomplishments. Other cultures, such as India, have a very precise social caste system where it is hard to move between different levels.

5.2.2 Cross-Cultural eMH or Telepsychiatry

The term cross-cultural telepsychiatry or culturally appropriate eMH care is in "real-time" synchronous telepsychiatry (STP; or videoconferencing) and/or asynchronous (formerly store-and-forward) telepsychiatry (ATP). The clinical service may include the interview, other assessment, psychiatric consultation between referring physicians and specialist, and other components [14]. eMH applications have been tested and developed over the last five to six decades, but most published reports of care to cultural populations are descriptive over the last 15 years.

Only one description – in the form of a case or letter – discussed *videoconferencing and culture*, that being a telepsychiatric consultation to primary care of a Hispanic patient [15]. It involved a 90-min diagnostic interview of a 56-year-old Mexican American woman conducted via videoconference by a Spanish-speaking psychiatrist located at an academic medical center 60 miles away. The local PCP spoke some Spanish, but there were no mental health (MH) providers in the vicinity, much less ones speaking Spanish, and the patient was concerned about seeing a MH provider anyway in her community for fear of being stigmatized.

A few years later, in 2004, on the other side of the globe, a cross-cultural telepsychiatry service was launched due to pilot project in order to overcome the burden of poor service access for ethnic minorities in Denmark and promote a new way of delivering mental health care by use of videoconference [16]. Thereafter, different approaches have been described [5, 17]. More specifically, the current sites face many challenges in terms of specific needs of Hispanics/Latinos and Asians [17–20], Native American [21, 22], Eastern European [23], and other populations (e.g., sign language) [24].

A few rigorous and many preliminary studies have evaluated diagnosis and treatment with cultural populations. Asynchronous telepsychiatry (ATP), formerly known as store-and-forward services, works at the patient end via taping a video recording of local providers and patients; it uses a basic questionnaire and uploaded videos and patient histories for a remote psychiatrist for review. The psychiatrist then evaluates the information, diagnoses the patient, and makes 2–3 treatment recommendations in a report. It was demonstrated to be feasible, valid, and reliable in English- and Spanish-speaking patients in primary care [25, 26]. In addition, it may obviate the need for real-time interpreters and be cost effective [27]. If an interpreter voice translates interview though, caution must be exercised to ensure that the affective tone is not lost; in this study, the historical information and video compensated for any of these impacts.

A model project is *The Little Prince Treatment Centre* in Copenhagen (Denmark), which has telepsychiatry cross-cultural expertise more than other places in Europe [28]. When the Centre launched the pioneer telepsychiatry pilot project in Denmark in 2004, ethnic minorities amounted to 8.6 % of the country's population [29], and MH care was burdened by long waiting times (3–6 months at private practitioners and even 12–36 months at specialized centers for treatment of refugees and torture victims); there was also a lack of bilingual resources and most services were provided via interpreters. Four stations (i.e., two hospitals, one asylum seekers center, and one social institution for rehabilitation of refugees and migrants) used bilingual clinicians at a distance that via video conference made possible to assess and/or treat patients via their own language, to enhance reliable assessment, and provide valid treatment for a

Table 5.1 Telepsychiatry user satisfaction questionnaire

Questions		Yes, in high degree (%)	Yes, in some degree (%)	No, only in less degree (%)	No, not at all (%)
1.	Did you get enough information about telepsychiatry?				
2.	Do you perceive "contact via TV" as uncomfortable?				
3.	Did you feel safe under telepsychiatry contact?				
4.	Have you been satisfied with sound quality?				
5.	Have you been satisfied with picture quality?				
6.	Did you achieve your goal via telepsychiatry / could you express everything you wanted to?				
7.	Would you recommend telepsychiatry to others?				
8	Would you prefer contact via translator in future?				
9.	What advantages did you perceive by telepsychiatry contact?				
10.	What disadvantages did you perceive by telepsychiatry contact?				

wide variety of psychiatric disorders. A patient satisfaction questionnaire was specially designed (Table 5.1) for completion at the end of the visit. High acceptance and satisfaction, regardless of their ethnicity or educational level, was noted [23].

Furthermore, all participants preferred "remote" contact with bilingual cinician i.e. via mother tongue, compared to in-person care with a translator, partly due to perceived higher anonymity, confidence/trust in providers, and self-efficacy to express intimate thoughts and feelings without a third person involved [23]. It was also believed that distance bilingual clinicians had additional experience with other frameworks of care, which was perceived as helpful, rather than a disadvantage of not knowing local or regional services. As expected, there was a clear correlation between the number of sessions, reported satisfaction level, and quality of care [23]. The patients' judgment of enhanced safety and comfort by telepsychiatry might also be due to less likelihood of meeting the doctor on the street and the risks of spreading rumors in the patients' neighborhood; this is similar to Native American populations in small tribes in the United States [30]. The telepsychiatry based service continued after the pilot project ended in 2007 and is still functioning between Psychiatric department on island Bornholm and The Little Prince Treatment Centre in Copenhagen. It is so far the only such service in EU where assessment and treatment of ethnic minorities is provided via bilingual specialists through videoconference mostly and not using of interpreters [28].

5.3   Culture, Language, and the Value of eMH

It has been reported that patients who face language barriers (i.e., refugees, asylum seekers, and migrants) are less likely than others to have a usual source of medical care, frequently receive preventive services at reduced rates, have an increased risk of non-adherence to medications, are less likely than others to return for follow-up appointments after visits to the emergency room, and have higher rates of hospitalization and drug complications [31]. Among many cultural differences regarding the use of mental health system, involuntarily admissions are relatively frequent among mentally ill ethnic minorities compared to domicile population. This might be due to poorer contact with general practitioners and outpatient psychiatric services, thereby causing greater risk of serious deterioration in mental health and mental illness before treatment is started [32–34].

One common theme in the literature for culture and language is the benefit of using the primary language for expression and more "comfort" in-person than by video [35]. As described above, many issues go through patients' minds. Those who are asylum seekers wandered if interpreters, depending on their nationality, would translate correctly (e.g., "One can never know whether they are translated correctly or not. That's why I prefer one that speaks my language." Or, "One can never trust them. Today I speak with the doctor and tomorrow the whole city knows everything about it." "They (Serbs/Albanians) have tortured me in Kosovo, so how can I trust them now?") [23].

Communication between providers (mental health professionals) and patients (ethnic minorities) is therefore more complicated with a third person involved as an interpreter. It is known that use of relatives or untrained interpreters miscommunicate medical complaints [36] or de-emphasize information [37], leading to calls for credentialing [38]. Nurses, too, do a little better with concrete medical complaints than capturing the narrative or cultural metaphors [39]. Culturally competent bilingual clinicians may have the same ethnic and cultural background as their respective patients (i.e., "ethnic matching"). Several studies have found that language barriers are associated with lower rates of patient satisfaction and poor care delivery in comparison with care received by patients who speak the language of the care provider [40, 41].

Language barriers are also likely to affect patients' trust in their providers. Patients who do not speak the language of respective care providers have reported feelings of being discriminated against in clinical settings, whereas communicating with health professionals in a common language is associated with increased trust and confidence [42]. Further, interpreter mediated communication is linked to increase risk of loss of confidentiality which is why the most refugees, asylum seekers, and migrants exposed for such kind of communication tend to be suspicious wondering, "How soon will everyone in this little city speak about my illness?" Nevertheless, the most ethnic minorities brought their stigma already from their respective home countries.

By a review of available scientific surveys one learns that: the presence of a third person (i.e., an interpreter) in a confidential relationship affects patient satisfaction, as it influences both transference and countertransference between individuals involved, with unavoidable consequences on a doctor-patient relationship [43]. Mistakes in interpretation (omissions, distorted questions, additions) occur frequently due to common practice where family members and non-trained interpreters involve as mediators in doctor-patient communication [36, 37, 39]. The use of a shared language (whether that of the patient or a third language shared by both patient and clinician) seems to be the most effective approach to ensure patient satisfaction and mutual comprehension [44]. There is no doubt that language-concordance plays significant role in building sustainable doctor-patient relationship. However, not only linguistic but also cultural and even racial concordance affect patient satisfaction as well as the satisfaction of the providers and are associated with better patient compliance, better adherence to treatment, and higher patient and provider satisfaction [45–49].

The use of professional interpreters is associated with improved clinical care and patient satisfaction more than the use of ad hoc interpreters [50]. Nevertheless, "ethnic matching" appears to be the most desirable model used in addressing language barriers and cultural disparities in mental health-care provision. Ethnic matching, supplemented by culture-competency training, has been proved as a common strategy to address a number of barriers in cross-cultural–related health-care provision [51, 52]. However, "ethnic matching" model is not that easy to implement. When the patient and the "matching" clinician are located in different places a consultation is likely to require travel, either for the patient or the clinician. This is where a videoconference becomes an obvious solution.

5.4   International Perspectives: Culturally Sensitive Collaborative Treatment of Ethnic Minorities Worldwide

The use of technology enables users and providers to be located in different parts of the world while still being connected via various applications of telecommunications technologies. eMH services/applications described in this book have a potential to provide efficient and cost-effective opportunity to reach individuals and groups with poor service access despite geographical distances and/or national borders.

5.4.1   International, Cross-Border Studies

When it comes to remote real-time eMH consultations via videoconferencing, there are only few studies describing international, cross-border studies, and none involve developing countries [53]:

- A consulting psychiatrist, who was licensed in Australia but living in New Zealand, provided care for two patients in a facility in Australia; one of the cases was a new consultation and the other was a follow up [54].
- A 6-month trial of telepsychiatric tertiary care from South London to the island of Jersey, reported five teleconsultations of a single second-opinion and four case reviews [55].

- International eMH and tele-education for Swedish medical students about cross-cultural issues in refugees with MH problems was conducted between Sweden, the United States, and Australia. There was one real patient at the American site and one simulated patient at the Australian site, with patient interviews by experts, while medical students exercised observation on videoconference and participated in the discussion [56].
- Videoconferencing provided psychoanalytic clinical care and training to psychoanalytic candidates in China by US psychoanalysts, and this involved 40 psychoanalytic and 30 psychodynamic psychotherapies [57].
- The most comprehensive international eMH service in the world was established via *The Little Prince Treatment Centre* in Denmark in mid 2006 as a part of the above-mentioned cross-cultural telepsychiatry project [58]. It became apparent that the lack of certain bilingual clinicians posed a greater problem than previously estimated. Bilingual clinicians from Sweden were employed to provide care due to their cross-cultural skills, including clinicians who spoke Arabic, Polish, Kurdish, and ex-Yugoslavian languages. Over a period of 18 months, 31 cross-cultural patients (i.e., refugees, migrants, and asylum seekers) were assessed and treated by videoconferencing from providers who spoke the patients' own language. Videoconferencing equipment connected the Swedish Department of the Little Prince Psychiatric Centre with two hospitals: one asylum seekers' center and one social institution in Denmark. The distances from the Swedish station located in Malmö to the Danish telepsychiatry stations were from 140 to 300 km. Overall, high patient satisfaction was reported and minor disadvantages of eMH were offset by doctor-patient language and cultural matching.

5.4.2 Development of International eMH Networks?

Experiences from the above-mentioned projects might pave the way for development of an International eMH Network within European Union (EU). Most of European countries have established rehabilitation and research centers for torture victims. eMH mediated collaboration between the centers will enable international exchange of expertise and enhance research in the field. Such network could, by the use of various eMH applications, improve assessment and/or treatment of primarily asylum seekers, refugees, and migrants within EU. At the same time, MH care of all other patient population groups could be improved as a result of increased access to specialized expertise, especially in outlying underserved areas and in urban communities with considerable limitations in access to specialized MH care (see also Chap. 12).

National implementation of cross-cultural telepsychiatry service predicts patients' acceptance as well. Religious patients are less likely to accept eMH when compared to those who are secular [59]. In recent study the author suggests that increasing public awareness of the use and effectiveness of technology may help facilitate patients' acceptance [60].

Table 5.2 Questions and policy implications for the intersection of TMH programs and culturally competent clinical care

Questions:
1. What kind of assessment methods and measures are needed to assess the clinical care and the roles of patients, providers, interpreters, and technology related to the provision of culturally appropriate or competent mental health (MH) care?
2. What are the intersections of culture, language, class, geography, and technology in our current MH system, and how do these intersections vary across racial/ethnic and class subgroups?
3. To what extent can technology be used to increase access to high quality MH services – along a continuum of options (e.g., web-based information, interactive sites, self-help assessment, and treatment strategies, evidence-based treatment with asynchronous interaction, asynchronous TMH, and fully synchronous treatments similar to in-person care)?
4. Can culturally and linguistically appropriate MH outcomes (acceptability, accessibility, utilization, continuity of care, improved MH status) be achieved electronically and if so, what types of electronic platforms work best for patients and providers?
5. Will patients' disorder, racial/ethnic identity, socioeconomic status, and geographic characteristics determine whether e-mental health or in-person care is more effective?
6. Should a hybrid model of in-person and electronic services provide more accurate diagnosis and a higher quality outcome?
7. Will patients' disorder, racial, or ethnic identity, or other factors determine whether e-mental health or in-person care is more effective?
Policy implications:
8. Should policy makers downplay the influence of culture on the use of technology and is it economically realistic to target e-mental healthcare toward existing monocultural clinics where it is common to have a clinic primarily focused on, for instance Asian Americans, North American Indians, or similar ethnic groupings?
9. What is the most cost-effective and logistically feasible way to provide language and interpreting support for e-mental health programs? How should policy makers maximize automated written translation services, now available on many Websites, which clearly could be used in the health industry to rapidly translate the written word for e-mail or instant messaging follow-up and treatment? What is the most effective way to link cultural interpreters to the language interpretation process?
10. What new approaches to care should be the core options and which others to be used, if needed?
11. How does one educate patients, providers, systems, and others on how to effectively participate in, and contribute to, culturally competent care?

Adapted from Yellowlees et al. [5]

It is certainly true, but … if the only alternative to videoconference via respective mother tongue is mental health-care provision via interpreters or no care at all, then the patient's acceptance of remote consultation is just a very logical choice, of course predicted by the service that includes cultural competent bilingual mental health providers. Further, the brief and easily understandable information received prior to the session, which is followed by reassurance that no one is listening, watching, or recording the sessions, and that the setting is absolutely private and confidential may contribute to increase acceptance of the model [23] (Table 5.2).

5.5   Discussion and Conclusions: Change from Within and Without

5.5.1   Changes from "Within" Patients and Providers?

There is a somewhat consistent pattern that many patients prefer eMH compared to in-person care with a translator [23], partly due to perceived higher anonymity, confidence/trust in providers (e.g., experience abroad), and self-efficacy to express intimate thoughts and feelings without a third person involved. The patients' judgment of enhanced safety and comfort by eMH might also be due to less likelihood of meeting the doctor on the street and the risks of spreading rumors in the patients' neighborhood; this is similar to Native American populations in small tribes in the United States [30].

Clinicians' attitudes and perceptions of eMH influence their intention to use the technology with their patients. The key predictor of the intention to use eMH is not clinicians' attitude toward it, but essentially how useful they expect it to be for their cross-cultural patients. Perceived usefulness will have a positive impact on attitudes toward this technology, and perceived ease of use will positively influence perceived usefulness [61]. Furthermore, mental health providers working with, e.g., Aboriginal and Torres Strait Islander clients show initially high level of acceptability of eMH application in provision of mental health [62]. Finally, clinicians do not share thoughts or feelings of incompetence about adapting too many cultures and languages, but the herald eMH as a tool capable of finding "other therapists" who match culturally, racially, linguistically, and even nationally and/or religiously. They may be aware of local limitations compared to remote consultation benefits?

As long as cross-cultural–related eMH applications are not seen as a substitute but as a supplement to existing system, the providers' acceptability level is likely to be high. Nevertheless, (un)expected resistance from the non-bilingual clinicians employed in centers for treatment of refugees, asylum seekers, and migrants occur the moment they feel threatened by being replaced and/or losing the control. Indeed, the introduction of an alternative means of treatment for ethnic minorities' base via telepsychiatry with professionals from other countries poses a number of threats and concerns. These threats included: accountability for care, consistency in the provision of care in accordance with the countries' medical policies and guidelines as well as the costs associated with treatment [63, 64].

5.5.2   From "Without"…Societal Perspectives?

A delicate issue in dealing with culture and language of patients is the tension between a goal generalizing an approach or the search for "standard" nuances of specific tribes, with the difficulty of stereotyping groups, and making clinical errors [5]. Meeting with members of the community, including the health clinic, in advance is recommended to understand cultural issues. In addition, some nuances are best learned "in vivo" (e.g., during a consultation with "real" patients). Ethnocentrism refers to the attitude that one's own culture is the "correct" one, while the relativist approach compares other cultures to one's own in a less punitive way. Adopting a relativist approach to providing e-mental healthcare to individuals from diverse backgrounds is a minimal, essential step toward culturally appropriate care.

Different cultural and ethnic groups value the role and perspective of the individual differently [5]. Certain cultural groups are highly individualistic, such as many individuals in the United States and in many western European countries. Other cultural groups, such as many Asian societies, value instead the goals and needs of the group/society as a whole. With regard to their mental healthcare, they may not see mental health problems as individual challenges that can be successfully treated, but as shameful or burdensome to themselves or to their families. The value of the individual should be a consideration when planning e-mental health interventions.

Refugees and asylum seekers are very often traumatized and are quite vulnerable when they seek therapy. Trust, confidentiality, and safety in therapeutic context decrease due to the presence of a third person, i.e., interpreter. However, majority of refugees and asylum seekers worldwide are still exposed for assessments and/or treatments provided via interpreters that very often belong to "wrong" nationality and even speak with "wrong" dialect. Decreased level of confidentiality leads consequently to a patient's unwillingness to divulge intimate personal information, thoughts and feelings to the interpreter. Professionals have a part of responsibility for such situations, as we must aim to match culture, language, and other differences between patients and providers, allied MH staff, and interpreters – all in our advocacy of those with mental illness, prone to stigma, and likely to have difficulty accessing services. We aim for this because every individual has a human right to health care.

It is estimated that by 2040 40 % of care will be virtual. This means that providers, hospitals, clinics, and other systems must be accessible, available, acceptable, be of good quality and make every effort to facilitate communication (e.g., preferably in the primary language). Or conversely, might we be able to use a computer – in a fashion that we currently use companies to find the "right" or most proximate language by simply dialing a 1–800 number or PubMed by typing in key words for a search – by entering culture, ethnicity, language, and other well-accepted diversity parameters? This could move us over or across national, regional, and local legislative, legal, or other bureaucratic barriers – probably, with only a few exceptions – those are people without access to money, Internet, or literally freedom (e.g., war contexts and other forms of significant discrimination or intolerance). Formal eMH guidelines and policies, while scarce internationally, are a start but do not overcome such barriers (Table 5.2).

Conclusion

Culturally sensitive care, with attention to differences, facilitates quality care, trust, safety, respect, and privacy – all essential when working with cross-cultural patient populations worldwide. Satisfaction is clearly tied to culture, ethnic, and (when possible) language matching. The literature, model programs, and others' descriptions give us good insight on successful programs and the ingredients involved. eMH certainly facilitates care and will continue to, as international collaboration and global networks of cross-cultural experts, address the MH and other health-care needs of ethnic minorities. Clinicians' attitudes, advocacy, and enhanced performance through supervision, tele-education, and "second opinion" service are essential, too. eMH has the potential to significantly impact – reduce – the burden of disease associated with mental illness worldwide.

Acknowledgments Ministry of the Interior and Health, the Egmont Foundation, and the Health Insurance Foundation for projects funded in Denmark from 2004 to 2012.

References

1. Shrestha LB, Heisler EJ. The changing demographic profile of the United States. Washington, DC: Congressional Research Service; 2011. February 28, 2015. At: http://fas.org/sgp/crs/misc/RL32701.pdf.
2. United States Census Bureau. An older and more diverse nation by midcentury [press release]. 2008. February 28, 2015. At: http://www.census.gov/newsroom/releases/archives/population/cb08-123.html.
3. Loue S, Wilson-Delfosse A, Limbach K. Identifying gaps in the cultural competence/sensitivity components of an undergraduate medical school curriculum: a needs assessment. J Immigr Minor Health. February 2014. At: http://link.springer.com/article/10.1007%2Fs10903-014-0102-z#
4. Office of the Surgeon General (US); Center for Mental Health Services (US); National Institute of Mental Health (US). Chapter 4: Mental health care for American Indians and Alaska Natives. In Mental health: culture, race, and ethnicity: a supplement to mental health: a report of the surgeon general. Rockville: Substance Abuse and Mental Health Services Administration (US); 2001. February 28, 2015. At: http://www.ncbi.nlm.nih.gov/books/NBK44242/.
5. Yellowlees PM, Marks SL, Hilty DM, et al. Using e-health to enable culturally appropriate mental health care in rural areas. Telemed J E Health. 2008;14(5):486–92.
6. Liaison Committee on Medical Education Competencies Revision, 2015. February 28, 2015. At: https://www.lcme.org/publications/2015-16-functions-and-structure-with-appendix.pdf.
7. Weissman JS, Betancourt J, Campbell EJ, et al. Resident physicians' preparedness to provide cross-cultural care. JAMA. 2005;294(9):1058–67.
8. Berger JT. Culture and ethnicity in clinical care. Arch Int Med. 1998;58(19):2085.
9. Beach MC, Price EG, Gary TL, et al. Cultural competency: a systematic review of health care provider educational interventions. Med Care. 2005;43(4):356.
10. Sherrill WW, Crew L, Mayo RM, et al. Educational and health services innovation to improve care for rural Hispanic communities in the US. Educ Health (Abingdon). 2005;18:356–67.
11. Walker KO, Moreno G, Grumbach K. The association among specialty, race, ethnicity, and practice location among California physicians in diverse specialties. J Natl Med Assoc. 2012;104(1–2):46–52.
12. Manetta A, Stephens F, Rea J, et al. Addressing health care needs of the Latino community: one medical school's approach. Acad Med. 2007;82(12):1145–51.
13. Galanti GA. Caring for patients from different cultures. 3rd ed. Philadelphia: University of Pennsylvania Press; 2004.
14. Hilty DM, Ferrer DC, Parish MB, et al. The effectiveness of telemental health: a 2013 review. Telemed J E Health. 2013;19:444–54.

15. Cerda GM, Hilty DM, Hales RE, et al. Use of telemedicine with ethnic groups. Psychiatr Serv. 1999;50(10):1364.
16. Mucic D. Telepsychiatry in Denmark: mental health care in rural and remote areas. J e-Health Tech Appl. 2007;5(3):426. February 28, 2015. At: http://dx.doi.org/10.1016/j.eurpsy.2007.01.1163.
17. Moreno FA, Chong J, Dumbauld J, et al. Use of standard webcam and Internet equipment for telepsychiatry treatment of depression among underserved Hispanics. Psychiatr Serv. 2012;63(12):1213–7.
18. Nieves JE, Stack KM. Hispanics and telepsychiatry. Psychiatr Serv. 2007;58(6):877.
19. Ye J, Shim R, Lukaszewski T, et al. Telepsychiatry services for Korean immigrants. Telemed E Health. 2012;18(10):797–802.
20. Chong J, Moreno F. Feasibility and acceptability of clinic-based telepsychiatry for low-income Hispanic primary care patients. Telemed J E Health. 2012;18(4):297–304.
21. Shore JH, Brooks E, Savin D, Orton H, Grigsby J, Manson SM. Acceptability of telepsychiatry in American Indians. Tel e-Health. 2008;14(5):461–6.
22. Weiner MF, Rossetti HC, Harrah K. Videoconference diagnosis and management of Choctaw Indian dementia patients. Alzheimers Dementia. 2011;7(6):562–6.
23. Mucic D. Transcultural telepsychiatry and its impact on patient satisfaction. J Telemed Telecare. 2010;16(5):237–42.
24. Lopez AM, Cruz M, Lazarus S, et al. Case report: use of American sign language in telepsychiatry consultation. Tel e-Health. 2004;10(3):389–91.
25. Yellowlees PM, Odor A, Patrice K, et al. PsychVACS: a system for asynchronous telepsychiatry. Telemed J E Health. 2011;17(4):299–303.
26. Yellowlees PM, Odor A, Iosif A, et al. Transcultural psychiatry made simple: asynchronous telepsychiatry as an approach to providing culturally relevant care. Tel e-Health. 2013;19(4):1–6.
27. Butler TN, Yellowlees P. Cost analysis of store-and-forward telepsychiatry as a consultation model for primary care. Tel e-Health. 2012;18(1):74–7.
28. http://www.denlilleprins.org/
29. Udlændingestyrelsen (Nøgletal på udlændingeområdet), 2004. At: https://www.nyidanmark.dk/NR/rdonlyres/B62D14EE-0264-46FF-AA4D-C1EE543EC8A2/0/talogfakta2004.pdf.
30. Hilty DM, Yellowlees PM, Tarui N, et al. Mental Health Services for California American Indians: usual service options and a description of telepsychiatric consultation to select sites. In Ramesh M, Shahram K, editors. Telemedicine, InTech Europe, Rijeka, Croatia; 2013. p. 75–104.
31. Flores G. Language barriers to health care in the United States. N Engl J Med. 2006;355:229–31.
32. Burnett R, Mallett R, Bhugra D, et al. The first con- tact of patients with schizophrenia with psychiatric services: social factors and path- ways to care in a multi-ethnic population. Psychol Med. 1999;29(2):475–83.
33. Parkman S, Davies S, Leese M, et al. Ethnic differences in satisfaction with mental health services among representative people with psychosis in south London: PRiSM study 4. Br J Psychiatry. 1997;171:260–4.
34. Tolmac J, Hodes M. Ethnic variation among adolescent psychiatric in- patients with psychotic disorders. Br J Psychiatry. 2004;184:428–31.
35. Hilty DM, Lim RF, Koike AK, et al. Planning for telepsychiatric consultation: a needs assessment for cultural and language services at rural sites in California. J Rural Mental Health. In Press.
36. Brooks TR. Pitfalls in communication with Hispanic and African-American patients: do translators help or harm? J Natl Med Assoc. 1992;84(11):941.
37. Brua C. Role-blurring and ethical grey zones associated with lay interpreters: three case studies. Commun Med. 2008;5(1):73.
38. Carlson J. Breaking down language barriers. Hospital interpreters get credentialed with new certification programs. Mod Healthc. 2010;40(46):32–4.
39. Elderkin-Thompson V, Silver RC, Waitzkin H. When nurses double as interpreters: a study of spanish-speaking patients in a US primary care setting. Soc Sci Med. 2001;52:1343–58.

40. Carrasquillo O, Orav EJ, Brennan TA, et al. Impact of language barriers on patient satisfaction in an emergency department. J Gen Intern Med. 1999;14:82–7.
41. Sarver J, Baker DW. Effect of language barriers on follow-up appointments after an emergency department visit. J Gen Intern Med. 2000;15:256–64.
42. Mutchler JE, Bacigalupe G, Coppin A, Gottlieb A. Language barriers surrounding medication use among older Latinos. J Cross Cult Gerontol. 2007;22:101–14.
43. Spiegel JP. Cultural aspects of transference and countertransference revisited. J Am Acad Psychoanal. 1976;4:447–67.
44. Riddick S. Improving access for limited English-speaking consumers: a review of strategies in health care settings. J Health Care Poor Underserved. 1998;9:40–61.
45. Freeman GK, Rai H, Walker JJ, et al. Non-English speakers consulting with the GP in their own language: a cross-sectional survey. Br J Gen Pract. 2002;52:36–8.
46. Pöchhacker F. Language barriers in Vienna hospitals. Ethn Health. 2000;5:113–9.
47. Saha S, Komaromy M, Koepsell TD, et al. Patient-physician racial concordance and the perceived quality and use of health care. Arch Intern Med. 1999;159:997–1004.
48. Bowen S. Language barriers in access to health care. Ottawa: Health Canada; 2001.
49. Perez-Stable EJ. Language access and Latino health care disparities. Med Care. 2007;45:1009–11.
50. Karliner LS, Jacobs EA, Chen AH, et al. Do professional interpreters improve clinical care for patients with limited English proficiency? A systematic review of the literature. Health Serv Res. 2007;42(2):727–54.
51. Ton H, Koike A, Hales RE, et al. A qualitative needs assessment for development of a cultural consultation service. Transcult Psychiatry. 2005;42:491–504.
52. Jerrell JM. Effect of ethnic matching of young clients and mental health staff. Cult Divers Ment Health. 1998;4:297–302.
53. Jefee-Bahloul H. Telemental health in middle east: overcoming the barriers. Front Public Health. 2014;2:86. doi:10.3389/fpubh.2014.00086.
54. Samuels A. International telepsychiatry: a link between New Zealand and Australia. Aust N Z J Psychiatry. 1999;33:284–6.
55. Harley J. Economic evaluation of a tertiary telepsychiatry service to an island. J Telemed Telecare. 2006;12(7H):354–7.
56. Ekblad S, Manicavasagar V, Silove D, et al. The use of international videoconferencing as a strategy for teaching medical students about transcultural psychiatry. Transcult Psychiatry. 2004;41:120–9.
57. Fishkin R, Fishkin L, Leli U, et al. Psychodynamic treatment, training, and supervision using internet-based technologies. J Am Acad Psychoanal Dyn Psychiatry. 2011;39:155–68.
58. Mucic D. International telepsychiatry: a study of patient acceptability. J Telemed Telecare. 2008;14:241–3.
59. Werner P. Willingness to use telemedicine for psychiatric care. Telemed J E Health. 2004;10:286–9310.
60. Jefee-Bahloul H, Moustafa MK, Shebl FM, et al. Pilot assessment and survey of Syrian refugees' psychological stress and openness to referral for telepsychiatry (PASSPORT Study). Telemed J E Health. 2014;20(10):977–9.
61. Monthuy-Blanc J, Bouchard S, Malano C, et al. Factors influencing mental health providers' intention to use telepsychotherapy in First Nations communities. Transcult Psychiatry. 2013;50(2):323–43.
62. Dingwall KM, et al. Like drawing into sand: acceptability, feasibility, and appropriateness of a new e-mental health resource for service providers working with Aboriginal and Torres Strait Islander People. Aus Psychol. 2015;50(1):60.
63. Mucic D. Telepsychiatry pilot-project in Denmark Videoconference by distance by ethnic specialists to immigrants/refugees. WCPRR. 2007;2(1):3–9.
64. Melaka A, Edirippulige S. Psych-technology: a systematic review of the telepsychiatry literature. Centre for Online Health Annual Report, 2009. February 28, 2015. At: http://www.docs-toc.com/docs/101738932/CENTRE-FOR-ONLINE-HEALTH-ANNUAL-REPORT-2009.

Part III

Clinical Care Models:
Stepped Care, Collaborative Care
and Integrated Care By Telepsychiatry

Donald M. Hilty

The Effectiveness of e-Mental Health: Evidence Base, How to Choose the Model Based on Ease/Cost/Strength, and Future Areas of Research

6

6

Donald M. Hilty, Peter M. Yellowlees, Kathleen Myers,
Michelle B. Parish, and Terry Rabinowitz

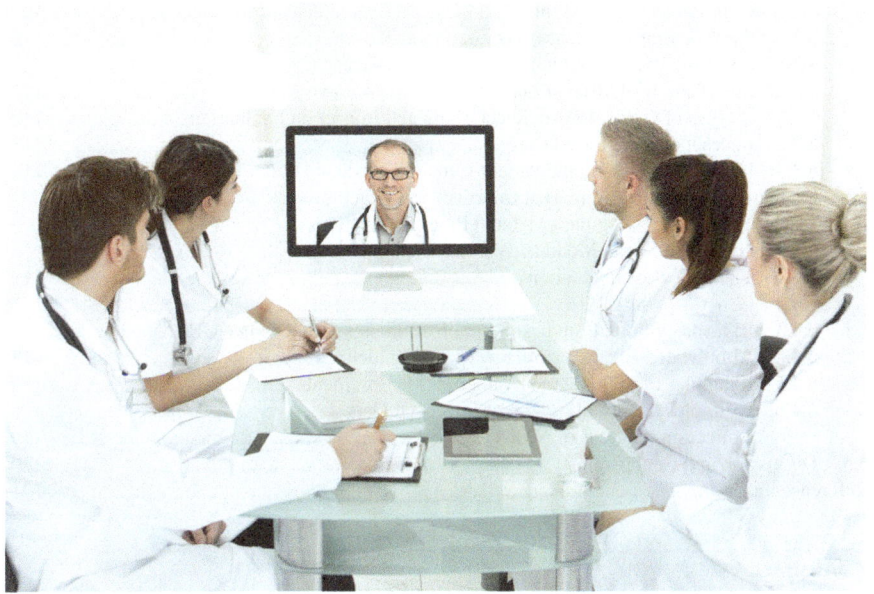

D.M. Hilty, MD (✉)
Keck School of Medicine, University of Southern California,
Los Angeles, CA, USA
e-mail: donh031226@gmail.com

P.M. Yellowlees, MD, MBBS
Health Informatics Graduate Program, University of California,
Davis Health System, Sacramento, CA, USA

© Springer International Publishing Switzerland 2016
D. Mucic, D.M. Hilty (eds.), *e-Mental Health*,
DOI 10.1007/978-3-319-20852-7_6

K. Myers, MD, MPH, MS
Telemental Health Service, Seattle Children's, University of Washington,
Seattle, WA, USA

M.B. Parish, MA
UC Davis Telepsychiatry and Health Informatics, University of California,
Davis School of Medicine & Health System, 2450 48th Street Suite 2800,
Sacramento, CA 95817, USA

T. Rabinowitz, MD
Psychiatry and Family Medicine, University of Vermont College of Medicine,
Burlington, VT, USA

Contents

6.1   Introduction   97
6.2   eMH is Effective and as Good as or Better Than In-Person Care   98
    6.2.1   Adult, Geriatric, and Other Populations   98
    6.2.2   Children and Adolescents   103
    6.2.3   Psychotherapy Evidence Base   112
6.3   Models of Care: The e-Continuum Toward Integrated
    and Stepped Care for Different Populations, Disorders, and Treatments.....................   112
    6.3.1   Models of Care: How to Select Them and Impact on Evaluation   112
    6.3.2   Internet or Web-Based Care..   115
    6.3.3   Integrated Care and the Patient-Centered Medical Home (PCMH)   116
6.4   Evaluating Options for Care That Improve It and Facilitate
    Tracking Outcomes: Regular eMH and Emerging Options
    (e.g., Texting and Social Media)..   116
    6.4.1   The "Do's" of Evaluation   117
    6.4.2   General "Don'ts"   117
    6.4.3   Rigorously Sound Studies: Sound Instruments Studied via eMH.......................   118
    6.4.4   Abbreviated Examples of How to Use Guidelines   118
    6.4.5   Examples of 360-Degree Evaluation Measurement   118
    6.4.6   Examples of New Research or Improved Data
        Collection in Areas of Need   119
6.5   Discussion and Conclusions...   120
References...   121

Abstract

The evidence base in e-Mental Health (eMH), especially telepsychiatry, is substantial, as we proceed in the third active decade of eMH services and sixth decade overall. eMH improves access to quality care for variety of disorders (e.g., depression, anxiety, dementia), treatments (evaluation, medication, therapy), and settings (psychiatric, primary care). It is as good as in-person care – and in some ways better. Some areas are being more thoroughly assessed (e.g., child and adolescent, service delivery models) by traditional research methodology. More work is needed in many areas, though, in terms of elementary quantitative and qualitative indices for the average or regular clinical service or how to implement and improve a program. Specifically, a semistructured approach to services and a practical evaluation approach are needed related to new innovations (digital connectivity between patients and doctors or social media).

6.1   Introduction

There is always room for improvement in the evidence base of most telemedicine work, including eMH, according to a systematic review of review articles [1–3]. The most commonly stated flaws are inadequately powered trials, a lack of consistency in clinical endpoints (which makes it difficult to consolidate evidence, overall), and a belief that clinical effectiveness alone is not sufficient evidence for implementing a telehealth system. Some believe that interim analysis should be used in studies to adjust design according to early results [4]. For example, if there is a multimodel intervention potentially affecting variables numbered 1–5, it would helpful early on to be able to identify variables changing more than others, in order to adjust the study and maximize use of resources. Another tact is the use of "adaptive" treatment strategies, which allow clinical flexibility at the level of the patient to maximize outcomes [5].

Evaluation of telepsychiatry has gone through three phases [6]. First, a review of telepsychiatry's effectiveness considered it effective in terms of increasing access to care, being well accepted, and having good educational outcomes [7]. Second, a transition moved into validity and reliability of clinical care compared to in-person services [6]. The building of rapport relies on detection of nonverbal cues and openly paced conversation. In addition to comparison (or "as good as") studies, telepsychiatric outcomes are not inferior to in-person care (i.e., noninferiority studies) [8]. Third, frameworks to approach its evaluation are helpful [9–11], though costs/economic assessments are very complex [12]. Adult American Telemedicine Association (ATA) videoconferencing guidelines are helpful [9] and steps are being taken toward a child and adolescent eMH guideline [12], based on the American Academy of Child and Adolescent Psychiatry Practice Parameter [13].

In eMH/telepsychiatry research and evaluation, there are areas that show steady progress (e.g., adult comparison to in-person care, models of care including asynchronous telepsychiatry (ATP), posttraumatic stress disorder (PTSD), cultural and language applications), some that are moving quickly (e.g., child and adolescent), and many that need much more emphasis (e.g., geriatric, emergency room (ER) eMH, forensic populations, inpatient) [14]. Areas needing more emphasis may be limited by many factors (e.g., size of the field, number of practitioners or researchers in that area, and system issues). Though it is not distinct from any of these above, the fastest moving area is the use of distance communication (i.e., texting) and social media options between consumers and between patients and doctors. Here, we need an evaluation framework to be put in place to somehow capture the qualitative, quantitative, and human factors that make these engagements so colorful.

This chapter will help the reader to learn in three primary ways:

1. Assess how eMH/telepsychiatry is effective, reliable, and valid and how does it compare to in-person care, including for different ages (e.g., geriatric) [15], disorders, cultures [16], and biopsychosocial treatments (e.g., preliminary work in the psychotherapies) [17, 18]

2. Weigh the pros and cons of models to add to practice, including curbside consultation (e.g., phone/e-mail), synchronous telepsychiatry (STP; video), asynchronous telepsychiatry (ATP) and other Web- and wireless-based systems [19–22], and hybrid models of care (i.e., using in-person and e-health methods), which is being done by many informally now and which may be the standard in the future [22–24]
3. Learn about future areas and opportunities for eMH research, and be able to apply an approach to implement and improve a eMH program, by prioritizing goals and evaluating all components of the program (e.g., participants are the patient, provider, system of care, and the community; treatment; outcomes; and other administrative)

6.2 eMH is Effective and as Good as or Better Than In-Person Care

For specifics of evaluating eMH outcomes, there are two main resources in the literature. First, ATA eMH expert consensus produced a lexicon for patient satisfaction (i.e., access, distance to service, use of), provider satisfaction, process of care (e.g., no-shows), communication (e.g., rapport, presence), reliability/validity (e.g., assessment, treatment vs. in-person), specific disorder measures, costs, and other factors (e.g., facility management, team staffing) [10]. Second, program evaluation assesses clinical, cost, outcomes and other issues to focus on how to prioritize and implement program change based on interactive feedback [11].

6.2.1 Adult, Geriatric, and Other Populations

Telepsychiatry simulates in-person experiences in terms of audio and video quality at 384+ kilobytes per second (KBPS) (Table 6.1). Comparison and noninferiority studies show telepsychiatry in adults is as good as in-person care in terms of diagnosis and treatment [8, 25, 26] and may reduce length of hospitalization and improve medication adherence [6], depression [27–30], panic disorder [31–33], PTSD [21, 34], and other anxiety [35] – as well as mixed anxiety and depression [36].

More studies are needed in geriatric telemedicine and eMH care. Obstacles include access to service, functional challenges, primary care provider attitudes, and lack of psychiatrists [15] and perhaps what could be called a lack of nursing home "ownership" by any one provider to formalize a clinical approach. Nursing home telepsychiatry studies show effectiveness for depression, dementia [37], psychiatric assessment, and cognitive interventions [38]. Acceptance of telepsychiatry appears equivalent to or better than adults [39]. A new development is telemonitoring of depression in the home [40].

Telepsychiatry has been studied in culturally diverse populations and other special populations/settings, as summarized elsewhere [6, 11]. This includes Hispanics/Latinos, Asians, Native American, Eastern Europeans, and other populations (e.g., sign language). Language is a key factor and a common practice is to use "interpreters" on

Table 6.1 Summary of clinical/outcome studies by population age, disorder, or culture

Study	N	Patients	KBS	Location	Comment(s)
Geriatic					
Lyketsos et al. (2001) [89]	NAP	Geriatric outpatients	NS	USA	Video reduced "unneeded" hospitalizations
Poon et al. (2005) [90]	22	Geriatric dementia patients	1.5 Mb	China	Significant, comparable cognitive improvement in video and in-person; high satisfaction; feasible assessment, intervention, and outcomes
Rabinowitz et al. (2010) [38]	106	Nursing home residents	384	USA	Reduced travel time, fuel costs, physician travel time, personnel costs
Weiner et al. (2011) [37]	85	Adult and Geriatric Dementia patients	NS	USA	Feasible alternative to face-to-face care in patients with cognitive disorders who live in remote areas
Adult					
Graham et al. (1996) [91]	39	Adult outpatients	768	USA	Video reduced "unneeded" hospitalizations
Zaylor et al. (1999) [92]	49	Adult depressed or schizoaffective outpatients	128	USA	Video equals in-person in GAF scores at 6-month follow-up
Hunkeler et al. (2000) [93]	302	Adult primary care outpatients	NS	USA	Video by nurses improved depressive symptoms, functioning, and had high satisfaction vs. in-person
Ruskin et al. (2004) [94]	119	Adult veterans	384	USA	Depression outcomes video and in-person equal, as were adherence, satisfaction, cost
Manfredi et al. (2005) [95]	15	Adult inmates	384	USA	Feasibility from an urban university to rural jail; less need for inmate transport
Sorvaniemi et al. (2005) [96]	60	Adult emergency patients	384	Finland	Minor technical problems occurred Assessment and satisfaction fine
Modai et al. (2006) [97]	24/15	Adult outpatients	NS	Israel	Video > in-person cost per service and more hospitalization cost (less available per usual care)
Urness et al. (2006) [98]	39	Adult outpatients	384	Canada	Video < in-person for encouragement; improved outcomes for both

(continued)

Table 6.1 (continued)

Study	N	Patients	KBS	Location	Comment(s)
O'Reilly et al. (2007) [25]	495	Adult outpatients	384	Canada	Video equal to in-person in outcomes, Satisfaction; 10 % less expensive per video
Yellowlees et al. (2010) [99]	60	Nonemergency adult patients	NAP	USA	First asynchronous telepsychiatry (ATP) to demonstrate feasibility
All ages					
De Las Cuevas et al. (2006) [26]	130	All ages – Outpatients	384–768	Spain	Video equals in-person, including those in remote areas with limited resources
Depression					
Ruskin et al. (2004) [94]	119	Adult veterans	384	USA	Video equals in-person for adherence, patient satisfaction, and cost
Fortney et al. (2007) [27]	177	Adult outpatients	NS	USA	Video can help adapt collaborative care model in small PC clinics and symptoms improved more rapidly in intervention group vs. usual care group
Moreno et al. (2012) [28]	167	Adult patients	NS	USA	Video may close gap in access to culturally and linguistically congruent specialists; improves depression severity, functional ability, and quality of life
Fortney et al. (2013) [21]	364	Adult patients	NS	USA	Video collaborative care group > reductions in severity than usual care
Titov et al. (2011) [36]	37	Adult patients	384+/Internet	USA	Depression reduction at 3-month follow-up after 8 weekly CBT sessions
Johnston et al. (2013) [35]	129	Adult patients	384+/Internet	USA	Both sole diagnosis and those with comorbid disorders had significant symptom reduction by CBT
Post-traumatic stress disorders (PTSD) or panic disorder					
Bouchard et al. (2004) [31]	21	Adults, panic disorder	384/NS	Canada	Video 81 % of patients panic-free posttreatment and 91 % at 6-month follow-up via CBT

Frueh et al. (2007) [34]	38	Adult male veterans, PTSD	384/NS	USA	Video equals in-person in clinical outcomes and satisfaction at 3 month follow-up Video < comfort vs. in-person in talking with therapist post-treatment and had worse treatment adherence
Morland et al. (2010) [56]	125	Adult male veterans, PTSD	384/NS	USA	Video CBGT for PTSD-related anger is feasible for rural/remote veterans, with reduced anger
Germain et al. (2009) [100]	48	Adult patients, PTSD	NS	Canada	Video equals in-person in reducing PTSD over 16–25 weeks
Hedman et al. (2014) [33]	570	Adult patients	384+	Sweden	Video CBT over 6 weeks significantly improved symptoms
Fortney et al. (2015) [21]	296	Adult patients in VA community clinics, PTSD	384+	USA	Cognitive processing therapy for the treatment group > usual care group over 12-month follow-up
Substance abuse					
Frueh et al. (2005) [101]	14	Adult male outpatients	384/NS	USA	Video had good attendance, comparable attrition and high satisfaction
Developmental disability					
Szeftel et al. (2012) [102]	45	Adolescents	NS	USA	Video led to changed Axis I psychiatric diagnosis (excluding developmental disorders) 70 % , and changed medication 82 % of patients initially, 41 % at 1 year and 46 % at 3 years Video helped PCPs with recommendations for developmental disabilities
Hispanic					
Moreno et al. (2012) [28]	167	Adult patients	NS	USA	Video lessens depression severity and raises functional ability, and quality of life; improves access to culturally and linguistically congruent specialists
Chong et al. (2012) [103]	167	Adult patients	NS	USA	Video acceptable to low-income depressed Hispanic patients, but its feasibility is questionable

(continued)

Table 6.1 (continued)

Study	N	Patients	KBS	Location	Comment(s)
Yellowlees et al. (2013) [16]	127	English- and Spanish-speaking patients	NS	USA	ATP equal for English- and Spanish speaking patients;
American Indian					
Shore et al. (2008) [104]	53	Male adult patients	NS	USA	Video equals in-person assessment, interaction, and satisfaction; comfort level high and culturally accepted
European					
Mucic (2010) [105]	61	Adult outpatients	2 Mbit (Denmark) 10 Mbit (Sweden)	Denmark	Video improved access, reduced waiting time and reduced travel to see bilingual psychiatrists; high satisfaction Video preferred via "mother tongue" rather than interpreter-assisted care
Asian					
Ye et al. (2012) [106]	19	Adult outpatients	NS	USA	Primary language facilitates expression of feelings, emotional discomfort, or social stressors
Sign language					
Lopez et al. (2004) [107]	1	Adult female, deaf since birth	NS	USA	Video communication fine with American Sign Language (ASL) interpreter and psychiatric symptoms improved

site, but sometimes relatives/family members or untrained interpreters miscommunicate medical complaints [41] or de-emphasize information [42]. Nurses, too, do a little better with concrete medical complaints than capturing the narrative or cultural metaphors [43], which is potentially very significant in psychiatric care.

Special settings and populations, as well as cost analysis, are areas of need for more data. Settings of interest include the involuntary, inpatient, and incarcerated – and those in emergency rooms – and adjustments may be needed to ensure quality of care, informed consent, and privacy. Preliminary guidelines for emergency telepsychiatry need to be evaluated [6, 44]. Cost and economic outcomes depend on the program and the measures used [6] or sites/settings [10]. There are different types of cost analyses: cost-offset, cost-minimization, cost-effectiveness, and cost-benefit analysis. Cost studies have differences in data sought, its collection, and how it is analyzed. Savings may be shown vs. in-person with high consultation rates, "breakeven" or other thresholds used (e.g., number of consultations/year), or when patient's travel, time, and food are included. ATP appears cost-effective [16, 45].

6.2.2 Children and Adolescents

Child telepsychiatry research is now beyond feasibility, acceptability, and good initial outcomes (Table 6.2) [46, 47]. Satisfaction has improved steadily in the last 10 years – part of that is the better technology (e.g., bandwidth) and part of it has to do with distinguishing satisfaction with eMH vs. system issues that posed problems in the process of care (e.g., lack of social support locally, family members expecting "too" much from a consultation). Some child populations, though, may do better with eMH than in-person care [48]. Major breakthroughs have been occurring in the primary care setting, first with routine eMH and then via systematic, integrated behavioral health programs that combined on-site screening, therapy, and primary care with telepsychiatric assistance [49, 50]. Another growth area has been in the treatment of attention deficit hyperactivity disorder (ADHD) at a distance in rural primary care – including the blockbuster use of combined synchronous and asynchronous collaborative care, partly using Web-based data systems, which significantly improved outcomes [22]. Caregiver distress has also been reduced by similar interventions [51].

Providing quality child and adolescent psychiatry care will require a higher level of organization and more planning before a patient visit [12]. Web- or phone-based questionnaires may prediagnose patients before a visit [52], and the mental health clinician may be able to gather useful collateral from the referring team prior to a visit [53]. The patient-side interview room will need to be large enough to accommodate the child, their family, and often a patient-side staff member [12]. The camera and microphone setup should be flexible to allow a wide view of the room (to catch patient–family interactions), and the room should be equipped with child-size furniture and toys. Ideally, should the consultant need to observe the child's play in order to inform their assessment, they could ask patient-side staff to play with/draw with the child [54]. Lastly, as with all child and adolescent psychiatry, the clinician should be very transparent as to who else is viewing the encounter on the provider's side, and whether the encounter is being videotaped.

Table 6.2 Summary of clinical outcome studies for child and adolescent eMH (not inclusive of satisfaction-only studies)

Citation (old to new)	Design	Sample	Assessment	Findings
Blackmon et al. (1997) [108]	Descriptive	43 Children Parents	Routine clinical	All children and 98 % of parents report satisfaction equal to in-person care
Elford et al. (2000) [109]	RCT	25 Children Various diagnoses	Diagnostic interviews	96 % concordance between Video and in-person evaluations; no difference in satisfaction
Elford et al. (2001) [110]	Descriptive	23 Children	Routine clinical	Diagnosis and treatment recommendation – equal to usual, in-person care
Glueckauf et al. (2002) [111]	Modified RCT Pre vs. post	22 Adolescents 36 Parents	Issue-specific measures of family problems Teen functioning (Social Skills Rating System – SSRS) Working Alliance Inventory Adherence to appointments	Improvement for problem severity and frequency in all conditions. Therapeutic alliance high; teens rated alliance lower for video
Nelson et al. (2003) [112]	RCT	28 Children Depression	Diagnostic interview and scale	Video=in-person for improvement of depressive symptoms in response to therapy
Myers et al. (2004) [113]	Comparative	159 Youth (age 3–18)	Comparison of patients evaluated through eMH vs. FTF in clinic	Video basically similar to in-person outpatients demographically, clinically, and by reimbursement Video > "adverse case mix"
Greenberg et al. (2006) [114]	Descriptive	NS Children 35 PCPs and 12 caregivers	Not specified Focus groups with PCPs, interviews with caregivers	PCP and caregiver satisfied video; frustrated with limitations of local supports Family caretakers and service providers frustrated with limitations of the video

Study	Design	Sample	Measure	Results
Myers et al. (2006) [115]	Descriptive	115 Incarcerated youth (age 14–18)	11-item Satisfaction Survey	80 % successfully prescribed medications and they expressed confidence in the psychiatrist by video; Youth expressed concerns about privacy
Myers et al. (2007) [116]	Descriptive,	172 Patients (age 2–21) and 387 visits	11-item Provider/PCP Satisfaction Survey	Video to patients at 4 PCP sites: high satisfaction with services; pediatricians > family physicians
Bensink et al. (2008) [117]	Descriptive	8 Youth Pediatric cancer	Feasibility and satisfaction ratings	Video (by phone) use to families with a child diagnosed with cancer: technically feasibility and high parental satisfaction
Clawson et al. (2008) [118]	Descriptive	15 Youth (age 8 months–10 year)	VC feasibility with pediatric feeding disorders	Video feasible and resulted in cost-savings
Fox et al. (2008) [119]	Pre-post	190 Youth in juvenile detention	Goal Attainment Scale (GAS)	Improvement in the rate of attainment of goals associated with family relations and personality/behavior
Morgan et al. (2008) [120]	RCT	27 Parents Child age ≤25 months	Video vs. telephone for children with congenital heart disease, anxiety ratings	Video > phone for reducing parent anxiety enabling significantly greater clinical information than phone
Myers et al. (2008) [121]	Descriptive	172 Patients Parental satisfaction	12-item Parent Satisfaction Survey	Parents with school-aged children endorsed higher satisfaction than those with adolescents; Adherence high for return appointments

(continued)

Table 6.2 (continued)

Citation (old to new)	Design	Sample	Assessment	Findings
Shaikh et al. (2008) [122]	Pre-/post	99 youth (age: 1–17)	Diagnostic assessment, weight measurement	Video consultations resulted in substantial changes/additions to diagnoses; subset with repeated consultations led to improved health behaviors, (e.g., weight maintenance or loss)
Wilkinson et al. (2008) [123]	RCT	16 youth (age not reported)	Children with cystic fibrosis Assessment of quality of life, anxiety, depression, service utilization.	Video = in-person for quality of life, anxiety levels, depression levels, admissions to hospital or clinic attendances, general practitioner calls or intravenous antibiotic use between the two groups
Witmans et al. (2008) [124]	Descriptive	89 Children Sleep disorders	Sleep diary Childhood Sleep Habits Questionnaire Pediatric QOL Questionnaire Client Satisfaction Quest.	Patients were very satisfied with the delivery of multidisciplinary pediatric sleep medicine services over video
Yellowlees et al. (2008) [50]	Pre-post	41 Children in rural primary care	Child Behavior Check List (CBCL)	At 3-month, improvements in the Affect and Oppositional Domains of the Child Behavior Checklist
Pakyurek et al. (2010) [48]	Descriptive	12 Children Autism-spectrum in primary care	Routine clinical	Video might actually be superior to in-person for consultation
Myers et al. (2010) [75]	Descriptive	701 patients, 190 PCPs	Collection of patient demographics, diagnoses, and utilization of services	Video feasible; psychiatrists adjust practice from in-person well
Lau et al. (2011) [125]	Descriptive and advanced assessment	45 Children/adolescent	Patient characteristics, reason for consultation and treatment recommendations	Video reaches a variety of children, with consultants providing diagnostic clarification and modifying treatment

Mulgrew et al. (2011) [126]	Descriptive	25 Children Pediatric obesity	Consulting providers' listening skills and ease of instruction to patients Comfort level of parents in discussing health concerns	Video = in-person for parent satisfaction between consultations for weight management
Stain et al. (2011) [127]	Descriptive and RCT	11 Adolescents/young adults	Diagnostic Interview for Psychosis Diagnostic Module (DIP-DM)	Strong correlation of assessments done in-person vs. video
Storch et al. (2011) [128]	RCT	31 Children and teenagers	Routine clinical and measures 1. ADIS-IV-C/P 2. Clinician-admin. CY-BOCS 3. Clinical Global Impressions Scales (CGI) 4. Others: obsessive, anxiety, depression inventory	Video was superior to in-person on all primary outcome measures, higher % meeting remission. Consultants providing diagnostic clarification and modifying treatment
Himle et al. (2012) [129]	RCT	20 Children Tourette's Disorder or Chronic Motor Tic Disorder	Routine clinical assessment with Yale Global Tic Severity Scale (YGTSS); Parent Tic Questionnaire (PTQ; Clinician Global Severity & Improvement Scales (CGI-S and CGI-I)	Both treatment delivery modalities resulted in significant tic reduction with no between group differences
Jacob et al. (2012) [130]	Descriptive	15 children (age 4–18; mean 9.73)	Routine clinical 12-item Parent Satisfaction Survey	Patient satisfaction high and PCPs found recommendations helpful; outcomes pending on follow-up

(continued)

Table 6.2 (continued)

Citation (old to new)	Design	Sample	Assessment	Findings
Nelson et al. (2012) [131]	Service utilization chart review	22 Children	Routine clinical	No factor inherent to the video delivery mechanism impeded adherence to national ADHD guidelines
Reese et al. (2012) [132]	Pre-post	8 Children; Asian	Routine clinical ADHD	Families reported improved child behavior and decreased parent distress via video format of Group Triple P Positive Parenting Program
Szeftel et al. (2012) [89]	Descriptive Chart review	45 Patients; 31 ≤ 18 yo	Routine clinical – medication changes, frequency of patient appointments, diagnostic changes, symptom severity and improvement	Video led to changed Axis I psychiatric diagnosis (excluding developmental disorders) 70 %, and changed medication 82 % of patients initially, 41 % at 1 year and 46 % at 3 years Video helped PCPs with recommendations for developmental disabilities
Heitzman-Powell et al. (2013) [133]	Pre-post	NS Youth 7 Parents	OASIS training program Problem Behavior Recording (PBR) Incidental Teaching Checklist (ITC)	Parents increased their knowledge and self-reported implementation of behavioral strategies
Xie et al. (2013) [134]	RCT	22 Children Behavioral disorder	Routine clinical Parent Child Relationship Questionnaire (PCQ-CA), Vanderbilt Assessment Scales, CGAS, CGIS	Parent training through video was as effective as in-person training and was well accepted by parents

Reese et al. (2013) [135]	Descriptive and RCT	21 Children; 90 % Caucasian	Autism Diagnostic Observation Schedule (ADOS) – Module 1 Autism Diagnostic Interview – Revised (ADI-R) Parent Satisfaction	No difference in reliability of diagnostic accuracy, ADOS observations, ratings for ADI-R parent report of symptoms, and parent satisfaction
Davis et al. (2013) [136]	Descriptive	58 Youth Pediatric obesity	Body Mass Index 24-h dietary recall ActiGraph – physical activity duration and intensity Child Behavior Checklist Behavioral Pediatrics Feeding Assessment Scale	Both groups showed improvements in BMI, nutrition, and physical activity, and the groups did not differ significantly on primary outcomes
Freeman et al. (2013) [137]	Descriptive	71 Youth Diabetes adherence	Baseline metabolic control Conflict Behavior Questionnaire Diabetes Responsibility and Family Conflict Scale – Parent and Youth Working Alliance Inventory	No differences were found in therapeutic alliance between the groups
Hommel et al. (2013) [138]	Descriptive	9 Youth Irritable Bowel Disease, adherence	Pill count Pediatric Ulcerative Colitis Activity Index Partial Harvey-Bradshaw Index Feasibility Acceptability Questionnaire	Video improved adherence and cost-savings across patients

(continued)

Table 6.2 (continued)

Citation (old to new)	Design	Sample	Assessment	Findings
Lipana et al. (2013) [139]	Descriptive	243 Youth Pediatric obesity	Review of medical records	Video > in-person in enhancing nutrition, increasing activity, and decreasing screen time
Rockhill et al. (2013) [51]	RCT	223 Children with ADHD ± ODD ± Anxiety	Caregiver distress assessed with Patient Health Questionnaire-9, Parenting Stress Index, Caregiver Strain Questionnaire, Family Empowerment Scale	Parents of children with ADHD and a comorbid disorder had significantly more distress than those with ADHD alone
Comer et al. (2014) [140]	Pre-/post	5 Children (age 4–8)	Behavioral intervention with child, facilitated by parent; OCD rating scale by parent	Child OCD symptoms and diagnoses declined; child global functioning improved
Myers et al. (2015) [22]	RCT	223 Children with ADHD ± ODD ± anxiety	CBCL screening, DISC-IV diagnostic assessment, ADHD rating scales (inattention, hyperactivity, combined, ODD, role performance) and Columbia Impairment Scale	Caregivers reported significantly greater improvement for inattention, hyperactivity, combined ADHD, ODD, role performance for video vs. those treated in primary care Teachers reported significantly greater improvement in ODD and role performance for video group, too

Tse et al. (2015) [141]	RCT Subsample	37 Caregivers of children with ADHD±ODD±anxiety	Caregiver Behavior Training (CaBT) delivered via. CBCL screening, DISC-IV diagnostic assessment, ADHD rating scales (inattention, hyperactivity, combined, ODD, role performance) and Columbia Impairment Scale	Caregivers reported comparable improvements for children's outcomes whether CaBT video=in person; no improvement in caregivers' distress when CaBT provided through video
Rockhill et al. [142; In press]	Descriptive; Telepsychiatrists in RCT	223 children with ADHD±ODD±Anxiety, the telepsychiatrists and PCPs	Telepsychiatrists' adherence to guidelines-based care, ADHD outcomes by prescriber based on comorbidity status	Telepsychiatrists adhered to guideline-based care, used higher medication doses than PCPs, and their patients reached target of 50 % reduction in ADHD symptoms more often than with PCPs

RCT randomized controlled trial, *NS* not specified, *PCP* primary care provider, *eMH* e-mental health, *ADHD* attention deficit hyperactivity disorder, *ODD* oppositional defiant disorder, *OCD* obsessive compulsive disorder, *DISC* diagnostic interview schedule for children, *CaBT* caregiver behavioral training (note: this acronym is not standard, but created to avoid first glance confusion with cognitive behavioral therapy)

6.2.3 Psychotherapy Evidence Base

The evidence base for therapy by eMH is growing and most data shows it to be as good as in-person treatment. Initial studies focused on satisfaction, working alliance between the patient and provider, and communication changes [6, 55], and it appeared that no significant problems were arising once the technology bandwidth had increased [6]. Early studies showed impact for PTSD [34, 56]. Reports on therapy and even more broadly defined "e-therapy" have been done [57]. Studies in adults generally involve patients with depression and anxiety – often military populations with posttraumatic stress disorder (PTSD) – and these studies show comparative efficacy of eMH to in-person services (see Table 6.3).

Some data are encouraging with new therapy modalities and suggest, also, that teletherapy may be better than in-person treatment. A preliminary study on therapeutic alliance and attrition among participants receiving anger management group therapy was basically equivalent to in-person; rapport with the group leader was not as substantial, though [58]. eMH is better than in-person care, in terms of adherence to treatment [59], reduced anxiety symptoms via exposure therapy at 6 weeks follow-up [60], less binge eating [61], and less PTSD symptoms at 6 and 12 months [21]. These studies are consistent with eMH for autistic spectrum adolescents mentioned above [48].

Guidelines for therapy by videoconferencing have been explored [17], as have systematic reviews [18]. We suggest three factors have a hand in this: (1) the "extra" preparation of eMH service (consent, discussions) may result in "readiness" for treatment; (2) the hands-on approach by the interdisciplinary team (e.g., telemedicine coordinator, nurse, others) may enhance the therapeutic alliance, and (3) access to treatment, in general, and "in-time" may empower the patient [14].

6.3   Models of Care: The e-Continuum Toward Integrated and Stepped Care for Different Populations, Disorders, and Treatments

6.3.1 Models of Care: How to Select Them and Impact on Evaluation

A summary of eMH models of care reviewed the pros and cons of each model [6, 19] and other models have been thoroughly studied and well articulated [62].

Low intensity
- Case review of diagnosis and follow-up after a discussion [63].
- Telepsychiatric consultation to primary care helps to align primary care practitioners' (PCPs) diagnosis/es and medication treatments [6], with an indirect benefit over time of improving PCPs' knowledge and skills [19, 64, 65].
- In-person, telephone, or e-mail doctor-to-doctor "curbside" consultations may arise during patient care in day-to-day practice [66] and meet

Table 6.3 Summary of clinical outcome studies for eMH vs. in-person psychotherapy (not including satisfaction-only studies)

Study	N	Sample	Intervention	Findings
Bastien et al. (2004) [143]	21	Adults, panic disorder	CBT for PD delivered via eMH compared to in-person	Significant reduction in PD symptoms and increase in the number of PD free patients at follow-up; equivalent to in-person
Grady and Melcer (2005) [59]	81	Active duty/ retired personnel and adult family members	Retrospective review of eMH care compared to in-person	Improved patient adherence for both, but *better follow-up adherence with eMH*
Cluver et al. (2005) [84]	9	Adults, terminally ill cancer, adjustment disorder or depression	Psychotherapy alternated between in-person and eMH	Therapy delivery mode made no difference in patient reports; eMH feasible
Frueh et al. (2007) [34]	38	Adults, combat related PTSD	CBT for PTSD delivered via eMH compared to In-person	No significant differences in clinical outcomes for eMH vs. in-person
Morgan et al. (2008) [144]	186	Adult male inmates	Therapy for mood disorder and psychosis via eMH compared to in-person	No significant differences in inmates' satisfaction, postsession mood, or work alliance with the MH professional
Ertelt et al. (2008) [145]	128	Adults, DSM-IV criteria for BN or eating disorder	CBT delivered for BN via eMH compared to in-person	Acceptable to participants and equivalent in outcome to therapy delivered in-person
Germain et al. (2009) [100]	48	Adults, PTSD	CBT delivered via eMH compared to in-person	Significant decline in symptoms in both groups; effectiveness same
Germain et al. (2010) [146]	46	Adults, PTSD	Therapeutic alliance via eMH compared to in-person	Equivalent in both groups on Working Alliance Inventory, Videoconference Telepresence Scale, and other measures
King et al. (2009) [147]	37	Adults, opioid-agonist treatment	Addiction counseling delivered via eMH compared to in-person	No significant difference between assistance in both groups
Marrone et al. (2009) [61]	116	Adults, BN	CBT delivered for BN via eMH compared to in-person	*Reduction in binge eating at week 6 eMH and week 8 for in-person*
Tuerk et al. (2010) [60]	47	Adult veterans, PTSD	Prolonged exposure therapy via eMH compared to in-person comparison group	*Statistically significant decreases in self-reported pathology for veterans eMH > in-person*

(continued)

Table 6.3 (continued)

Study	N	Sample	Intervention	Findings
Morland et al. (2010) [56]	125	Adult male veterans, PTSD	CBT for anger management via eMH compared to in-person	eMH viable; does not compromise a therapist's ability to effectively structure and manage patient care
Gros et al. (2011) [148]	89	Veterans, PTSD	Exposure therapy for trauma via telemedicine compared to in-person	Findings support the utility of eMH services to provide effective, evidence-based psychotherapies
Yuen et al. (2013) [149]	24	Adults, social anxiety disorder	12 sessions of weekly CBT for generalized social anxiety via eMH	Significant improvements in social anxiety, depression, disability, quality of life, and experiential avoidance
King et al. (2014) [150]	85	Adults, substance use	Addiction counseling delivered via eMH compared to in-person	Similar rates of counseling attendance and drug-positive urinalysis results
Khatri et al. (2014) [151]	18	Adults, depression and anxiety	CBT for depression anxiety via eMH compared to in-person	Pre–post intervention scores for depression comparable in-person vs. eMH
Fortney et al. (2015) [21]	133	Veterans, PTSD	Collaborative care, therapy, psychiatry via eMH compared to in-person	*Significant decrease in PTSD symptoms eMH > in-person at 6 and 12 months.* Participation in cognitive processing therapy predicted improvement

VC videoconferencing, *eMH* e-mental health, *CBT* cognitive behavioral therapy, *BN* bulimia nervosa, *PD* panic disorder, *PTSD* posttraumatic stress disorder

approximately 33 % of informational PCPs' needs "in-time" [67]. Both telephone and face-to-face contacts occur; the former are purposeful and timely and that latter are random and prone to delays. More recently, e-mail consultations that do not include patient evaluations are valuable, inexpensive, brief, and more readily available [68], including a multispecialty phone and e-mail consultation system to PCPs for the care of adults and children with developmental disabilities [69].
- Cultural consultation to rural primary care using telemedicine [16].

Moderate intensity
- An integrated program of mental health screening, therapy on site, telepsychiatric consultation (phone, e-mail, or video), continuing medical education (CME), and staff training on screening questionnaires has improved patient outcomes and site-based staff skills [49, 50].
- A randomized controlled trial (RCT) for depression in adults using disease management and telepsychiatric consultation vs. usual care over 12 months improved the care of both groups; the latter group benefitted from the

Hawthorne effect and providers' application of skills from the intervention group [39].

- Asynchronous telepsychiatry (ATP) is feasible, valid, reliable, and cost-effective in English- and Spanish-speaking patients in primary care [16, 45]. (Similar methods are used in radiology, dermatology, ophthalmology, cardiology, and pathology.) One ATP model uses a basic questionnaire for screening by the provider of the patient, video capture of that interview, and uploading of patient histories for a remote psychiatrist to review in a HIPAA-adherent manner [20].

High intensity
- Collaborative care, which has now been more formally applied to telemedicine [21, 27, 29, 70], has encouraging results. The virtual collaborative care team was able to produce better outcomes than the traditional "gold standard" methodology of primary care psychiatry [29].
- Child collaborative care for children with ADHD at a distance used STP and ATP (i.e., Web-based) approaches for further training, data collection and monitoring showed positive clinical outcomes [22].

6.3.2 Internet or Web-Based Care

Patients benefit from tools for self-directed habit, lifestyle or illness changes, prompts for appointments, and evidence-based treatments via the Internet (e.g., anxiety disorders). "Fear Fighter," a computer guided self-exposure approach to treat phobia/panic fills a hole when qualified and trained therapists are scarce [71]. Another is PTSD Coach, which is designed to help veterans learn about and manage symptoms that commonly occur after trauma – not as a substitute for treatment, but to support MH interventions – including symptom assessment, illness-specific education, treatment resource location, and tracking of treatment progress [72, 73]. Recent patient-centered strategies to increase patient compliance are simple mail, telephone, or SMS reminders that have shown to be an effective way to support patient attendance to follow-up appointments [74]. Internet-based CBT (ICBT) interventions are as effective as traditional in-person care and a 30-month follow-up study for treatment of social phobia and panic disorder [75–77]. ICBT combined with monitoring by text messages (mobile CBT or mCBT) and minimal therapist support by e-mail and telephone helps prevent depression relapse [77]. Interestingly, a review of virtual reality reports it has been used in the treatment of many MH conditions [78], including eating disorders, autism spectrum disorders, stress management, pain management, and diagnosis and treatment of neurological conditions such as stroke. Finally, avatar therapy is a novel therapy that may significantly reduce the frequency and intensity of the voices, their omnipotence and malevolence, as a schizophrenic can create a virtual representation of the scary voices, then work with a therapist in real time to manage the avatar speaking the voices [79].

Caregivers, too, may benefit by the use of telecommunication technology. A review of Internet-based interventions for medical and MH disorders showed that approximately two-thirds of open or randomized controlled trials reduced stress and improved quality of life – at least significantly in terms of specific measured outcomes [80]. Family caregivers located in rural areas found e-health support to be beneficial in comparison with conventional caregiver support [81]. The interventions include interactive communities, bulletin board chatting, and therapy groups [80]. Patient populations included MH (dementia, schizophrenia, anorexia) and medical (older adults/aging, heart transplant, traumatic brain injury, hip fracture, cancer, stroke). Caregivers' outcomes improved and they are satisfied and comfortable with support services delivered by cell phones [82].

6.3.3   Integrated Care and the Patient-Centered Medical Home (PCMH)

Integrated care and stepped care models provide efficient expertise to the point of service – eMH further enhances that (see also Chap. 7). These services are in development and need to be better studied, although costs are dramatically decreasing. PCMH is founded on the presence of inadequate treatment in primary care and/or an inability to access needed services [83]. Under oversight of the primary care provider, PCMH allows telepsychiatric input at home and has been shown to improve patient care and health [84, 85]. Desk-mounted video systems offer great convenience for therapy to cancer patients to avoid travel, but the cost used to be prohibitive for most consumers [84, 85]. Stepped care models may be the most cost-effective models in health system where the effectiveness of the intervention is maximized by making the best use of resources adequately available at the right time [86, 87].

6.4   Evaluating Options for Care That Improve It and Facilitate Tracking Outcomes: Regular eMH and Emerging Options (e.g., Texting and Social Media)

Prioritization of outcomes and evaluation in the provision of clinical (eMH) services is important – not just after you start, but preferably before you start [12]. Process, procedures, levels of depth, and do's and don'ts are offered to give the reader options. Fundamentals about evaluation are necessary for clinical managers and clinicians because the approach and processes that guide "good" evaluation may require a fundamental shift in philosophy – from seeing what happens to designing the services in advance to achieve outcomes. The process and content of evaluation can be lumped into program, research/evaluation, and clinical care and other adjunct measures (e.g., models, guidelines). These areas can be stratified across a level of complexity/level of planning/time to achieve/rigor of targeted outcomes – so there are basic, intermediate, and advanced options.

Parameters and methods fall into three basic frameworks that naturally overlap with one another:

1. Research/evaluation measures, in the form of feasibility, validity, reliability, satisfaction, costs, and outcomes – fortunately, many of these have already been studied previously or are built-in to your clinical mindset.
2. Section on clinical care measures (e.g., PHQ, Beck Depression Inventory).
3. Supplemental "adjunct" measures (e.g., clinical guidelines on assessment or prescribing).

6.4.1   The "Do's" of Evaluation

- Pick an outcome that is "sexy" or at least has high heuristic value (e.g., ADHD study above looked at caregiver distress…that is meaningful in trying to parent 1–2 kids with that illness, much less comorbid ODD).
- Adopt standardized measures already used in in-person or eMH care published projects; they typically have undergone multiple iterations, levels of review, and sometimes psychometric testing.
- Use specific measures unless generalized measures with different parts are efficient. This arises. The Beck Depression Inventory could be used to grade severity of depression, unofficially, but the PHQ-9 is available in many languages, shorter and easier to score (unless you employ a BDI-13 or −7).
- Check for disorders that are commonly comorbid as they confound outcome measures. For substance abuse, use the Alcohol Use Disorders Identification Test (AUDIT).
- Have self-report/patient completion, if it is accurate. This comes down to time and money. The clinician has limited time. But, some things are not measured well by self-report (e.g., mania).
- Collect data and do the evaluation prospectively rather than retrospectively. Why? If you look back and analyze data, it will double or triple your administration/staff time and there will be "holes" in what was collected compared to what you really "want" or need.
- Make sure you know (or someone knows) what you are doing. Get a consultation?
- Evolve from nascent to specific targets from…determine if eMH works in rural primary care settings for depression to…determine the effectiveness of collaborative care by eMH in rural primary care settings will significantly decrease depressive symptoms as measured by PHQ-9 self-report questionnaire at 3, 6, and 12 months after starting treatment.

6.4.2   General "Don'ts"

- Collect "extra" data. If it is not immediately relevant, do not spend time on it. Folks put too much in front of patients to self-report, have clinicians fill out too many needless surveys, and have more data that they never get to it.
- Measure things needed for clinical care decisions and documentation (e.g., hospital standards or grant data); do not measure obvious things like satisfaction, as

it is usually so high there is no point to doing so. Measure satisfaction, though, if are doing a new treatment like Internet-based therapy.

- Automatically assume that in-place electronic health record (EHR), quality improvement (QI) and other processes can easily be used to save time/money.
- Evaluate cost, unless you have a big sample size and access to someone who is an expert in cost/health services.

6.4.3 Rigorously Sound Studies: Sound Instruments Studied via eMH

Many scales have been studied for adults and children/adolescents via videoconferencing [8, 9, 12]. These include the Brief Psychiatric Rating Scale (BPRS), Scales for the Assessment of Negative and Positive Symptoms (SANS; SAPS), the Structured Clinical Interview for DSM (SCID; Diagnostic and Statistical Manual), Hamilton Depression Rating Scale (HDRS), Diagnostic Interview Schedule (DIS), the Abnormal Involuntary Movement Scale (AIMS), and the Yale Brown Obsessive Compulsive Scale (semistructured, YBOCS) [12]. For children/adolescents, the DSM-IV, Schedule for the Assessment of Depression and Schizophrenia (K-SADS), and DIS Child (DISC) have been used. The Geriatric Depression Scale (GDS) and many neuropsychiatric scales like the Mini-Mental Status Examination (MMSE), CAMCOG (neuropsychiatric test, computerized), National Adult Reading Test Quick Test (NARTQT), and Adult Memory and Information Processing Battery are effective. The reliability and validity of asynchronous telepsychiatry has been shown using English and Spanish versions of the SCID and Mini-International Neuropsychiatric Interview (MINI) [12].

6.4.4 Abbreviated Examples of How to Use Guidelines

- Example 1: Use of ADHD guidelines for multicenter child telepsychiatry initiatives [47, 88]. The strength of the research is better when telepsychiatry clinical care uses validated instruments, of course, but also when the care/research evaluation uses standard treatments or follows guidelines that are nationally and internationally accepted.
- Example 2: Response of depression to primary care consultation to Indian Health population [6]. The study below in the next section under Program/Project A describes PCP changes in prescribing due to consultation. While change is good in and of itself, it is even better when it is in, or moves within, national standards for PCPs.

6.4.5 Examples of 360-Degree Evaluation Measurement

- Example 1: Satisfaction with care. Satisfaction is colloquially used in relationship to life, purchases, work, relationships, and other common experiences. It is affected by culture, personality, state (e.g., depression), trait (i.e., personality), values, past experiences, expectations and other factors. Many firms are interested in understanding what their customers thought about their shopping or purchase experience, because finding new customers is generally more costly and difficult than servicing existing or repeat customers. eMH has cued patients to think about things they should have (or had) already thought about the following:

– What do I expect with seeing the doctor by telemedicine?
– What experiences, good or bad, have I had with technology?
– I missed the handshake, handing of a tissue for my tears, or my doctor's sigh.

Whose satisfaction should we measure?

– Patient's subjective satisfaction: Did the service meet her/his health needs? Would patient do this again? Would patient refer others to this service?
– Provider satisfaction: The extent to which the provider values telehealth when interacting with patients (e.g., Do I prefer a clinic over another as I have better access to specialist providers by eMH, or did a consultation help with a technical competency (e.g., psychopharmacology)?)
– Clinic/system of care: Was wait time reduced, was it easy to schedule, and was it easy enough to staff the setup?

• Example 2: ADHD evaluation of outcomes. Who is the real "patient" … this bears some reflection on the example of treating it in primary care via the hybrid model of eMH [22].
    – The child or adolescent: Do I feel better, will I go to the visit, and do I like the Web part?
    – The parent: Is he/she improving at home, at the mall, and at school (less active, fewer fights)? And am I less stressed?
    – The teacher: Is he/she improving school (less active, less disruptive, and fewer fights)?
    – The primary care provider: Is this whole eMH thing worth it?

6.4.6   Examples of New Research or Improved Data Collection in Areas of Need

• Example 1: Clinical care with adolescent patients with depression using text, telephone, e-mail, and video in addition to in-person care (e.g., weekly therapy with the other modalities allowed for nonemergencies during business hours).
    – Identify the primary outcome measure (e.g., PHQ) for baseline and regular (e.g., monthly) follow-up assessment for a duration (e.g., year).
    – Stratify groups: log # of comorbid diagnoses in a binary fashion as it is easier to standardize groups with single, dual and triple diagnosis(es) to compare outcomes and perform rudimentary statistical analyses.
    – Quantify the # of clinical care exchanges (i.e., texts, telephone calls, e-mails, and video (if any) and in-person).
    – Use a 1-page questionnaire with one question on overall satisfaction, ability to connect with the provider (specific to texts, telephone calls, e-mails, video, and in-person), and 2–3 other factors, preferably with a 7-point Likert-like

scale (1 (low) to 7 (high); consider a blank text box for improvements, key events, and other reactions as an iterative feedback loop for the next survey (following year).

- Example 2: How eMH affects service delivery in an ER, using telepsychiatric consultation to a rural emergency room (modeled after study of eMH to primary care) [19].
  - Administrative structure to service: semistructure format, suggested duration, categorize consultation question (e.g., SI, psychosis, drug intoxication, or other), and "interventions"
  - Intervention options: patient education, provider education, assessment/additional work-up (e.g., collateral information, social work, labs), diagnosis, triage, treatment option 1, treatment option 2, and outcome of consultation
  - Follow-up evaluation (if possible)
  - Composite or aggregate analysis: first 25–50 consultations, patient/consultation mix, and outcomes

6.5   Discussion and Conclusions

The evidence base – or effectiveness – in eMH, especially telepsychiatry, is substantial and it appears as good or better than in-person care. More work is needed in many areas, though, in terms of elementary quantitative and qualitative indices for the average or regular clinical service or how to implement and improve a program. Specifically, a semistructured approach to services and a practical evaluation approach are needed related to new innovations (digital connectivity between patients and doctors or social media). Most clinicians, administrators and leaders want to ensure "good" care, do it professionally, and be remunerated for it. The characteristic of time-tested "quality" care in psychiatry is largely unchanged: a good patient–doctor engagement, the therapeutic relationship, shared decision-making, use of stories/narratives, and biopsychosocial treatment [6]. Folks are accepting eMH handily now, as the "innovation represents a potential efficacy in solving a perceived need or problem" [76].

Video/synchronous eMH and even ATP are being more thoroughly assessed by traditional research methodology, but we do not have a standard approach or framework for looking at the pros and cons of texting, Web and other mobile/wireless, and social media options. Since even the best research studies have the shortcomings of inadequately powered trials and a lack of consistency in clinical endpoints (which makes it difficult to consolidate evidence, overall), maybe we approach the rapid-paced emergence of these new technologies with a basic assessment, clinical outcome measure, standard period of reassessment, an automatically determined "study" duration, and a basic measure of evaluation (if fortunate, it would be 360° and iteratively aid in quality improvement).

We may be at a tipping point in which all the "little" things that eMH makes possible start adding up – and changing our framework and approach to healthcare – as we move from a new way to practice and a new standard of practice [14]. If we can disseminate evidence-based treatments and new modalities of treatment for a number of psychiatric disorders delivered at a distance, why not do it in combination with high quality in-person care – a so-called "hybrid care" model [9, 24]? This hybrid, combined with different levels of technological complexity (i.e., from low intensity e-mail and phone to high intensity videoconferencing) and stepped and integrative care models, seems like the new standard.

Acknowledgments American Telemedicine Association Telemental Health Interest Group

References

1. Law LM, Wason JM. Design of telehealth trials–introducing adaptive approaches. Int J Med Inform. 2014;83(12):870–80.
2. Ekeland AG, Bowes A, Flottorp S. Effectiveness of telemedicine: a systematic review of reviews. Int J Med Inform. 2010;79:736–71.
3. Ekeland AG, Bowes A, Flottorp S. Methodologies for assessing telemedicine: a systematic review of reviews. Int J Med Inform. 2012;81:1–11.
4. Collins LM, Murphy SA, Strecher V. The multiphase optimization strategy (MOST) and the sequential multiple assignment randomized trial (SMART): new methods for more potent e-health interventions. Am J Prev Med. 2007;32 Suppl 5:112–8.
5. Buyze J, Goetghebeur E. Evaluating dynamic treatment strategies: does it have to be more costly? Pharm Stat. 2013;12:35–42.
6. Hilty DM, Ferrer D, Callahan EJ, et al. The effectiveness of telemental health: a 2013 review. Telemed J E Health. 2013;19(6):444–54.
7. Hilty DM, Liu W, Marks SL, et al. Effectiveness of telepsychiatry: a brief review. Can Psychiat Assoc Bull. 2003;35(5)10–17.
8. Richardson LK, Frueh BC, Grubaugh AL, et al. Current directions in videoconferencing telemental health research. Clin Psychol (New York). 2009;16(3):323–8.
9. Yellowlees PM, Shore JH, Roberts L, et al. Practice guidelines for videoconferencing-based telemental health. Telemed J E Health. 2010;16(10):1074–89.
10. Shore JH, Mishkind MC, Bernard J, et al. A lexicon of assessment and outcome measures for telemental health. Telemed J E Health. 2013;3:282–92.
11. Hilty DM, Yellowlees PM, Nasatir SEH, et al. Program evaluation and practical, step-by-step program modification in telemental health. In: Behavioral telehealth series volume 1- clinical video conferencing: program development and practice. Springer Press: New York, NY; 2014. p. 105–34.
12. Hilty DM, Shoemaker EZ, Myers KM, et al. Issues and steps toward a clinical guideline for telemental health for care of children and adolescents. J Child Adol Psychopharm. In Press.
13. Myers K, Cain S, Work Group on Quality Issues; American Academy of Practice parameter for telepsychiatry with children and adolescents. Practice parameter for telepsychiatry with children and adolescents. J Am Acad Child Adolesc Psychiatry. 2008;47(12):1468–83.
14. Hilty DM, Yellowlees PM, Chan S, et al. Telepsychiatry: effective, evidence-based and at a tipping point in healthcare delivery. Psychol Clin North Am. In Press.
15. Sheeran T, Dealy J, Rabinowitz T. Geriatric telemental health. In: Myers K, Turvey CL, editors. Telemental health. New York: Elsevier; 2013. p. 171–95.
16. Yellowlees PM, Odor A, Iosif A, et al. Transcultural psychiatry made simple: asynchronous telepsychiatry as an approach to providing culturally relevant care. Telemed J E Health. 2013;19(4):1–6.
17. Nelson EL, Duncan AB, Lillis T. Special considerations for conducting psychotherapy via videoconferencing. In: Myers K, Turvey CL, editors. Telemental health: clinical, technical

and administrative foundations for evidenced-based practice. San Francisco: Elsevier; 2013. p. 295–314.

18. Backhaus A, Agha Z, Maglione ML, et al. Videoconferencing psychotherapy: a systematic review. Psychol Serv. 2012;9(2):111–31.

19. Hilty DM, Yellowlees PM, Cobb HC, et al. Models of telepsychiatric consultation-liaison service to rural primary care. Psychosomatics. 2006;47(2):152–7.

20. Yellowlees PM, Odor A, Patrice K, et al. PsychVACS: a system for asynchronous telepsychiatry. Telemed J E Health. 2011;17(4):299–303.

21. Fortney JC, Pyne JM, Kimbrell TA, et al. Telemedicine-based collaborative care for post-traumatic stress disorder: a randomized clinical trial. JAMA Psychiatry. 2015;72(1):58–67.

22. Myers KM, Vander Stoep A, Zhou C, et al. Effectiveness of a telehealth service delivery model for treating attention-deficit hyperactivity disorder: results of a community-based randomized controlled trial. J Am Acad Child Adolesc Psychiatry. 2015;54(4):263–74.

23. Yellowlees PM, Nafiz N. The psychiatrist-patient relationship of the future: anytime, anywhere? Rev Psychiatry. 2010;18(2):96–102.

24. Hilty DM, Yellowlees PM. Collaborative mental health services using multiple technologies – the new way to practice and a new standard of practice? J Am Acad Child Adolesc Psychiatry. 2015;54(4):245.

25. O'Reilly R, Bishop J, Maddox K, et al. Is telepsychiatry equivalent to face to face psychiatry: results from a randomized controlled equivalence trial. Psychiatr Serv. 2007;258:836–43.

26. De Las Cuevas C, Arrendondo MT, et al. Randomized controlled trial of telepsychiatry through videoconference versus face-to-face conventional psychiatric treatment. Telemed J E Health. 2006;12:341–50.

27. Fortney JC, Pyne JM, Edlund MJ, et al. A randomized trial of telemedicine-based collaborative care for depression. J Gen Intern Med. 2007;22(8):1086–93.

28. Moreno FA, Chong J, Dumbauld J, et al. Use of standard webcam and Internet equipment for telepsychiatry treatment of depression among underserved Hispanics. Psychiatr Serv. 2012;63(12):1213–7.

29. Fortney JC, Pyne JM, Mouden SP, et al. Practice-based versus telemedicine-based collaborative care for depression in rural federally qualified health centers: a pragmatic randomized comparative effectiveness trial. Am J Psychiatry. 2013;170(4):414–25.

30. Huffman JC, Mastromauro CA, Beach SR, et al. Collaborative care for depression and anxiety disorders in patients with recent cardiac events: the Management of Sadness and Anxiety in Cardiology (MOSAIC) randomized clinical trial. JAMA Intern Med. 2014;174(6):927–35.

31. Bouchard S, Paquin B, Payeur R, et al. Delivering cognitive-behavior therapy for panic disorder with agoraphobia in videoconference. Telemed J E Health. 2004;10(1):13–25.

32. Wims E, Titov N, Andrews G, et al. Clinician-assisted internet-based treatment is effective for panic: a randomized controlled trial. Aust N Z J Psychiatry. 2010;44(7):599–607.

33. Hedman E, Ljótsson B, Rück C, et al. Effectiveness of internet-based cognitive behaviour therapy for panic disorder in routine psychiatric care. Acta Psychiatr Scand. 2013;128(6):457–67.

34. Frueh BC, Monnier J, Yim E, et al. Randomized trial for post-traumatic stress disorder. J Telemed Telecare. 2007;13:142–7.

35. Johnston L, Titov N, Andrews G, et al. Comorbidity and internet-delivered transdiagnostic cognitive behavioural therapy for anxiety disorders. Cogn Behav Ther. 2013;42(3):180–92.

36. Titov N, Dear BF, Schwencke G, et al. Transdiagnostic internet treatment for anxiety and depression: a randomised controlled trial. Behav Res Ther. 2011;49(8):441–52.

37. Weiner M, Rossetti H, Harrah K. Videoconference diagnosis and management of Choctaw Indian dementia patients. Alzheimers Dement. 2011;7:562–6.

38. Rabinowitz T, Murphy KM, Amour JL, et al. Benefits of a telepsychiatry consultation service for rural nursing home residents. Telemed J E Health. 2010;16(1):34–40.

39. Hilty DM, Marks SL, Wegeland JE, et al. A randomized controlled trial of disease management modules, including telepsychiatric care, for depression in rural primary care. Psychiatry. 2007;4(2):58–65.

40. Sheeran T, Rabinowitz T, Lotterman J, et al. Feasibility and impact of telemonitor-based depression care management for geriatric homecare patients. Telemed J E Health. 2011;17:620–6.
41. Brooks TR. Pitfalls in communication with Hispanic and African-American patients: do translators help or harm? J Natl Med Assoc. 1992;84(11):941.
42. Brua C. Role-blurring and ethical grey zones associated with lay interpreters: three case studies. Commun Med. 2008;5(1):73.
43. Elderkin-Thompson V, Silver RC, et al. When nurses double as interpreters: a study of Spanish-speaking patients in a US primary care setting. Soc Sci Med. 2001;52:1343–58.
44. Yellowlees PM, Burke MM, Marks SL, et al. Emergency telepsychiatry. J Telemed Telecare. 2008;14:277–81.
45. Butler TN, Yellowlees P. Cost analysis of store-and-forward telepsychiatry as a consultation model for primary care. Telemed J E Health. 2012;18(1):74–7.
46. Pesamaa L, Ebeling H, Kuusimaki ML, et al. Videoconferencing in child and adolescent telepsychiatry: a systematic review of the literature. J Telemed Telecare. 2004;10:187–92.
47. Myers KM, Palmer NB, Geyer JR. Research in child and adolescent telemental health. Child Adolesc Psychiatr Clin N Am. 2011;20(1):155–71.
48. Pakyurek M, Yellowlees PM, Hilty DM. The child and adolescent telepsychiatry consultation: can it be a more effective clinical process for certain patients than conventional practice? Telemed J E Health. 2010;16(3):289–92.
49. Neufeld JD, Bourgeois JA, Hilty DM, et al. The e-mental health consult service: providing enhanced primary care mental health services through telemedicine. Psychosomatics. 2007;48:135–41.
50. Yellowlees PM, Hilty DM, Marks SL, et al. A retrospective analysis of child and adolescent e-mental health. J Am Acad Child Adolesc Psychiatry. 2008;47(1):1–5.
51. Rockhill C, Violette H, Vander Stoep A, et al. Caregivers' distress: youth with attention-deficit/hyperactivity disorder and comorbid disorders assessed via telemental health. J Child Adolesc Psychopharmacol. 2013;23(6):379–85.
52. Brondbo H, Mathiassen B, Martinussen M, et al. Agreement on web-based diagnoses and severity of mental health problems in a Norwegian child and adolescent mental health Service. Clin Pract Epidemiol Ment Health. 2012;8:16–21.
53. Glueck DA. Telepsychiatry in private practice. Child Adolesc Psychiatr Clin N Am. 2011;20(1):1–11.
54. Savin D, Glueck DA, Chardavoyne J, et al. Bridging cultures: child psychiatry via videoconferencing. Child Adolesc Psychiatr Clin N Am. 2011;20:125–34.
55. Hilty DM, Nesbitt TS, Marks SL, et al. How telepsychiatry affects the doctor-patient relationship: communication, satisfaction, and additional clinically relevant issues. Primary Psychiatry. 2002;9(9):29–34.
56. Morland LA, Greene CJ, Rosen CS, et al. Telemedicine for anger management therapy in a rural population of combat veterans with posttraumatic stress disorder: a randomized noninferiority trial. J Clin Psychiatry. 2010;71:855–63.
57. Postel MG, de Haan HA, DeJong CA. e-Therapy for mental health problems: a systematic review. Telemed J E Health. 2008;14(7):707–14.
58. Greene CJ, Morland LA, Macdonald A, et al. How does tele-mental health affect group therapy process? Secondary analysis of a noninferiority trial. J Consult Clin Psychol. 2010;78(5):746–50.
59. Grady BJ, Melcer TA. Retrospective evaluation of telemental healthcare services for remote military populations. Telemed J E Health. 2005;11(5):551–8.
60. Tuerk PW, Yoder M, Ruggiero KJ, et al. A pilot study of prolonged exposure therapy for posttraumatic stress disorder delivered via telehealth technology. J Trauma Stress. 2010;23(1):116–23.
61. Marrone S, Mitchell JE, Crosby R, et al. Predictors of response to cognitive behavioral treatment for bulimia nervosa delivered via telemedicine versus face-to-face. Int J Eat Disord. 2009;42(3):222–7.

62. World Health Organization. Telemedicine opportunities and developments in member states. Results of the second global survey on eHealth. Geneva: WHO Press; 2011.
63. Dobbins ML, Roberts N, Vicari SK, et al. The consulting conference: a new model of collaboration for child psychiatry and primary care. Acad Psychiatry. 2011;35:260-2.
64. Hilty DM, Yellowlees PM, Nesbitt TS. Evolution of telepsychiatry to rural sites: change over time in types of referral and PCP knowledge, skill, and satisfaction. Gen Hosp Psychiatry. 2006;28(5):367-73.
65. Hilty DM, Nesbitt TS, Kuenneth TA, et al. Telepsychiatric consultation to primary care: rural vs. suburban needs, utilization and provider satisfaction. J Rural Health. 2007;23(2):163-5.
66. Manian FA, Janssen DA. Curbside consultations. JAMA. 1996;275:145-6.
67. Dee C, Blazek R. Information needs of the rural physician. A descriptive study. Bull Med Libr Assoc. 1993;81:259-64.
68. Bergus GR, Sinift D, Randall CS, et al. Use of an e-mail curbside consultation service by family physicians. J Fam Pract. 1998;47(5):357-60.
69. Hilty DM, Ingraham RL, Yang RP, et al. Multispecialty phone and email consultation to primary care providers for patients with developmental disabilities in rural California. Telemed J E Health. 2004;10:413-21.
70. Richardson L, McCauley E, Katon W. Collaborative care for adolescent depression: a pilot study. Gen Hosp Psychiatry. 2009;31:36-45.
71. Kenwright M, Liness S, Marks I, et al. Reducing demands on clinicians by offering computer-aided self-help for phobia/panic. Feasibility study. Br J Psychiatry. 2001;179(5):456-9.
72. National Center for Telehealth and Technology. PTSD Coach [Internet]. PTSD Coach, t2health, 2013. February 28, 2015. At: http://www.t2.health.mil/apps/ptsd-coach.
73. Luxton DD, McCann RA, Bush NE, et al. mHealth for mental health: integrating smartphone technology in behavioral healthcare. Prof Psychol Res Practice Hu C, Kung S, Rummans TA, et al. Reducing caregiver stress with Internet-based interventions: a systematic review of open-label and randomized controlled trials. J Am Med Inform Assoc. 2014. doi:10.1136/amiajnl-2014-002817.
74. Kunigiri G, Gajebasia N, Sallah D. Improving attendance in psychiatric outpatient clinics by using reminders. J Telemed Telecare. 2014;20(8):464-7.
75. Carlbring P, Nordgren LB, Furmark T, et al. Long-term outcome of Internet-delivered cognitive-behavioural therapy for social phobia: a 30-month follow-up. Behav Res Ther. 2009;47(10):848-50.
76. Kiropoulos LA, Klein B, Austin DW, et al. Is internet-based CBT for panic disorder and agoraphobia as effective as face-to-face CBT? J Anxiety Disord. 2008;22(8):1273-84.
77. Kok G, Bockting C, Berger H, et al. Mobile cognitive therapy: adherence and acceptability of an online intervention in remitted recurrently depressed patients. Internet Intervent. 2014;1(2):65.
78. Yellowlees PM, Holloway KM, Parish MB. Therapy in virtual environments—clinical and ethical issues. Telemed J E Health. 2012;18(7):558-64.
79. Leff J, Williams G, Huckvale M, et al. Avatar therapy for persecutory auditory hallucinations: what is and how does it work? Psychosis. 2014;6(2):166-76.
80. Hu C, Kung S, Rummans TA, et al. Reducing caregiver stress with internet-based interventions: a systematic review of open-label and randomized controlled trials. J Am Med Inform Assoc. 2014. doi:10.1136/amiajnl-2014-002817.
81. Blusi M, Dalin R, Jong M, et al. The benefits of e-health support for older family caregivers in rural areas. J Telemed Telecare. 2014;20(2):63-9.
82. Chi NC, Demiris G. A systematic review of telehealth tools and interventions to support family caregivers. J Telemed Telecare. 2015;21(1):37-44.
83. Rosenthal TC. The medical home: growing evidence to support a new approach to primary care. J Am Board Fam Med. 2008;21(5):427-40.
84. Cluver JS, Schuyler D, Frueh BC, et al. Remote psychotherapy for terminally ill cancer patients. J Telemed Telecare. 2005;11:157-9.
85. Hollingsworth JM, Saint S, Hayward RA, et al. Specialty care and the patient-centered medical home. Med Care. 2011;49(1):4-9.

86. van't veer-Tazelaar N, van Marwijk H, van Oppen P, et al. Prevention of anxiety and depression in the age group of 75 years and over: a randomized controlled trial testing the feasibility and effectiveness of a generic stepped care program among elderly community residents at high risk of developing anxiety and depression versus usual care. BMC Public Health. 2006;6:186.

87. Yesavage JA, Brink TL, Rose TL, et al. Development and validation of a geriatric depression scale: A preliminary report. J Psychiatr Res. 1983;17:37–49.

88. Myers KM, Vander Stoep A, McCarty CA, et al. Child and adolescent telepsychiatry: variations in utilization, referral patterns and practice trends. J Telemed Telecare. 2010;16:128–33.

89. Lyketsos C, Roques C, Hovanec L. Telemedicine use and reduction of psychiatric admissions from a long-term care facility. J Geriatr Psychiatry Neurol. 2001;14:76–9.

90. Poon P, Hui E, Dai D, et al. Cognitive intervention for community-dwelling older persons with memory problems: telemedicine versus face-to-face treatment. Int J Geriatr Psychiatry. 2005;20:285–6.

91. Graham MA. Telepsychiatry in Appalachia. Am Behav Sci. 1996;39:602–15.

92. Zaylor C. Clinical outcomes in telepsychiatry. J Telemed Telecare. 1999;5:59–60.

93. Hunkeler EM, Meresman JF, Hargreaves WA, et al. Efficacy of nurse telehealth care and peer support in augmenting treatment of depression in primary care. Arch Fam Med. 2000;9:700–8.

94. Ruskin PE, Silver-Aylaian M, Kling MA, et al. Treatment outcomes in depression: comparison of remote treatment through telepsychiatry to in in-person treatment. Am J Psychiatry. 2004;161:1471–6.

95. Manfredi L, Shupe J, Batki S. Rural jail telepsychiatry: a pilot feasibility study. Telemed J E Health. 2005;11(5):574–7.

96. Sorvaniemi M, Ojanen E, Santamäki O. Telepsychiatry in emergency consultations: a follow-up study of sixty patients. Telemed J E Health. 2005;11(4):439–41.

97. Modai I, Jabarin M, Kurs R, et al. Cost effectiveness, safety, and satisfaction with video telepsychiatry versus face-to-face care in ambulatory settings. Telemed J E Health. 2006;12:515–20.

98. Urness D, Wass M, Gordon A, et al. Client acceptability and quality of life – telepsychiatry compared to in-person consultation. J Telemed Telecare. 2006;12(5):251–4.

99. Yellowlees PM, Odor A, Burke MM, et al. A feasibility study of asynchronous telepsychiatry for psychiatric consultations. Psychiatr Serv. 2010;61(8):838–40.

100. Germain V, Marchand A, Bouchard S, et al. Effectiveness of cognitive behavioural therapy administered by videoconference for posttraumatic stress disorder. Cogn Behav Ther. 2009;38(1):42–53.

101. Frueh BC, Henderson S, Myrick H. Telehealth service delivery for persons with alcoholism. J Telemed Telecare. 2005;11(7):372–5.

102. Szeftel R, Federico C, Hakak R, et al. Improved access to mental health evaluation for patients with developmental disabilities using telepsychiatry. J Telemed Telecare. 2012;18(6):317–21.

103. Chong J, Moreno FA. Feasibility and acceptability of clinic-based telepsychiatry for low-income Hispanic primary care patients. Telemed J E Health. 2012;18(4):297–304.

104. Shore JH, Brooks E, Savin D, et al. Acceptability of telepsychiatry in American Indians. Telemed J E Health. 2008;14(5):461–6.

105. Mucic D. Transcultural telepsychiatry and its impact on patient satisfaction. J Telemed Telecare. 2010;16(5):237–42.

106. Ye J, Shim R, Lukaszewski T, Yun K, et al. Telepsychiatry services for Korean immigrants. Telemed J E Health. 2012;18(10):797–802.

107. Lopez AM, Cruz M, Lazarus S, et al. Use of American sign language in telepsychiatry consultation. Telemed J E Health. 2004;10(3):389–91.

108. Blackmon LA, Kaak HO, Ranseen J. Consumer satisfaction with telemedicine child psychiatry consultation in rural Kentucky. Psychiatr Serv. 1997;48:1464–6.

109. Elford R, White H, Bowering R, et al. A randomized, controlled trial of child psychiatric assessments conducted using videoconferencing. J Telemed Telecare. 2000;6:73–82.

110. Elford DR, White H, St John K, et al. A prospective satisfaction study and cost analysis of a pilot child telepsychiatry service in Newfoundland. J Telemed Telecare. 2001;7:73–81.
111. Glueckauf RL, Fritz SP, Ecklund-Johnson EP, et al. Videoconferencing-based family counseling for rural teenagers with epilepsy: phase 1 findings. Rehabil Psychol. 2002;47(1):49–72.
112. Nelson EL, Barnard M, Cain S. Treating childhood depression over videoconferencing. Telemed J E Health. 2003;9:49–55.
113. Myers KM, Sulzbacher S, Melzer SM. Telepsychiatry with children and adolescents: are patients comparable to those evaluated in usual outpatient care? Telemed J E Health. 2004;10(3):278–85.
114. Greenberg N, Boydell K, Volpe T. Pediatric telepsychiatry in Ontario: caregiver and service provider perspectives. J Behav Health Serv Res. 2006;33(1):105–11.
115. Myers K, Valentine J, Morganthaler R, et al. Telepsychiatry with incarcerated youth. J Adolesc Health. 2006;38(6):643–8.
116. Myers KM, Valentine JM, Melzer SM. Feasibility, acceptability, and sustainability of telepsychiatry for children and adolescents. Psychiatr Serv. 2007;58:1493–6.
117. Bensink M, Armfield N, Irving H, et al. A pilot study of videotelephone-based support for newly diagnosed paediatric oncology patients and their families. J Telemed Telecare. 2008;14(6):315–21.
118. Clawson B, Selden M, Lacks M, et al. Complex pediatric feeding disorders: using teleconferencing technology to improve access to a treatment program. Pediatr Nurs. 2008;34(3):213–6.
119. Fox KC, Conner P, McCullers E, et al. Effect of a behavioural health and specialty care telemedicine programme on goal attainment for youths in juvenile detention. J Telemed Telecare. 2008;14(5):227–30.
120. Morgan GJ, Craig B, Grant B, et al. Home videoconferencing for patients with severe congential heart disease following discharge. Congenit Heart Dis. 2008;3(5):317–24.
121. Myers KM, Valentine JM, Melzer SM. Child and adolescent telepsychiatry: utilization and satisfaction. Telemed J E Health. 2008;14(2):131–7.
122. Shaikh U, Cole SL, Marcin JP, et al. Clinical management and patient outcomes among children and adolescents receiving telemedicine consultations for obesity. Telemed J E Health. 2008;14(5):434–40.
123. Wilkinson OM, Duncan-Skingle F, Pryor JA, et al. A feasibility study of home telemedicine for patients with cystic fibrosis awaiting transplantation. J Telemed Telecare. 2008; 14(4):182–5.
124. Witmans MB, Dick B, Good J, et al. Delivery of pediatric sleep services via telehealth: the Alberta experience and lessons learned. Behav Sleep Med. 2008;6(4):207–19.
125. Lau ME, Way BB, Fremont WP. Assessment of SUNY Upstate Medical University's child telepsychiatry consultation program. Int J Psychiatry Med. 2011;42(1):93–104.
126. Mulgrew KW, Shaikh U, Nettiksimmons J, et al. Comparison of parent satisfaction with care for childhood obesity delivered face-to-face and by telemedicine. Telemed J E Health. 2011;17(5):383–7.
127. Stain HJ, Payne K, Thienel R, et al. The feasibility of videoconferencing for neuropsychological assessments of rural youth experiencing early psychosis. J Telemed Telecare. 2011;17(6):328–31.
128. Storch EA, May JE, Wood JJ, et al. Multiple informant agreement on the anxiety disorders interview schedule in youth with autism spectrum disorders. J Child Adolesc Psychopharmacol. 2012;22(4):292–9.
129. Himle MB, Freitag M, Walther M, et al. A randomized pilot trial comparing videoconference versus face-to-face delivery of behavior therapy for childhood tic disorders. Behav Res Ther. 2012;50(9):565–70.
130. Jacob MK, Larson JC, Craighead WE. Establishing a telepsychiatry consultation practice in rural Georgia for primary care physicians: A feasibility report. Clin Pediatr (Phila). 2012;51(11):1041–7.
131. Nelson EL, Duncan AB, Peacock G, et al. Telemedicine and adherence to national guidelines for ADHD evaluation: a case study. Psychol Serv. 2012;9(3):293–7.

132. Reese RJ, Slone NC, Soares N, et al. Telehealth for underserved families: an evidence-based parenting program. Psychol Serv. 2012;9(3):320–2.
133. Heitzman-Powell LS, Buzhardt J, Rusinko LC, et al. Formative evaluation of an ABA outreach training program for parents of children with autism in remote areas. Focus Autism Dev Disabl. 2013;29(1):23.
134. Xie Y, Dixon JF, Yee OM, et al. A study on the effectiveness of videoconferencing on teaching parent training skills to parents of children with ADHD. Telemed J E Health. 2013;19(3):192–9.
135. Reese RM, Jamison R, Wendland M, et al. Evaluating interactive videoconferencing for assessing symptoms of autism. Telemed J E Health. 2013;19(9):671–7.
136. Davis AM, Sampilo M, Gallagher KS, et al. Treating rural pediatric obesity through telemedicine: outcomes from a small randomized controlled trial. J Pediatr Psychol. 2013;38(9):932–43.
137. Freeman KA, Duke DC, Harris MA. Behavioral health care for adolescents with poorly controlled diabetes via Skype: does working alliance remain intact? J Diabetes Sci Technol. 2013;7(3):727–35.
138. Hommel KA, Greenley RN, Maddux MH, et al. Self-management in pediatric inflammatory bowel disease: a clinical report of the North American Society for Pediatric Gastroenterology, Hepatology, and Nutrition. J Pediatr Gastroenterol Nutr. 2013;57(2):250–7.
139. Lipana LS, Bindal D, Nettiksimmons J, et al. Telemedicine and face-to-face care for pediatric obesity. Telemed J E Health. 2013;19(10):806–8.
140. Comer JS, Furr JM, Cooper-Vince CE, et al. Internet-delivered, family-based treatment for early-onset OCD: a preliminary case series. J Clin Child Adolesc Psychol. 2014;43(1): 74–87.
141. Tse YJ, McCarty CA, Vander Stoep A, et al. Teletherapy delivery of caregiver behavior training for children with attention-deficit hyperactivity disorder. Telemed J E Health. 2015;21(6):451–8.
142. Rockhill C, et al. Telepsychiatrists' adherence to guidelines-based care, ADHD outcomes by prescriber based on comorbidity status. Tel e-Health. In Press.
143. Bastien CH, Morin CM, Ouellet MC, et al. Cognitive-behavioral therapy for insomnia: comparison of individual therapy, group therapy, and telephone consultations. J Consult Clin Psychol. 2004;72(4):653–9.
144. Morgan RD, Patrick AR, Magaletta PR. Does the use of telemental health alter the treatment experience? Inmates' perceptions of telemental health versus face-to-face treatment modalities. J Consult Clin Psychol. 2008;76(1):158–62.
145. Ertelt TW, Crosby RD, Marino JM, et al. Therapeutic factors affecting the cognitive behavioral treatment of bulimia nervosa via telemedicine versus face-to-face delivery. Int J Eat Disord. 2011;44(8):687–91.
146. Germain V, Marchand A, Bouchard S, et al. Assessment of the therapeutic alliance in face-to-face or videoconference treatment for posttraumatic stress disorder. Cyberpsychol Behav Soc Netw. 2010;13(1):29–35.
147. King VL, Stoller KB, Kidorf M. Assessing the effectiveness of an internet-based videoconferencing platform for delivering intensified substance abuse counseling. J Subst Abuse Treat. 2009;36:331–8.
148. Gros DF, Price M, Strachan M, et al. Behavioral activation and therapeutic exposure: an investigation of relative symptom changes in PTSD and depression during the course of integrated behavioral activation, situational exposure, and imaginal exposure techniques. Behav Modif. 2012;36(4):580–99.
149. Yuen EK, Herbert JD, Forman EM, et al. Acceptance based behavior therapy for social anxiety disorder through videoconferencing. J Anxiety Disord. 2013;27(4):389–97.
150. King VL, Brooner RK, Peirce JM. A randomized trial of Web-based videoconferencing for substance abuse counseling. J Subst Abuse Treat. 2014;46:36–42.
151. Khatri N, Marziali E, Tchernikov I, et al. Comparing telehealth-based and clinic-based group cognitive behavioral therapy for adults with depression and anxiety: a pilot study. Clin Interv Aging. 2014;7(9):765–70.

How e-Mental Health Adds to Traditional Outpatient and Newer Models of Integrated Care for Patients, Providers, and Systems

7

Donald M. Hilty, Barb Johnston, and Robert M. McCarron

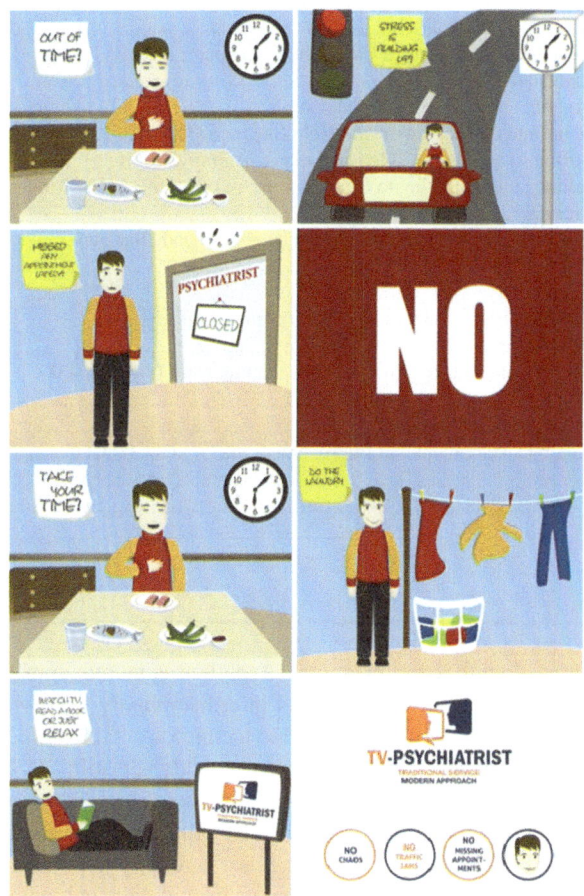

© Springer International Publishing Switzerland 2016
D. Mucic, D.M. Hilty (eds.), *e-Mental Health*,
DOI 10.1007/978-3-319-20852-7_7

D.M. Hilty, MD (✉)
Keck School of Medicine, University of Southern California, Los Angeles, CA, USA
e-mail: donh031226@gmail.com

B. Johnston, RN
HealthLinkNow, Sacramento, CA, USA

California Telemedicine and e-Health Center, Sacramento, CA, USA

R.M. McCarron, DO
Department of Anesthesiology and Pain Medicine, University of California, Davis Health System, Sacramento, CA, USA

Contents

7.1   Introduction 131
7.2   Patient-Centered and Integrated Care: The Participants,
      Quality Care, and Evaluation.. 134
      7.2.1   Program Evaluation and Leadership 135
7.3   Telemedicine and eMH: How It Can Help Integrate Care 136
7.4   The Interdisciplinary Team: Role Definitions, Training Needs,
      Cross-Training, and Adapting to New Stepped and Integrated Care Models 139
      7.4.1   Overview 139
      7.4.2   Best Practice for Integrated Care: Depression and Diabetes
            (or Heart Disease or Other) 139
      7.4.3   Treatment Options 140
      7.4.4   Best Practice for Integrated Care: Training/Education
            for Integrated Care 141
      7.4.5   Project Consultation: Program Development and Improvement
            via Organizational Consultation.. 141
7.5   Discussion and Conclusions... 142
Appendix: Program Development and Improvement via Organizational Consultation 144
      Overview 144
      Logistics... 144
References.. 146

Abstract

Contemporary health care promotes a patient-centered approach, integrates health/mental health care, emphasizes interdisciplinary teamwork, and adopts innovations such as communications technology. Telemedicine, including e-Mental Health (eMH), e.g., telepsychiatry, adds versatility to service delivery by improving access to care, leveraging expertise of key disciplines to the point-of-service, and disseminating education. Key disciplines in integrated care that provide mental health services into primary care are the psychiatrist, mid-level professionals, and nurses. These clinicians provide clinical, administrative, and care coordination expertise or oversight. A more recent addition to this integrated team is the care navigator who essentially coordinates care across all other team members and the patients. Overall, telemedicine, cross-training, stepped care roles, and use of clinically "versatile" clinicians – all of these help to fill "holes" in services for patients. Evidence-based treatment becomes more accessible, better disseminated, and in "real time" with use of health technologies. Best practices for clinical care, education, and program development are needed for integrated care and e-health.

7.1 Introduction

Health care is being confronted with questions on how to deliver quality, affordable, and timely care to patients in a variety of settings [1]. Increased clinical operating efficiency gets the clinician with expertise to the point-of-service and emphasizes teamwork for clinical, administrative, and informal care coordination (see Table 7.1). Specifically, this involves many disciplines working at the "top of one's license." For psychiatry, this is facilitated by having non-MD mental health professionals seeing the less complex cases and reserving the psychiatrist's direct clinical time judiciously; this may include management of more complicated cases or providing clinical oversight and review of cases seen by others. Psychiatric disorders/illnesses significantly impact primary care, as those with psychiatric illness (e.g., schizophrenia, bipolar disorder, recurrent major depression) have higher mortality primarily due to socioeconomic factors, poor access to effective primary/preventative care, and the burden of chronic health conditions [2].

One of the best options for integrated care appears to be using eMH/telepsychiatry for clinical care, education, and other interventions [3]. In its sixth decade, telepsychiatry has increased access to care in urban, suburban, and rural settings – with patients, clinicians, and health care systems very satisfied with it for a wide variety of services and cultures [3, 4]. Telepsychiatry has been shown effective for diagnosis and assessment across many populations (e.g., adult, child, geriatric, and ethnic), for psychiatric disorders in many settings (e.g., emergency, home health), and been found to be comparable to in-person care. It has been used with a variety of models of care (i.e., collaborative care, asynchronous, mobile, telemonitoring) with equally positive outcomes [3]. eMH has been shown to assist health care professionals by providing timely access to specialty care [5, 6] and also for education/lifelong learning opportunities [7, 8].

Integrated care provides an approach to psychiatric illness in a general medical setting, and though not quite as well known, providing general medical care in a primary psychiatric clinical setting (i.e., "reverse integration"). The *seven core characteristics/levels* of integrated care first include responsibility, decision-making, and oversight of patient care; this is true along the entire interdisciplinary team from physicians to care coordinators. A second characteristic is co-location of services, both literally and/or virtually – that applies to both inpatient and outpatient sector care. Characteristics three to five are integrated funding, evaluation, and outcome measurement. We contend that two additional characteristics are needed:

Table 7.1 Health care innovation and evolution: the changing ecosystem

Stressors/changes/trends to health care and "global" parties involved	Changes, trends, and stressors in the healthcare ecosystem	Challenges moving from traditional practice to a new model/ecosystem of health care
$		
% GNP	1/6 of the GNP is more than other countries spend, not sustainable, and contains duplication/inefficiency/waste	Change is the primary obstacle, assuming that a new paradigm could be agreed upon and integration could occur
Recession and unbalanced budget	Economic times are not good and most likely, over time, more "pressure" will arise	Short-term costs, fear and loss of existing frameworks will be used as reasons to not change
National leadership		
Accountability	Leaders want more accountability from providers and institutions Medicine leaves itself vulnerable by "blind spots" (e.g., lack of self-policing, COIs) and an ineffective, unintegrated lobby	Fiefdoms, systems in isolation and even private practices are being assailed The "rich" get richer and the "poor" get poorer at least in research and AHC grants
Control vs. free market tension	The current system has "ballooned" as much as it can, it will deflate, parties will "leave" due to inadequate profits and reform will cut costs, and technology goes "around" current obstacles for those with means	Cost will be cut in a "good" or "worse" ways =>there is incentive to look at this for patients, payees, and payors? Obama care will re-sort populations e-Health will re-distribute care
Decrease disparities	Many Americans support better access and the costs of SES determinants (e.g., lack of education) for uninsured are more obvious	Many parties' dissatisfaction will unite toward reform; ACA and 2014; communities are mobilizing
Payors/reimbursement		
Metrics are changing or need to shift	Reimbursement based on non-outcomes (e.g., a trainee providing care, service delivered) do not result in the "best" outcomes	The movement for quality, affordability, access, portability, safety, and other indices is strong
MD-centered to patient-centered		
What should be the unifying or organizing model of service delivery?	The AHC or clinic model of care works for only a few, not efficient, costly, and not patient-centered	How do we partner with patients to share decisions (better), work with communities, and define goals based on populations?

Table 7.1 (continued)

Stressors/changes/trends to health care and "global" parties involved	Changes, trends, and stressors in the healthcare ecosystem	Challenges moving from traditional practice to a new model/ecosystem of health care
Parameters of "good" care are?	Systems were set up on "best" care models what were defined by AHCs or specialties, not always tested in all populations and not accessible to many	The "best" care by "best" provider "Fast," timely, portable Cheap/inexpensive or affordable Culturally and linguistically sensitive
Provider/team satisfaction		
How do we define it and what are our values?	"Traditional" metrics were "good" care, expert-based (now EBM), training the new generation, making scientific advances and knowledge My career is not everything to me?	Additions or reform questions: How can I see impact better, enjoy what I do, be helpful to high utilizers or those with differences, make a good living, be independent and team up?
AHC-centered to patient- or community-centered systems		
What is the difference, really? We already work to help patients, right?	We (AHCs) "know" best and are the leaders – why do we need help? Why do things have to change? Do our skills need to change? Translational research is a "good" idea but not for everything Of course we want quality and safe care...we do that already	If we do include others, who should they be and what do we have to change? How to "stay" a doctor and shift from knowledge → skills → leadership and improvis'n? We have to do translational education, clinical care, and administration too? How do I learn to collect different data, enter it, analyze it, and measure outcomes?
Transformed training: quality, safe		
Other		
	Medicine moves slowly to maintain the patient-doctor relationship, ensure validity of diagnosis and treatments, and preserve the profession	How do we... Use technology for integration and access Vertically and horizontally integrate care Make care transparent and predictable Shift evaluation to a primary role Maintain privacy, confidentiality, and such

sixth, an e-platform, and seventh, reimbursement. Reimbursement is variable in the USA as it may align (e.g., a capitated or sole "Medicare" population) or not align (i.e., mixed populations) with one or more payers.

This chapter will help the reader to: (1) use a patient-centered, integrated approach to facilitate access to quality and affordable care, in general, and for comorbid conditions (e.g., depression/diabetes); (2) learn how telehealth is a versatile option for stepped and integrated care models; and (3) evaluate role definitions, telehealth and integrated care training needs, cross-training and interdisciplinary teamwork that help with integrated care.

7.2   Patient-Centered and Integrated Care: The Participants, Quality Care, and Evaluation

Integrated models of care (IMC) are patient-centered and usually have a psychiatrist as a consultant with co-location of psychiatric and medical service [9]. IMC improve *medical* outcomes in primary care settings [10], via mental health (MH) case managers [11, 12], in terms of patient functional improvement [13], reduced disability days [14], increased quality-adjusted life years [15], and increased adherence to medication [14] when compared with other models of care. IMC psychiatric outcomes may include improved global assessment of function (GAF), geriatric depression scale (GDS) scores, or mini-mental status examination (MMSE) scores.

Patients are generally stratified in quadrants – with the setting pre-determining those quadrants. In outpatient care, there are four quadrants [16]:

- I: Low medical and mental health (MH)
- II: Low medical and high MH
- III: Low MH and high medical
- IV: High for both

In the medical inpatient setting, the quadrants are as follows:

- I: Medium-to-high psychiatric acuity and none-to-low medical acuity
- II: Medium-to-high medical acuity and none-to-low psychiatric acuity
- III: Medium-to-high psychiatric acuity and low-to-medium medical acuity
- IV: Medium-to-high psychiatric acuity and medium-to-high [17]

Poor outcomes for patients with psychiatric and medical comorbidity have been alarming. In addition to poor medical outcomes mentioned above, patients with major depression are also at higher risk of medical illness, such as diabetes mellitus and ischemic heart disease [18, 19] and there may be increased risk of diabetes, metabolic syndrome, cardiovascular disease, and stroke associated with atypical antipsychotics [20]. A recent review measured the outcomes in the literature, systematically, in terms of the participants, description of the IMC, interventions, and outcomes [21].

Outcomes can be stratified by who is designated the primary service and the secondary consultant, which is usually the model except for fully integrated units. The history and recent trends in the literature are best summarized as:

- Medical outpatient: Historically, it went from the 1980s with no/little psychiatric/MH care to "curbside" consultations [22], to one-time psychiatric consultation one time usually off-site, to consultation on-site, to 1995 with a collaborative care model [23], to the late 1990s with a telepsychiatry consultation and disease management [24, 25]; email and phone consultation [26] to traditional integrated behavioral health on-site (above) and now collaborative care by telepsychiatry [25, 27].
- Medical inpatient: Historically, it went from no/little psychiatric/MH care to "curbside" consultations, one-time psychiatric consultation one time or ongoing, to liaison for education role and support, and eventually to medical-psychiatric units; only recently has a collaborative care model been applied to the inpatient setting.
- Psychiatric outpatient setting: Historically, it went from none/little to "curbside" consultations, one-time medical evaluation/consultation usually off-site, but very rarely to consultation or a collaborative care model; no reverse integration by telepsychiatry consultation has been described to date.
- Psychiatric inpatient/hospital setting: Historically, it went from none/little to "curbside" consultations, one-time medical evaluation in the emergency room (ER; either "medical clearance" or medicine consultation in psychiatry ER) or at admission, but very rarely to consultation or a collaborative care model; no reverse integration by telepsychiatry consultation has been described to date. Ironically, dietetics/nutrition is often co-located on the unit, and an additional medical initial or PRN evaluation may occur.

In addition to traditional psychiatric consultation to medicine or primary care and integrated or joint units, there are as follows: (1) multidisciplinary joint treatment by a geriatric team in addition to the usual care on a general medicine ward [28]; (2) a "Type IV" integrated medicine and psychiatry treatment program with the provisions of an acute medicine as well as a psychiatric ward administered through the department of internal medicine [17]; and a (3) nurse-led mental health liaison service in addition to usual care on internal medicine [29].

7.2.1   Program Evaluation and Leadership

Program evaluation has become increasingly important to meet program, patient, provider, and externally driven (Joint Commission, reimbursement) needs. Its roots, therefore, are founded in a clinical care, business, quality improvement, and organizational leadership. Alignment of participants' missions from the top to the bottom cannot be overstated – is there support for infrastructure, short- and long-term planning, competency development for participants, adequate funding, and fitness?

Good evaluation of outcomes related to eMH begins with a program and its fitness: organization, function (e.g., adaptability, change management), leadership (i.e., vision, operations), team members (e.g., interdisciplinary with overlapping roles or cross-training), experience with growth, and many other parameters. Programmatic changes are based on evaluation of all participants and an iterative feedback loop.

Contemporary program evaluation itself and integration of MH and medical services are both *substantial shifts* in philosophical approach for many and adding an e-services component adds versatility but complexity [30, 31]. The potential for misunderstanding among large teams is tremendous unless a shared mental model of expectation, roles, and outcomes is created [32]. For integrated care, questions are the starting place and the point to return to, since few programs are built proactively to do this work. Questions fall into four main domains:

- Leadership and decision-making: Is there a common goal? Is there joint responsibility? Are the medical and MH sides well represented and collaborative? This is from the big (i.e., program design) to the small (when to discharge, clinical goals).
- Structure: How are the services co-located physically/virtually? Is the reporting among the clinical, administrative, and other academic/practice bodies well aligned?
- Stepped care with a range of in-person and e-service options: Do folks practice at "the top of their license"? Can the patient access care many ways or places? Is telemedicine facilitating or delivering the services/expertise efficiently?
- Are outcomes for clinical services (i.e., medically and MH-based), team players' education/training [33], and program goals in harmony and measurable?

7.3 Telemedicine and eMH: How It Can Help Integrate Care

E-platforms have traditionally distributed academic networks of like-minded researchers and clinicians into regional health information organizations (RHIOs). These RHIOs empower consumers and clinicians in day-to-day health care delivery by improving access to evidence-based information at the point of care; facilitate the delivery of a wider range of health services, particularly to primary and community care; provide accurate data to support research and clinical policy and governance arrangements; and ensure a sustainable, secure, reliable electronic environment, underpinned by strong, policy-driven privacy protection [34]. Previously, the single most important technical innovation was broadband distribution, which enables high-quality videoconferencing, multimedia-based applications, and other options particularly doctor's desk. The contemporary e-platform adds the electronic medical record (EMR), integration of in-person and eMH care administration (i.e., scheduling, documentation, payment, and other), enhanced patient to doctor or system engagement/communication (e.g., HIPAA compliant email "into" the EMR e.g., Relay Health), and leveraging the expertise at a distance (phone, email, video, asynchronous and other methods).

eMH models of clinical care and education have pros and cons [3, 35, 36], including their level of overall intensity, cost, feasibility, and depth of the relationship between the eMH provider, the primary care practitioner (PCP), and patient. *Low intensity* models include tele-education, formal case review and in-person, telephone or email doctor-to-doctor "curbside" consultations. A systematic approach was a multi-specialty phone and email teleconsultation system for adults and children with developmental disabilities [37]. *Moderate intensity* models include an integrated program of mental health screening, therapy on-site, and tele-psychiatric consultation (phone, email, or video), with continuing medical education (CME) and training on screening questionnaires [38, 39] or asynchronous telepsychiatry (ATP) to primary care in English and Spanish-speaking patients in primary care [4, 40, 41]. *High-intensity* models are typically the ones previously mentioned, including collaborative care [27, 42–44] (Table 7.2).

Stepped care models may be the most cost-effective models in health system where the effectiveness of the intervention is maximized by making the best use of resources adequately available at the right time [44, 45]. The stepped care model seems to be a logical approach from both clinical and economic perspectives and several countries [46]; England and New Zealand have implemented guidelines for stepped care model for managing common mental disorders, including depression and anxiety. The first trial on 170 older adults recruited in primary care found the stepped care program halved the incidence of depression and anxiety disorders from 24 to 12 % in 12 months [47] with demonstrated cost-effectiveness [48] and the positive effects were sustained at 24 months [49].

The patient-centered medical home (PCMH) is a concept founded on the presence of inadequate treatment in primary care and/or an inability to access needed services [50]. Under oversight of the primary care provider, PCMH allows telepsychiatric input at home and has been shown to improve patient care and health [51, 52]. Desk-mounted video systems offer great convenience for therapy to cancer patients to avoid travel, but the cost used to be prohibitive for most consumers [51, 52].

HealthLinkNow, in the USA, with funding from the Center for Medicaid and Medicare Innovation, has integrated telepsychiatry services into multiple primary care clinics across three states. This PCMH model employs care navigators (CNs) who are key to coordination for patients, primary care providers, and the psychiatrists. These CNs also provide training on the telemedicine and electronic health record (psychiatrist use) and personal health record (patients use) – all of this is done remotely. The CNs do the initial patient intakes and follow-up with patients after consultations to promote adherence to the treatment plan.

There are populations, settings, and other issues that add complexity. One consideration is geographic, with rural/remote populations, though these are better online with broadband pipelines now. Another is the urban underserved, who face obstacles of lack of money, transportation, health care coverage, and "easy" access to in-person or telemedicine access points (going ten blocks without a bus is no easier than 2 miles via three buses). Culturally diverse populations of many ethnicities, cultures, and languages – even sign language – have been aided [3, 30, 53]. Caution is merited for using relatives or untrained interpreters, who may

Table 7.2 Training/education for synchronous and asynchronous telepsychiatry to primary care: Competencies, goals, and objectives

Outline of annual curriculum
1. *Basic* skills, knowledge, and attitudes. Areas: clinical; psychosomatic medicine-based; other subspecialty applications; culture; and technology
2. *Advanced* skills, knowledge, and attitudes. Areas: problem analysis; feedback; depression; and difficult situations
3. *Additional* advanced skills, knowledge, and attitudes and *consultation* skills. Areas: management of complex clinical cases; stepped care; planning for system limitations; and self-identification of strengths and weaknesses
4. Advanced skills, knowledge, and attitudes. Areas: cultural formation and clinical consultation to other providers
Overview of needs for mental health services
Skill objectives
Overview of models, training, and services by telepsychiatry
Model of services
Sample training clinic model for residents and students
1. Services provided
2. Psychiatric (Regular) clinical
3. Medical
4. Psychosomatic medicine or consultation-liaison
5. Subspecialty basics
6. Technology
Knowledge objectives
1. Primary care
2. Regular areas
3. Subspecialty basics
4. Technology
5. Alternative treatments
Attitude objectives
6.1 Administrative objectives Leadership 6.2 Documentation
Teaching and learning objectives: faculty, fellows, residents, mss, and interdisciplinary team members
Readings
1. Primary care
2. Psychiatric disorders
3. System issues
4. Subspecialty-related
5. Technology and communication
6. Other

miscommunicate medical complaints [54] or de-emphasize information [55]. Other special settings and populations also include involuntary, inpatient, and incarcerated; the old and young; and those in emergency rooms, schools, or other settings.

7.4 The Interdisciplinary Team: Role Definitions, Training Needs, Cross-Training, and Adapting to New Stepped and Integrated Care Models

7.4.1 Overview

One place to start with this discussion is considering a three-dimensional cube with three axes: team member/provider of care, method of service delivery, and medical/ MH complexity. The *team member/provider of care* would be a range of care coordinators or point persons of contact for basic entry into care. This could mean fielding emails from patients, checking in patients at the clinic, or data management staff. On the other end of the spectrum would be your psychiatrist /family physician/internist complemented by additional specialists. The members in-between would be medical assistants, licensed vocational nurses, registered nurses, nurse practitioners, physician assistants (i.e., mid-level providers who are readily available and manage basic and some advanced clinical problems), and MH clinicians. The *method of service delivery* would include a range of Website to in-person to tele-transported expertise, starting with education Websites, brochures, kiosks, and local support networks/ groups (e.g., Depression and Bipolar Support Alliance or American Diabetes Association) – to in-person individual or group education with a coordinator (e.g., diabetes or depression/grief group) – to tele-based groups (e.g., for those in a remote area or with an uncommon illness) – to video capture and data stored/organized in a "digital packet" then forwarded to an expert for review (i.e., asynchronous telepsychiatry) – to the top synchronous teleconsultant evaluation and/or management tier (i.e., the Rolls Royce of technology). The medical/MH complexity may pre-determine where the patient enters the above axes and where in the cube he/she spends the most time (i.e., the least ill as a small bottom cube and the most ill in a top smaller cube), proportionally, in the total three-dimensional cube.

7.4.2 Best Practice for Integrated Care: Depression and Diabetes (or Heart Disease or Other)

7.4.2.1 ID Info
A 49-year-old Native American male with diabetes, obesity, and alcohol use presents to the rural clinic with obesity, "I need medication" and a mother that reports "he eats too many sweets." He was referred to a telepsychiatric consultation at an academic center 175 miles away.

7.4.2.2 Background

Patients with diabetes mellitus (DM) have high rates of psychiatric disorders, particularly depression, with a 14 % mean range of 8.5–27 % [56], with higher rates in Native Americans [57]. Depression contributes to poor adherence to diabetic regimens, feelings of helplessness related to chronic illness and poor outcomes. DM and mental illness cause significant disability and increase risk for one another, as well as other disorders like coronary artery disease (CAD) [18, 58–60]. Patients with co-morbid depression and diabetes fare worse than those with diabetes who are not depressed. Depressed patients with diabetes are less adherent to self-care regimens. Moreover, depression is associated with poorer glycemic control [61, 62] and increased cardiovascular risk factors [63]. Depression is also associated with increased complications from diabetes such as retinopathy, nephropathy higher rates of disability, dementia, and mortality [64].

7.4.2.3 HPI

This patient has been seen, as his entire family as, at the reservation's internal medicine service as an adult, and he was described as "irritable, angry...and lacking hope." A substance abuse counselor is concerned about him drinking "3–4 beers per day." He was referred to an adjacent city's psychiatrist (45 miles; 70 min away to the coast) but did not go. He is referred to a psychosomatic medicine service via telemedicine 140 miles away.

7.4.2.4 Evaluation

A psychiatrist met with all parties – the patient/mother first and then the PCP came in, with discussion of depression as a new diagnosis and alcohol use that was maladaptive

7.4.3 Treatment Options

1. "Regular" care
   (a) Substance treatment with family attending
   (b) Dietary consultation for patient and family, to include itemized groceries (good and bad), co-shopping, and meal plans
   (c) One-time telepsychiatric consultation leading to an antidepressant treatment and access to brief CBT; both are effective for depression and may lower Hg1Ac levels [65].
   (d) Diabetic and weight education, Website, and support group in neighboring city.
2. "Better" integrated care
   (a) Administrative: Ignoring limitation for one doctor visit per day (federal reimbursement) → internist and teleconsultant same day. The PCP and psychiatrist can work with the patient to address the depression and how it directly contributes to both the alcohol misuse and the uncontrolled diabetes. The psychiatrist can model targeted motivational interviewing techniques that can be used in the PC setting.

(b) Transportation to health care visits locally and to neighboring city.

(c) Joint (or juxtaposed) tele-endocrinology and psychiatric consultations for integrated data, decision-making, and follow-up planning.

(d) Multisite, nurse-based diabetic coordinator support group by telemedicine (within or across cultures; in English).

7.4.4   Best Practice for Integrated Care: Training/Education for Integrated Care

Training/education programs vary in their approach (from low to higher levels in parentheses) in terms of the center of the learning process (curriculum to patient or learner); outcomes (knowledge, attitudes, and skills); individual vs. teamwork (spontaneous vs. shared mental models); teaching methods (case/practice vs. lecture/didactic), and perhaps most importantly level of supervision for feedback, encouragement of reflection, and developing lifelong habits.

"Good" integrated training uses milestone-based learning with didactics temporally mirroring clinical experiences, when possible, and combined training it an outcome to shoot for [66]. This pedagogical approach is longitudinal in nature, ideally beginning in postgraduate year 1 or 2 (PGY-1 or 2) and extending through PGY-4. It has an online curriculum with modules on integrated and collaborative care and the curriculum shifts from core medical topics in year 2 (key systems, geriatrics, pain, and some prevention) to MH topics in year 3 (epidemiology, collaborative care, integrated care models) to year 4 (being a consultant, team-based learning, brief therapies, and advocacy skills).

Telehealth has increased both education of and service delivery by rural doctors and nurses. A review of effectiveness of videoconference-based tele-education for medical and nursing education showed high satisfaction with videoconferencing education and that it is equivalent or better than in-person education knowledge acquisition and integration [67]. Clinically, the evidence base is growing on nursing interventions like coaching via telehealth [68]. Simulated patients at a distance are used to teach general clinical skills, how to work as part of a team, how to gain experience in previously unfamiliar work settings, and how to get on the same page across disciplines (i.e., how to develop mental models) for the care of a patient [30, 31].

7.4.5   Project Consultation: Program Development and Improvement via Organizational Consultation (see Appendix)

7.4.5.1 Overview
The director of a rural health network of 10 clinics that shared resources sought help from an academic medical center to access a telepsychiatry service. The original idea, primarily, was to use the service as a part of MH care for the clinics. It was

thought this would boost likelihood to obtain funding from external agencies, as part of a community-wide project.

7.4.5.2 Original Plan

The original proposal was a good start and well researched in terms of rural health, underserved populations, and mental health services (see Appendix). It had a list of services to be provided: in-person on-site and telepsychiatric consultation. There was no budget for evaluation.

7.4.5.3 Evaluation/Consultation

The consultant suggested an evaluation plan/budget and rewrite the project description three times, before arriving at a plan for direct services, training/education, community collaboration, and an evaluation budget (see Appendix). Specifically, it had outcomes for patients, PCP skills, and administrative/clinic functions.

7.4.5.4 Summary/Results

A number of services were provided: on-site – including MH screening with questionnaires, therapy/"warm" handoffs, education for all levels of staff and at a distance – telepsychiatric consultation, data collection/analysis, and written summaries.

- The rural health network used the consultation to the following:
  - Improve health service delivery and outcomes [37, 38]
  - Recruitment MH providers and PCPs to site
  - Employ screening, diagnostic and outcome questionnaires/clinician-administered short scales (e.g., Child Behavioral Checklist or CBCL)
  - Learning integrated care principles
- Four academic publications occurred and other reports were disseminated, including the case mix population of patients served by telepsychiatry and another specific to child.

7.5   Discussion and Conclusions

Contemporary health care is patient-centered approach and integrates health and mental health care. eMH facilitates this process by leveraging expertise of key disciplines to the point-of-service. It is mostly used to provide mental health care to the medical setting, and it has not been used much to provide medical care to mental health settings. Good programs emphasize teamwork and have clinical, administrative, and care coordination oversight.

There is little doubt that integrated care with integration on the seven levels described above – responsibility (decision-making, oversight of patient care), co-location of services, funding, evaluation plan, outcome measurement, an e-platform, and reimbursement – is the new "gold standard" for patient-centered care. This model for quality care must undergo further integration with the patient/consumer movement, academic health center (AHC), and community missions. A salient question becomes: "Is it easier to deconstruct and rebuild the traditional academic health center "culture" and structure, or build a new AHC that is more progressive (e.g., Mayo Clinic model)?"

A question also remains on where to go from there, in terms of minimal standards for medical and psychiatric care dependent on the setting and who provides the care? Outpatient psychiatric clinics "should" have VS, weight, and other staples of medical clinics; in-patient ones need medical clearance, medical co-management, and specialty consultation – rarely is that the case, though. In terms of who provides what care, is there a way to reasonably update PCP training in MH/psychiatry (e.g., ½ proctored/supervised tracks like a fellowship rather than full-time ones that disrupt clinical and other life arrangements)? Or, could a psychiatrist provide basic medical care, e.g., screening, education, prescribing for routine or chronic but stable conditions (e.g., hypertension) as part of a theoretically three-tiered medical acuity system?

And, what are the training best practices of the future? Will training evolve from separate undergraduate medical education (UME) to graduate medical education (GME) and lifelong continuing medical education (CME) streams – linked by throwing the participants in clinical settings – to a more purposeful framework that emphasizes team care, with shared models, team-based learning and practicing at the top of the license? Will tele-education leverage resources better, will simulation be more of a fundamental method, and how much will we practice before performing examinations/procedures/other work with patients?

Acknowledgment American Telemedicine Association Telemental Health Interest Group

Appendix: Program Development and Improvement via Organizational Consultation

Overview

The Director of a rural health Network of 10 clinics that shared resources sought help from an academic medical center to access a telepsychiatry service. The original idea, primarily, was to use the service as a part of MH care for the clinics. It was thought this would boost likelihood to obtain funding from external agencies, as part of a community-wide project.

Logistics

- Assessment of initial proposal. The proposal was a good start and well researched in terms of rural health, underserved populations, mental health services, and a plan of services to be covered. There was no budget for evaluation. The original proposal was outlined as follows:

Project component	Objective	Outcome
Direct service delivery	Provide 7,000 h of mental health services at seven primary care sites in NSRHN region (28 h a month clinical, 4 h on data) per site. Mid-level provider 1 day a week	Increase assessment for mental illness by 50 % at each site. Decrease depression via treatment in 65 % of diagnosed consumers accepting care
Telepsychiatry consultation	Provide 600 h of psychiatrist services via on-site care and telemedicine	Assure high-quality assessment and knowledgeable prescription of psychotropic medication for diagnosed consumers in need of medication

- The consultant suggested an evaluation plan/budget and rewrite the project description three times, before arriving at the following outline.

Project components	Objectives	Outcomes
1. Direct service delivery	50 % more consumers at six primary care clinics will be screened for behavioral illness	Increased identification and treatment of behavioral health problems
	Consumers treated for depression will show a 25 % reduction in depression	Increased consumer health and well-being
	90–100 % of the consumers who are receiving inadequate psychotropic medication doses will be identified so that interventions can take place	Improved consumer behavioral health outcomes
	25 % improvement in consumer satisfaction with primary behavioral health care services	Increased consumer health and well-being

Project components	Objectives	Outcomes
2. Training and technical assistance	Increase by 25 % primary care providers' knowledge and skills in assessment, diagnosis, and treatment of mental illness	Improved service delivery and increased consumer access to behavioral health care services delivered at their primary care clinic
	Increase by 25 % the knowledge and understanding of all clinic staff about how to integrate behavioral health into primary care practices	Full integration of behavioral health care services into six primary care clinic sites
	Development of integrated care protocols, policies and procedures, and use of outcomes data to inform quality improvement activities at each site	Full integration of behavioral health care services into six primary care clinic sites
3. Collaborate along the continuum of BH/MH services	Identify and document the entire continuum of care in each county	Improved knowledge of available care for consumers
	Hold a minimum of 10 interdisciplinary team meetings for didactics, case-based discussions, and collaboration on difficult cases. Teams will solicit consumer and front-line provider recommendations to alleviate barriers to care	Improved referral relationships, case management, and better informed service providers along the behavioral health care continuum
4. Policy development	Make recommendations to decision makers based on outcome data and clinical provider and consumer identified barriers	Increased awareness of service delivery barriers and identification of policies to improve access to care
	Develop options to address service delivery concerns	Improved systems of care. Increased access to consumer-focused, collaborative services

The final evaluation plan was formatted into three groups:

1. Patients: objectives, methods, and outcomes for diagnosis, treatment of depression, and satisfaction.
2. PCPs: skills and knowledge objectives, methods, and outcomes.
3. Administrative/clinic function: (a) integrated care protocols, policies, and procedures, and use of outcomes data to inform quality improvement activities at each site; (b) and documentation of the continuum of care in each county; (c) interdisciplinary team meetings for didactics, case-based discussions and collaboration on difficult cases; and (d) policy development.

Summary/Results of Project

- A number of services were provided: on-site – including MH screening with questionnaires, therapy/"warm" handoffs, education for all levels of staff; and at a distance – telepsychiatric consultation, data collection/analysis, and written summaries.
- The rural health network used the consultation to the following:

- Improve health service delivery and outcomes [38, 39]
- Recruitment MH providers and PCPs to site
- Employ screening, diagnostic and outcome questionnaires/clinician-administered short scales (e.g., Child Behavioral Checklist or CBCL)
- Learning integrated care principles
- Four academic publications occurred and other reports were disseminated, including the case mix population of patients served by telepsychiatry and another specific to child.

References

1. Akinci F, Patel PM. Quality improvement in healthcare delivery utilizing the patient-centered medical home model. Hosp Top. 2014;92(4):96–104.
2. Druss BG, Zhao L, Von Esenwein S, et al. Understanding excess mortality in persons with mental illness: 17-year follow up of a nationally representative US survey. Med Care. 2011;49:599–604.
3. Hilty DM, Ferrer D, Parish MB, et al. The effectiveness of telemental health: a 2013 review. Telemed J E Health. 2013;19(6):444–54.
4. Yellowlees PM, Odor A, Iosif A, et al. Transcultural psychiatry made simple: asynchronous telepsychiatry as an approach to providing culturally relevant care. Telemed J E Health. 2013;19(4):1–6.
5. Phillips BC. Healthcare reform and the future of nursing and nurse practitioner. Nurse practitioners business blog, 2010. 15 Mar 2015. At: http://npbusiness.org/health-care-reform-future-nursing-nurse-practitioners/.
6. Health and Human Services. The 2008 report to the secretary: rural health and human services issues: twentieth anniversary report. 15 Mar 2015. At: ftp://ftp.hrsa.gov/ruralhealth/commit-tee/NACreport2008.pdf.
7. Hilty DM, Yellowlees PM, Nesbitt TS. Evolution of telepsychiatry to rural sites: change over time in types of referral and PCP knowledge, skill, and satisfaction. Gen Hosp Psychiatry. 2006;28(5):367–73.
8. Hilty DM, Nesbitt TS, Kuenneth TA, et al. Telepsychiatric consultation to primary care: rural vs. suburban needs, utilization and provider satisfaction. J Rural Health. 2007;23(2):163–5.
9. Druss BG, Rohrbaugh RM, Levinson CM, et al. Integrated medical care for patients with serious psychiatric illness: a randomized trial. Arch Gen Psychiatry. 2001;58:861.
10. Dobscha SK, Corson K, Perrin NA, et al. Collaborative care for chronic pain in primary care. JAMA. 2009;301:1242–51.
11. Unützer J, Katon W, Callahan CM, et al. Collaborative care management of late-life depression in the primary care setting. JAMA. 2002;288:2836–4285.
12. Bower P, Gilbody S. Managing common mental health disorders in primary care: conceptual models and evidence base. Br Med J. 2005;330:839–42.
13. Katon WJ, Seelig M. Population-based care of depression: team care approaches to improving outcomes. J Occup Environ Med. 2008;50:459–67.
14. Simon GE, Katon WJ, Lin EHB, et al. Cost-effectiveness of systematic depression treatment among people with diabetes mellitus. Arch Gen Psychiatry. 2007;64:65.
15. Wang PS, Patrick A, Avorn J, et al. The costs and benefits of enhanced depression care to employers. Arch Gen Psychiatry. 2006;63:1345.
16. Davis MH, Everett A, Kathol R, et al. American Psychiatric Association ad hoc work group report on the integration of psychiatry and primary care, 2011. 15 Mar 2015. At: http://naapimha.org/wordpress/media/Integration-of-Psychiatry-and-Primary-Care.pdf.

17. Kishi Y, Kathol RG. Integrating medical and psychiatric treatment in an inpatient medical setting: the type IV program. Psychosomatics. 1999;40:345–55.
18. Mezuk B, Eaton W, Albrecht S, et al. Depression and type 2 diabetes over the lifespan. Diabetes Care. 2008;31:2383–90.
19. Van der Kooy K, van Hout H, Marwijk H, et al. Depression and the risk for cardiovascular diseases: systematic review and meta-analysis. Int J Geriatr Psychiatry. 2007;22:613–26.
20. American Diabetes Association, American Psychiatric Association, American Association of Clinical Endocrinologists, North American Association for the Study of Obesity and Diabetes. Consensus development conference on antipsychotic drugs and obesity and diabetes. Diabetes Care. 2004;27:596–601.
21. Hussain M, Seitz D. Integrated models of care for medical inpatients with psychiatric disorders: a systematic review. Psychosomatics. 2014;55(4):315–25.
22. Manian FA, Janssen DA. Curbside consultations. JAMA. 1996;275:145–6.
23. Katon W, Von Korff M, Lin E, et al. Collaborative management to achieve depression treatment guidelines. J Clin Psychiatry. 1997;58 Suppl 1:20–4.
24. Hilty DM, Servis ME, Nesbitt TS, et al. The use of telemedicine to provide consultation-liaison service to the primary care setting. Psychiatr Ann. 1999;29:421–7.
25. Hilty DM, Marks SL, Wegeland JE, et al. A randomized controlled trial of disease management modules, including telepsychiatric care, for depression in rural primary care. Psychiatry. 2007;4(2):58–65.
26. Hilty DM, Yellowlees PM, Cobb HC, et al. Use of secure e-mail and telephone psychiatric consultations to accelerate rural health care delivery. Telemed J E Health. 2006;12(4):490–5.
27. Fortney JC, Pyne JM, Mouden SP, et al. Practice-based versus telemedicine-based collaborative care for depression in rural federally qualified health centers: a pragmatic randomized comparative effectiveness trial. Am J Psychiatry. 2013;170(4):414–25.
28. Slaets J, Kauffmann R, Duivenvoorden H, et al. A randomized trial of geriatric liaison intervention in elderly medical inpatients. Psychosom Med. 1997;59:585–91.
29. Baldwin R, Pratt H, Goring H, Marriott A, Roberts C. Does a nurse-led mental health liaison service for older people reduce psychiatric morbidity in acute general medical wards? A randomized controlled trial. Age Ageing. 2004;33:472–8.
30. Hilty DM, Yellowlees PM, Nasatir SEH, et al. Program evaluation and practical, step-by-step program modification in telemental health. In Behavioral telehealth series volume 1- clinical video conferencing: program development and practice. Springer Press, New York, NY. 2014. p. 105–34.
31. Rutledge CM, Haney T, Bordelon M, et al. Telehealth: preparing advanced practice nurses to address healthcare needs in rural and underserved populations. Int J Nurs Educ Scholarsh. 2014;11(1):1–9.
32. Ross S, Allen N. Examining the convergent validity of shared mental model measures. Behav Res. 2012;44:1052–62.
33. Armstrong EG, Mackey M, Spear SJ. Medical education as a process management problem. Acad Med. 2004;79(8):721–8.
34. Yellowlees PM, Hogarth MA, Hilty DM. The development of distributed academic networks in America. Acad Psychiatry. 2006;30(6):451–5.
35. Hilty DM, Yellowlees PM, Cobb HC, et al. Models of telepsychiatric consultation-liaison service to rural primary care. Psychosomatics. 2006;47(2):152–7.
36. Hilty DM, Marks SL, Urness D, et al. Clinical and educational applications of telepsychiatry: a review. Can J Psychiatry. 2004;49(1):12–23.
37. Hilty DM, Ingraham RL, Yang RP, et al. Multispecialty phone and email consultation to primary care providers for patients with developmental disabilities in rural California. Telemed J E Health. 2004;10:413–21.
38. Neufeld JD, Bourgeois JA, Hilty DM, et al. The e-Mental Health Consult Service: providing enhanced primary care mental health services through telemedicine. Psychosomatics. 2007;48:135–41.
39. Yellowlees PM, Hilty DM, Marks SL, et al. A retrospective analysis of child and adolescent e-mental health. J Am Acad Child Adolesc Psychiatry. 2008;47(1):1–5.

40. Yellowlees PM, Odor A, Patrice K, et al. PsychVACS: a system for asynchronous telepsychiatry. Telemed J E Health. 2011;17(4):299–303.
41. Butler TN, Yellowlees P. Cost analysis of store-and-forward telepsychiatry as a consultation model for primary care. Telemed J E Health. 2012;18(1):74–7.
42. Richardson L, McCauley E, Katon W. Collaborative care for adolescent depression: a pilot study. Gen Hosp Psychiatry. 2009;31:36–45.
43. Myers KM, Vander Stoep A, Zhou C, McCarty CA, Katon W. Effectiveness of a telehealth service delivery model for treating attention-deficit hyperactivity disorder: results of a community-based randomized controlled trial. J Am Acad Child Adolesc Psychiatry. 2015;54(4):263–74.
44. Haaga DA. Introduction to the special section on stepped care models in psychotherapy. J Consult Clin Psychol. 2000;68:547–8.
45. van't Veer-Tazelaar N, van Marwijk H, et al. Prevention of anxiety and depression in the age group of 75 years and over: a randomized controlled trial testing the feasibility and effectiveness of a generic stepped care program among elderly community residents at high risk of developing anxiety and depression versus usual care. BMC Public Health. 2006;1:186.
46. NICE. NICE clinical guidelines 90 and 91 depression: treatment and management of depression in adults, including adults with a chronic physical health problem, 2009. 15 Mar 2015. At: http://www.nice.org.uk/nicemedia/live/12329/45890/45890.pdf.
47. van't Veer-Tazelaar PJ, van Marwijk HW, van Oppen P, et al. Stepped-care prevention of anxiety and depression in late life: a randomized controlled trial. Arch Gen Psychiatry. 2009;66:297–304.
48. van't Veer-Tazelaar P, Smit F, van Hout H, van Oppen P, van der Horst H, et al. Cost-effectiveness of a stepped care intervention to prevent depression and anxiety in late life: randomized trial. Br J Psychiatry. 2010;196:319–25.
49. van't Veer-Tazelaar PJ, van Marwijk HWJ, van Oppen P, et al. Prevention of late-life anxiety and depression has sustained effects over 24 months: a pragmatic randomized trial. Am J Geriatr Psychiatry. 2011;19:230–9.
50. Rosenthal TC. The medical home: growing evidence to support a new approach to primary care. J Am Board Fam Med. 2008;21(5):427–40.
51. Hollingsworth JM, Saint S, Hayward RA, et al. Specialty care and the patient-centered medical home. Med Care. 2011;49(1):4–9.
52. Cluver JS, Schuyler D, Frueh BC, et al. Remote psychotherapy for terminally ill cancer patients. J Telemed Telecare. 2005;11:157–9.
53. Yellowlees PM, Shore JH, Roberts L, et al. Practice guidelines for videoconferencing-based telemental health. Telemed J E Health. 2010;16(10):1074–89.
54. Brooks TR. Pitfalls in communication with Hispanic and African-American patients: do translators help or harm? J Natl Med Assoc. 1992;84(11):941.
55. Brua C. Role-blurring and ethical grey zones associated with lay interpreters: three case studies. Commun Med. 2008;5(1):73.
56. Gavard JA, Lustman PJ, Clouse RE. Prevalence of depression in adults with diabetes: an epidemiological evaluation. Diabetes Care. 1993;16(8):1167–78.
57. Thackeray R, Merrill RM, Neiger BL. Disparities in diabetes management practice between racial and ethnic groups in the United States. Diabetes Educ. 2004;30(4):665–74.
58. Wells K, Stewart A, Hays R, et al. The functioning and well being of depressed patients: results from the Medical Outcomes Study. JAMA. 1989;262:914–9.
59. Campayo A, de Jonge P, Roy JF, et al. Depressive disorder and incident diabetes mellitus: the effect of characteristics of depression. Am J Psychiatry. 2010;167:580–8.
60. Carnethon MR, Biggs ML, Barzilay JI, et al. Longitudinal association between depressive symptoms and incident type 2 diabetes mellitus in older adults: the cardiovascular health study. Arch Intern Med. 2007;167(8):802–7.
61. Lustman PJ, Anderson RJ, Freedland KE, et al. Depression and poor glycemic control: a meta-analytic review of the literature. Diabetes Care. 2000;23:934–42.

62. Katon W, Lyles CR, Parker MM, et al. Association of depression with increased risk of dementia in patients with type 2 diabetes: the diabetes and aging study. Arch Gen Psychiatry. 2012;69:410–7.
63. Katon WJ, Von Korff M, Lin EH, et al. The pathways study: a randomized trial of collaborative care in patients with diabetes and depression. Arch Gen Psychiatry. 2004;61:1042–9.
64. Rustad JK, Musselman DL, Nemeroff CB. The relationship of depression and diabetes: pathophysiological and treatment implications. Psychoneuroendocrinology. 2011;36:1276–86.
65. Lustman PJ, Griffith LS, Freedland KE, et al. Cognitive behavior therapy for depression in type 2 diabetes mellitus. A randomized, controlled trial. Ann Intern Med. 1998;129(8):613–21.
66. McCarron RM, Bourgeois JA, Chwastiak LA, et al. Integrated Medicine and Psychiatry (IMAP) curriculum for psychiatry residency training: a model designed to meet growing mental health workforce needs. Acad Psychiatry. In Press.
67. Chipps J, Brysiewicz P, Mars M. A systematic review of the effectiveness of videoconference-based tele-education for medical and nursing education. Worldviews Evid Based Nurs. 2012;9(2):78–87.
68. Young H, Miyamoto S, Ward D, et al. Sustained effects of a nurse coaching intervention via telehealth to improve health behavior change in diabetes. Telemed J E Health. 2014;20(9):828–34.

Social Media and Clinical Practice: What Stays the Same, What Changes, and How to Plan Ahead?

8

Christopher E. Snowdy, Erica Z. Shoemaker, Steven Chan, and Donald M. Hilty

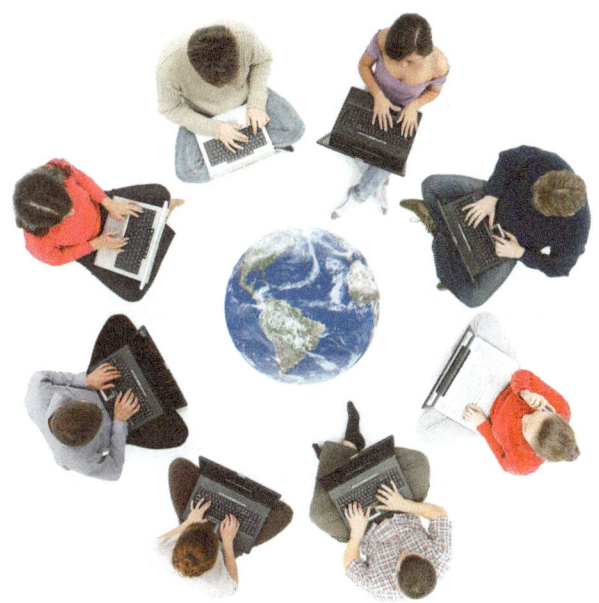

C.E. Snowdy, MD • E.Z. Shoemaker, MD, MPH
Department of Psychiatry and Behavioral Sciences, Keck School of Medicine at USC and LAC+USC Medical Center, 2250 Alcazar Street, CSC, Suite 2200, Los Angeles, CA 90033, USA

D.M. Hilty, MD (✉)
Keck School of Medicine, University of Southern California, Los Angeles, CA, USA
e-mail: donh031226@gmail.com

S. Chan, MD, MBA
Department of Psychiatry and Behavioral Sciences, University of California, Davis School of Medicine & Health System, 2150 Stockton Boulevard, Sacramento, CA 95817, USA

© Springer International Publishing Switzerland 2016
D. Mucic, D.M. Hilty (eds.), *e-Mental Health*,
DOI 10.1007/978-3-319-20852-7_8

Contents

8.1 Introduction 152
8.2 eMH: The Intersection of Communication, Technology, and MH Care 153
    8.2.1 The Evolution of Psychiatric Practice 153
    8.2.2 Verbal and Nonverbal Communication 154
    8.2.3 The eMH Evidence Base 155
8.3 Social Media and MH Care Evolution 155
    8.3.1 Facebook/Social Media Sites 156
    8.3.2 Impact on the Therapeutic Relationship 157
    8.3.3 Patient Privacy 158
    8.3.4 Provider and Patient Privacy 159
    8.3.5 Professionalism and Provider Image 159
    8.3.6 Patient Safety 161
8.4 Guidelines for Patient Care with eMH and Other Technologies 162
    8.4.1 Adult Guidelines for eMH: Clinical and Outcome Assessment 162
    8.4.2 Child and Adolescent eMH: Steps Toward a Guideline 162
    8.4.3 Guidelines for Social Media Use, Particularly in Child
         and Adolescent Populations 163
8.5 Discussion 166
Conclusions 167
References 167

Abstract

While the patient-centered healthcare movement, like traditional medicine movements, aims to deliver quality, affordable, and timely care in a variety of settings, the consumer movement on new technologies is passing it by with emerging technologies and new ways of communicating with others (text, e-mail, Twitter, Facebook). This chapter builds on what we know about e-Mental Health (eMH), technology and communication progress over the past 50 years in maintaining the tenets of "good" quality care, adjusting slightly to telemedicine models, and considering more significant adjustments for use of social media. The areas of challenges include privacy and confidentiality, health and personal practice, having "good" interpersonal/clinical boundaries, awareness of what information is out there about you, and discussing clear expectations about online communication between doctors and patients as part of the informed consent process. Guidelines, strategies, and tips for the clinician are offered.

8.1 Introduction

Patient-centered healthcare confronts us with a question about how to deliver quality, affordable, and timely care in a variety of settings [1, 2]. Our traditional, though innovative approach is the patient-centered medical home (PCMH), which is founded on the absence of adequate treatment or access to it in primary care [3]. The Affordable Care Act (ACA), funding/health care financing folks [4] and increased input from patients/the communities – all support this movement. Other models include collaborative, integrated, and stepped care. Participant satisfaction is high with eMH as a way to supplement in-person care and disseminate care in these models [5, 6]. eMH appears to be as good as in-person care [7]. The pilots exist on integrating both models – and providing this care with sensitivity to culture and diversity [5, 8, 9].

The field of child and adolescent psychiatry also has dual movements: (1) traditional progress, and (2) emerging social media trajectories. Traditional progress is occurring in research (e.g., neurobiology, autism, genomics) and clinical care initiatives (dyadic therapy for woman/infant; Institute for Healthcare Improvement's Triple Aim for perinatal care and the Baby Triple P (Positive Parenting Program) [10–12]. In addition, the consumer movement is seeking sources of information immediately available and clinical care options at multiple points-of-service [6, 13]. Emerging models of care are sprouting quickly and they impact clinical boundaries, communication, and engagement [14]. The American Psychiatric Association has a guideline on e-prescribing [15], and educators are seeking advice on how to teach professionalism [16].

The adolescent population and their generation are highly captivated by media, technology, and communication trends. As of January of 2014, 90 % of adults have a cell phone and 58 % have a smartphone [17]; the rate is probably higher on the smartphones for teenagers. Aside from entertainment purposes, those aged 13–54 years in the United States use a majority of their smartphone time to socialize and interact with others, manage themselves including their health, and research information [18]. New digital communication includes: e-mail, standard message service (SMS) text messaging, multiple message service (MMS) messaging, instant messaging; proprietary networks like Twitter direct messages, Facebook Messenger, Epic MyChart electronic medical record messaging, My HealtheVet electronic medical record messaging; and social media communication platforms that transmit from one to many users. Patients want to engage others and their doctors and they employ low-grade synchronous communication (i.e., videoconferencing) for relationships across the country [5].

This chapter will help the reader to consider:

1. What is same for both in-person and technology-based care (i.e. importance of clinical boundaries, privacy, confidentiality, and other)?
2. What is different are the options for connecting with your provider or patient (e.g., texting, a posting on Facebook like "Let's talk…I will text you" and googling)?
3. What planning can be done in advance and how can you adapt quickly to the unexpected for the best (and the worst)?

8.2 eMH: The Intersection of Communication, Technology, and MH Care

8.2.1 The Evolution of Psychiatric Practice

Our field emerged in part to help patients overcome the stigma of mental illness (e.g., psychiatric and neurologic patients were in prisons in the late eighteenth and early nineteenth centuries) and it remained tucked away from traditional medicine, until traumatic disorders became prominent through World War II (later renamed post-traumatic stress disorder). It was observed that healing occured by listening to patient stories and this led to the further development of the field of psychoanalysis and eventually the sub-specialty area of consultation-liaison or psychosomatic medicine.

The biopsychosocial model put the presenting problem in the context of the patient's life, identifying determinants of the symptoms/psychopathology [19]; more importantly, it was a compromise between the biomedical and analytic groups. We explore beliefs, norms, values, and to a greater degree than most in medicine, the ethnic, culture and language issues that affect health. The culture of the patient includes symptoms, presentation, meaning, causation, family factors, coping styles, treatment seeking, mistrust, stigma, immigration, and overall health status. Oftentimes, in order to better understand a patient's perspective, we need to hear him tell his story in his own words. Stories, though subjective, are well described in their role in healing, conveying abstract meaning (myths), moving people to change, and teaching learners to apply knowledge and learn skills [20].

Time-tested "quality" care in psychiatry is mostly attributed to the patient-doctor engagement, the therapeutic relationship, shared decision-making, and biopsychosocial treatment [21]. Shared decision-making equalizes the informational and power symmetry between doctors and patients – both parties share information and develop consensus in a decision [22]. Psychiatry is a good model of early and contemporary shared decision-making. When patients were allowed to choose between different treatment options for depression rather than being randomly allocated to treatment groups, patients chose psychotherapy more often than pharmacotherapy with no significant difference in patient satisfaction or outcomes.

Neurobiology informs us on how we learn [23] and how we adapt, mainly through synaptic efficacy between the presynaptic cell's repeated and persistent stimulation of the postsynaptic cell [24]. Injury and mental illness disrupt this, particularly during adolescence. Cognitive psychology and psychiatry have illuminated perceptual biases: why we think as we think, when our decisions are prone to error, and how to reduce those errors [25]. Our work with patients encourages reflection, tolerating ambiguity, and dealing with the unexpected.

8.2.2 Verbal and Nonverbal Communication

The assessment of telepsychiatry's impact on the doctor–patient relationship is complicated by the many types of patients, settings, and practice styles for which it is employed. Patient types vary by disorder, age, culture, and setting. A critical variable in communication is telemedicine's ability to simulate real-time experiences in terms of image and interaction. Another concept that bears on communication is "presence" [26]. Presence is defined as "… the fact or condition of being at the specified or understood place" [27]. In a physical environment, informational cues are incorporated without conscious awareness (e.g., a patient is seen walking in a reticent way). Participants need to be aware that the virtual environment created by telemedicine may be missing cues from the in-person physical environment.

A few studies evaluated the effect of telemedicine on nonverbal communication, which regardless of limitations, fundamentally establishes mutual connections and understanding. Examples are eye contact, gestures, posture, fidgeting, nods, grins, smiles, frowns, and lip-reading [28]. Decreased ability to detect nonverbal cues has been reported during videoconferencing for patient interviews. This has been previously described as the "cuelessness" phenomena [29, 30]. A task-oriented focus with a depersonalized content may occur [31]. A comparison of communication behaviors between 6 physicians and 6 patients using in-person, telephone, hands-free telephone, and low-cost telepsychiatry (KBS not specified) modes revealed higher levels (75 % of the time) of mutual gaze for the visual modes (in-person and telepsychiatry) [32], which exceeded usual interpersonal interactions (approximately 50 %) [33].

On a spectrum of detecting cues, telepsychiatry may be in the middle between telephone and in-person communication [34]. Currently, it is assumed that the videoconferencing provides "enough" of the physical environment for good decision-making. Cukor et al. reported that telepsychiatry facilitates a "social presence" that permits participants to share a virtual space, get to know one another, and discuss complex issues, even when low-cost systems are used [35]. The nature of what is exchanged also varies depending on the mode used. Information exchange takes place primarily on an audio channel rather than a video channel [35–37]. Participants respond in a "conservative" or "stilted" way when audio delay occurs with videoconferencing [28], resulting in more interruptions of the interview than with video disruption. For the same conversation, in-person takes less time than telephone, which in turn, takes less time than videoconferencing [36, 37].

The core issues are the impact of technology, patient education, exploring the virtual connection [38], and adjusting some behaviors (e.g., handing a tissue box, sighing, pat on the shoulder, handshake) to verbal statements conveying the same thing (e.g., empathy).

8.2.3   The eMH Evidence Base

Telehealth and eMH have been shown to assist healthcare professionals in underserved areas by providing timely access to specialty care in communities that lack specialty expertise locally [5]. Telepsychiatry and other services are in these sixth decade, and they have increased access to care in urban, suburban, and rural settings – with high participants satisfaction for a wide variety of services. Telepsychiatry is effective for diagnosis and assessment across many populations (e.g., adult, child, geriatric, and ethnic) and appears to be comparable to in-person care [5, 39, 40]. It has been used with a variety of models of care (i.e., collaborative care, asynchronous, mobile, telemonitoring; integrated care; stepped care; interdisciplinary care) with equally positive outcomes [5, 6, 41–43].

8.3   Social Media and MH Care Evolution

The expanding use of social media and advances in digital connectivity dictate that we must, once again, contemplate how best to account for and integrate new trends in technology with existing clinical practice. Social networking has been defined as "web-based services that allow individuals to (1) construct a public or semi-public profile within a bounded system, (2) articulate a list of other users with whom they share a connection, and (3) view and traverse their list of connections and those made by others within the system" [44]. Much as with the integration of eMH into existing psychiatric practice over the past 50 years, the ultimate goal of providing high-quality care to patients may include social media, but we must be mindful of those components and principles of effective mental health care that we can ill-afford to compromise.

The importance of the therapeutic alliance in successful treatment is well established across disciplines. In mental health treatment, the relationship between the provider and patient is unlike any other in one's personal life. Efforts to establish rapport, but with consistent attention to boundaries, allow the provider to be seen not as a friend (importantly) but as a professional to whom patients can feel confident revealing themselves [45]. Effective communication facilitates such disclosure. When the parameters of the therapeutic frame are significantly and repeatedly blurred, the trust that previously long-held secrets will be handled appropriately and with benefit to treatment begins to erode. The introduction of social media and other digital communications bring with them multiple opportunities to unintentionally jeopardize this process.

The impact of new technology on how we go about formulating an assessment and plan should also be considered. For example, the components of a thorough formulation, to include the biopsychosocial model, should remain the same. Questions arise, however, from increasingly facilitated access to information on our patients through social media applications and the ability to quickly search the Internet for data. At what point does the obligation to thoroughly inform our understandings begin to conflict with a patient's right to privacy? How do we define that data which is "fair game" and that which should remain privileged? We must also protect patient autonomy and ensure that limitations imparted by new modalities of communication do not infringe upon the principles of collaboration and informed consent. Finally, treatment planning that includes any new technology must still account for patient safety, appropriate follow-up, and attention to the management of emergency situations.

8.3.1 Facebook/Social Media Sites

The number of people who use social media is on the rise, and the data is staggering. For the month of December 2014, Facebook reported 1.39 billion at-least-monthly users and 890 million daily active users on average [46]. Contrast that to 360 million total users just 5 years prior [46]. It is also clear that social networking is also less-frequently tied to the home computer, but that smartphone apps and mobile Internet access mean people take their networks with them wherever they go. Facebook estimates that 745 million people access their accounts from mobile devices on a daily basis [46].

The sheer power and ease-of online networking platforms piques our interests with regard to how they might be used in healthcare. With similar motivations to those behind eMH, one can envision dramatically increasing the access to good quality patient information, promoting and de-stigmatizing mental health treatment, facilitating connections to online support groups and more, all with a few clicks of a button. One might consider the ability to advocate for patients and the profession in-line with one's personal views, à la the Facebook group Doctors for Obama, which rallied support in 2008 for the US president's campaign and continued to maintain dialogue with his administration post-election through the strength of the group's network [47]. Others who treat adolescents and young adults might be attracted to the idea of "meeting them where they are," with the opportunity to engage them in a "hip" and familiar medium. A provider's initial intentions for this latter idea might range from a separate professional page, with no intent for interaction, all the way to plans to engage patients therapeutically through tools built into the social networking site. All of the above offer exciting possibilities, each with a number of potential caveats to consider in practice.

8.3.2 Impact on the Therapeutic Relationship

Consider the hypothetical case of the therapist, who, while browsing her own Facebook account one evening, comes across a "friend request" from a current patient with whom she is engaged in therapy. The therapist must now consider the implications behind the request, choose whether or not to accept, and determine how best to respond to the patient regarding her decision. Does this request reflect a desire on the part of the patient to push the boundaries of the therapeutic frame, perhaps related to some aspect of his presenting problem or in response to an unfolding dynamic in session [48]? A recent study at Rouen University Hospital in France found 73 % of residents in multiple specialties had Facebook profiles, 6 % of whom had friend requests from patients, 4 of which were accepted [49].

By avoiding dual-relationships with patients, we establish that we are now, and even after therapy, only in the treating role. Patients are empowered to reveal shameful or painful details to their providers, in part through the trust that doing so will have little consequence on any outside relationship [50]. While we understand that a true friendship entails a more equal exchange of private information and confidences [45], patients may not have the same understanding. After all, the newly accepted provider now appears on the same list as the rest of the patient's friends and family. One can see how this sudden integration might impact the ability and willingness to self-disclose.

It is also worth noting the effect on the amount of information available to both parties following an affirmation of "friend" status. Many privacy settings on Facebook are dependent on this designation. That is to say, the ability to view pictures, wall-posts, send messages, and access various bits of personal information may be granted to "friends," while potentially forgetting the sheer range of acquaintances one has included in that same friends list (perhaps to include one's closest friends, one's family members, an old classmate with whom one no longer really associates, a friend of a friend one met at a function once). Aside from issues of privacy (to be discussed in short order), patients may now find themselves privy to many details of their providers' personal lives. While many argue that some self-disclosure on the part of the therapist can be useful when strategically applied, most agree that a great deal of disclosure is rarely advised and can become an obstacle [45]. For cases in which examining transference might be valuable to the treatment, the ability to maintain a somewhat neutral presence might be compromised.

8.3.3 Patient Privacy

Social media sites were not designed with protected doctor-patient interactions in mind; rather, they were designed for social networking. Hence, they are not equipped with the various protective measures, which are required of, for example, an electronic medical record [51]. At the same time, the provider has a responsibility to extend considerations of privacy to interactions with patients online. Something as simple as a patient forgetting to log-off his profile could lead to a breach in confidentiality when a family member stumbles upon therapeutic communications. At a minimum, providers need to protect their electronic devices with the same level of security as their paper charts [52].

Considerations should also be made to local regulations with regard to storing and transmitting identifiable health information. In the United States, this would include assessing whether those communications are considered HIPAA-compliant. Regulations and/or risk-management policies may also dictate the need to document communications with patients. In this case, one must determine which information collected and disseminated online belongs in the patient's chart, and the patient must be made aware of those intentions.

Less-obvious issues relating to patient privacy might also arise. Acquaintances of the patient might wonder about the new connection with a known psychiatrist, or vice versa, a therapist's friends might be able to deduce that the new addition (whose origin the therapist will not divulge upon asking) is indeed a patient. In rural communities with relatively few people, this may be an even bigger issue, especially if the patient expressly desires to keep her involvement in treatment a secret.

Finally, providers should ask themselves what information about the patient is ethically appropriate to access. After all, a new friend designation suddenly opens up the contents of many patients' accounts for perusal. Such a quandary applies to the notion of performing Internet searches on patients as well [53]. Frankish et al. suggested a novel approach to considering a particular piece of information's privacy [45]. They suggest dividing information into the categories of public-public (that which was clearly designated for public consumption, to include newspapers, opinion blogs, and public registries), public-private (that which might be available publicly, but which was clearly not intended for the general public, to include content commonly found in one's social media account), and private-private (that which is not easily publicly accessible and is not intended as such, to include a private face-to-face conversation or a private e-mail). While public-public information is generally considered acceptable to access, and private-private information is not, they illustrate the issue of public-private information with the example of walking past a patient's home with the intent to peek into their window. They argue that the failure of a patient to implement the intended privacy settings on a social media account (or in the above case, not having considered the implications of friending their provider) is akin to a patient neglecting to close the blinds on their window, and thus, still constitutes an intrusion on patient privacy [45].

8.3.4   Provider and Patient Privacy

While providers should strive to respect the privacy of their patients online, it is unlikely that most patients will employ the same standards in reverse. In 2010, approximately 140 million Americans were thought to use the Internet for healthcare each year [51]. While the anonymity afforded to those who search for information about their providers makes quantifying such activities difficult, the expansion of sites featuring physician information and consensus from the literature suggests this is common practice [50, 51, 53, 54]. Available information is seemingly endless and can include profession-related things like reviews from patients (accurate or not), educational background, professional affiliations, and one's CV, but also more personal items like one's political contributions, family genealogy, and even how much was paid for one's home. Since the average user views 1.9 pages of results per search term, it may be prudent for providers to search themselves and be familiar with at least the first few pages of results [54]. Providers should also be aware that information voluntarily posted online is likely permanent and use discretion accordingly [55].

8.3.5   Professionalism and Provider Image

Much like their patients, many providers across the world enjoy their own private social media accounts outside of work. Not all practitioners, however, routinely monitor their privacy settings (or set them in the first place) and some are shown engaging in behavior, that might influence the perceptions of others with regard to their character and, perhaps, their professions as a whole. A survey conducted in 2006 and 2007 of then-recent medical graduates in New Zealand found that 65 % of graduates had Facebook accounts. Around 63 % of those had implemented privacy settings, while 37 % of those remaining (those which were readily visible to the public) revealed private details such as sexual orientation, religious views, and relationship status. Another 10 % showed images of the users apparently intoxicated [56].

Another study in 2008 involving medical students at the University of Florida found that 68.3 % of medical students and 12.8 % of residents had Facebook accounts. A random subset of 10 profiles found that 7 included pictures involving alcohol and 3 had depictions of unprofessional conduct including drunkenness, foul language, overt sexuality, and patient-privacy violations. A small proportion of students had joined online Facebook groups with racially charged or sexist titles [57].

Finally, a survey including 78 US medical schools in 2009 yielded 60 % who reported incidents of students posting unprofessional content online. Discriminatory language (48 %), depiction of sexually suggestive material (38 %), use of profanity

(52 %), and violations of patient privacy (13 %) were among the incidents reported. Policies on online conduct already in place were reported by 38 %, with another 11 % actively developing them [58].

The understandable need for providers to live personal lives outside the public's eye can clash most unfortunately with the accessibility of information available online and the aforementioned patient desire to be informed about one's provider. Problems might even arise for those who choose not to contribute content. With the ability to "tag" other people in photos posted online, providers might learn they were featured in professionally unbecoming photographs long after many others have seen them [50]. Privacy settings may be insufficient to prevent such content from being seen by the particularly earnest or technologically savvy users [55].

Content found online can have far-reaching consequences. Some employers are beginning to utilize Internet and social media searches to screen potential candidates. There have been several news reports depicting medical board reprimands and even dismissals following patient privacy violations [59]. Another man found his career in jeopardy after content was found linking him to illicit drug use and male prostitution [59]. Public sentiment seems to suggest that many take notice of what professionals post online and hold medical providers to a higher standard of conduct. While combing through the lay public's comments on a story about unprofessional online behavior by medical students, Greysen et al. found the comments "Anybody who isn't smart enough to figure out what's OK to post on the Internet has absolutely no business being in charge of other people's health," and "As professionals, doctors, teachers, lawyers, etc., are held to a certain standard. If that's not your cup of tea, find a different job" [60].

On its face, being held to an expected level of decorum might seem unfair. Providers who lead stressful practices might feel constantly under the microscope without room for reprieve. Others might cite limits on free speech and self-expression. It is helpful, however, to consider the amount of deference afforded to physicians by many (with some cultures more than others) and the responsibility that might entail. People might look to a psychiatrist or therapist for cues in how to respond to a natural disaster or perhaps an interpersonal conflict. On the flip side, those with little contact with mental health providers might see certain conduct as affirming a particular stigma or personal belief (e.g., that psychiatrists are simply pill-pushers who don't actually care about their patient's individually). Or perhaps more disturbing, consider the parent of a child in need of mental health care, whose hesitancy to engage available resources is further heightened by witnessing crass and boorish behavior by a psychiatrist online.

The general consensus is mental health providers do have a duty to maintain a certain level of decorum and professionalism when in the public eye (a duty which is perhaps owed to the profession as a whole and to all those whose health might be otherwise negatively affected). With the nature and reach of social media, the concept of "in the public eye" may extend to anything, that is posted online, particularly when efforts to protect that information are nonexistent or fail. This notion is replicated in many institutional policies as well as in the American Medical Association's Policy on professionalism in the use of social media [55]. The latter also dictates a physician's responsibility to identify and bring to their attention the unprofessional behavior of other providers.

8.3.6   Patient Safety

As stated previously, providers wishing to introduce new technologies into clinical practice must do so while continuing to account for the patient's safety, an appropriate plan for follow-up and monitoring, and a clear plan for responding to emergency situations. This would certainly hold true when engaging patients via social media (or via text messaging, chat platforms, e-mail, or any other form of digital communication for that matter). On Facebook, contacts have the ability to send messages directly to one another, to post messages on another contact's personal page (or "wall"), which may then be seen by any audience member fitting criteria of the page owner's privacy settings, and to also post "status updates", which are then displayed to other contacts in a running "newsfeed" on Facebook's homepage.

Consider a psychiatrist who has accepted contacts from several patients for the purpose of organizing an online medication group. Suppose one of her patients leaves a post on the psychiatrist's wall to the effect of "Thanks SO much for all your stupid advice. Don't worry, you won't ever hear from me again. By the time you read this, I will be dead!" Existing literature is lacking for clear guidelines on how to handle such an event [61]. What should the psychiatrist's response be in this case? What if the post had been left 2 days prior and the psychiatrist was not in the habit of routinely checking her personal page? Alternately, are the psychiatrist's responsibilities the same if the patient voiced suicidal thoughts in a status update that went unnoticed? It would certainly seem unreasonable to expect her to monitor all of her patient's personal pages (bringing into question again issues of patient privacy). It is also worth mentioning that the above scenario could conceivably occur while using both one's personal account and with a separate professional account, as suggested in the AMA Policy.

Other types of discovery may prove similarly problematic. In many jurisdictions, licensed providers are required by law to report suspicions of child abuse and neglect. If evidence of such presented itself via a patient's photo in the provider's newsfeed, it may be her professional responsibility to investigate further or report her concerns to the appropriate agency. Similarly, the Tarasoff law in the United States assigns psychiatrists a duty to help protect potential targets from harm when their patients issue threats of violence. Similarly to the threat of suicide, the psychiatrist would need to consider how best to respond and to do so in an emergent manner. To throw an additional element into the mix, can we be sure the person we are interacting with online is truly our patient, and not an imposter with access to login information [51]?

These situations are not straightforward, and yet, it is prudent to consider them ahead of time (as much as is possible), rather than scramble in the moment to determine the best course of action. At a minimum, it would seem that establishing clear expectations and rules for communication online with one's patients is essential before entering into such an arrangement. Things to cover might include the frequency at which the provider will check his or her account, the expected time-frame for response, and what types of emergent information may be inappropriate to communicate online. In addition to a signed contract, a provider might reiterate the rules in print in strategic locations online. Of course, this still may not prevent an angry or attention-seeking patient from violating these rules and precipitating the same levels of distress and frustration nevertheless.

Drawing from previous sections of this chapter, other things to agree upon beforehand might be establishing what constitutes a boundary crossing or disruption of the frame, rules for things like "tagging" the provider in posts or pictures, and measures to protect privacy, such as agreements not to interact with people in each other's contact lists. A discussion about potential implications for the patient's privacy as well as the potential impact to the therapeutic relationship may also be apropos. Ultimately, the decision regarding how and if to implement social media into clinical practice is an individual one, based in part upon how the unique characteristics of one's practice, patient-base, and intended online endeavor combine to inform the potential risks and benefits. Consultation from a trusted source would likely be worth the effort and highly advised.

8.4 Guidelines for Patient Care with eMH and Other Technologies

8.4.1 Adult Guidelines for eMH: Clinical and Outcome Assessment

The ATA adult guidelines [7] review scope, clinical applications, and clinical/administrative/technical procedures for practice. Assessments (i.e., obtaining a history, mental status examination), treatments (e.g., psychotherapy), and other factors such as cultural competency are described. The ATA Outcomes Guideline was particularly well done [62]. Other guidelines may be evidence-based, but they are unofficial, that is, not done in a long-term, consensus building fashion (e.g., Nelson et al. 2013) [63]. There are no specific guidelines for groups of patients, but steps toward a child and adolescent eMH one is imminent [14]. The AACAP "Practice Parameter for Telepsychiatry With Children and Adolescents" practice parameter offered "strategies" for information on starting a service and reviewed administrative issues [64]. The AACAP Telepsychiatry Committee Minimal Standards (MSs) emphasized consistency with AACAP practice parameters, and discussed the specifics of patient appropriateness, site locations, therapeutic space, technology, how to select a model of care, and risk management.

8.4.2 Child and Adolescent eMH: Steps Toward a Guideline

Child and adolescent psychiatry practice poses significant differences in terms of scope of practice, the variety of providers, and the variety of specialized settings. First, child and adolescent psychiatry clinicians contend with additional disorders (e.g., autism/learning/cognitive disorders) and more often include family and systems work. Treatment modalities like play therapy require site- and technology-based improvisation (e.g., remote site room design, position of camera, camera options like zoom/control/tracking). Second, types of providers vary more widely, including psychiatrists, psychologists, social work, marriage/family/individual counseling, cognitive testing fields, and others. Finally, some patient populations require specialized expertise by providers (i.e., corrections/juvenile hall, school settings, and consultation-liaison or psychosomatic medicine for medical settings).

Specific steps toward guidelines for child and adolescent eMH have been focused in clinical, administrative, and regulatory dimensions [14]. Clinical issues may include the selection of eMH vs. in-person care, age of the patient, parent/family work, therapeutic engagement techniques, assessment and treatment (e.g., social media's impact on care, therapy, psychopharmacology, case management). Administrative issues include health services management, pre- and post-visit logistics, technology, plant/room issues, and hybrid models of care. Regulatory issues include reimbursement, scope of practice, adapting regular care to specialized settings, and privacy/confidentiality. Suggestions for clinicians and administrators are in Table 8.1.

If anything, eMH gets clinicians and clinics more organized in terms of planning before a visit and in selecting a model of care [14]. Web- or phone-based questionnaires may pre-diagnose patients without a visit [65]. Clinicians or coordinators may make pre-emptive calls to collateral sources of information, if consent was obtained for clinically (e.g., vital signs, palpation for EPS, olfactory data) [66]. The plant/room, participants, and roles may require some adjustment [14]. At the patient site, the space should be large enough to include the youth, a parent, and one to two other individuals, and to allow the camera to scan an area large enough to adequately observe children's motor skills as they move about the room, play, and separate from their parents. A table should be available to provide a surface for the child to draw or play while the parent relates the history. Some simple toys should be provided both to occupy the child based on age-appropriateness and child safety standards. Family members may need basic preparatory education; older adults tend to adapt better than expected. The clinician at a distance may direct all of the session or co-direct specific events with someone on-site [67].

8.4.3 Guidelines for Social Media Use, Particularly in Child and Adolescent Populations

The American College of Physicians released a comprehensive overview of physician online professionalism [68], focusing on communication with patients, gathering information, online education, and other topics. Although numerous papers insist on the separation of personal and professional [68, 69], others have argued how difficult it can be to separate both types of presence online [70]. In fact, physicians should assume that one's private profile could be found.

More recently, the Journal of Medical Internet Research provided the following guidelines for healthcare providers to more proactively take advantage of social media based on a review of over 100 articles, Websites, policies, and reports [71]: maintain professionalism, be authentic within the scope of practice, and follow general etiquette but adapt for professional care. Additional guidelines are available for youth patients [72] and privacy issues [73]. Additional ethics codes from the American Psychological Association, American Counseling Association, and the

Table 8.1 Practical considerations when designing eMH services for children and adolescents: the approach, patient selection, scope, technical, and other administrative issues

Category	Considerations	Citation
Approach		
Role definition and financial concerns	Limiting eMH practice to consultation to another prescribing provider will require less investment in technological, administrative, and staff resources from hub (eMH provider) and spoke (consultee or patient-side) sites	Glueck (2011) [66]
	Direct care via eMH (assessment and treatment) will require more investment from both sites	Spaulding
	The eMH provider is more likely to need to perform collateral activities and interact with agencies at the patient location (including child protective services) in a direct care arrangement	Savin et al. (2011) [67]
Patient selection and family issues		
Family involvement	Expect that each individual in the family will have their own level of comfort with and concerns about eMH. The provider will need to get buy-in from each family member before treatment proceeds smoothly	Savin et al. (2011) [67]
Patient-side staff, physical site, technical-based considerations		
Staff	Tasks:	Barretto et al. (2006) [78]
	Gather collateral data and rating scales prior to appointment	
	Able to gather consent forms when parent signatures are required (consent for evaluation/treatment, consent for medication, consent for release of information)	
	Obtain height/weight, vital signs	
	Monitor for extrapyramidal symptoms, rash	
	Maintain safe behavior during session	Nelson et al. (2013) [63]
	Comfortable playing with younger children so that provider may observe	
	Follows procedures for highly confidential information in the electronic medical record	Savin et al. (2011) [67], Barretto et al. (2006) [78]
	Liaison with outside agencies: school, juvenile justice, child protective services, pediatric medical care)	Nelson et al. (2013) [63]
	Maintain confidentiality of the family and between family members	
	Attitudes	
	Local staff attitude toward eMH may be essential at persuading reluctant family members (particularly if family members are older and uncomfortable with this technology)	
	Local staff must appreciate the highly sensitive and confidential information obtained during a child and adolescent psychiatry evaluation (as opposed to general medical evaluation)	Savin et al. (2011) [67]

Table 8.1 (continued)

Category	Considerations	Citation
Site	Local site needs interview room big enough to accommodate a family (3–5 people)	Nelson et al. (2013) [63]
	If local room has play supplies (puppets/action figures, drawing materials, board games, ideally a doll house), it will allow for better behavioral control and better observations for initial assessment/treatment response	Savin et al. (2011) [67]
	Must be interview room and waiting room set up so that when one member is being interviewed alone, family members waiting can't hear	
Technology	eMH provider must have control over the camera in patient room in order to be able to "pan" the room and zoom in on faces	Nelson et al. (2013) [63]
	If both sides have the ability to use split screens, this will facilitate play (e.g., YouTube viewing, playing online videogames together), and patient education (i.e., one screen projects the camera image and the other displays web-based information on resources)	
	If the eMH provider is able to view images from more than one patient-side camera, this will facilitate viewing multiple members of the family at once	
	In order to facilitate naturalistic conversations between eMH provider and family, multiple high-quality microphones placed throughout the room will allow the eMH provider to hear when many members of family talk at once or engage in side conversations	
Confidentiality		
	As with in-person child and adolescent psychiatric practice, the eMH provider and patient-side staff must attend to:	Standard child and adolescent psychiatry practice
	Confidentiality of family as a whole	
	Confidentiality of the medical record ("secure notes" in the electronic medical record)	
	Confidentiality between family members: The eMH provider must orient family to standards of confidentiality as in an in-person interview. This will include explanation of what will remain confidential and what will be told to parents and should also include explanation of what will result in report to child protective services or result in involuntary psychiatric commitment	
	For patients especially concerned about confidentiality, it may be useful for patient-side staff to demonstrate to the child/adolescent that no one is listening/can hear outside the room on patient side. Likewise, the eMH provider can use their camera to pan the provider's room, so as to reassure the patient no one is watching or listening on provider's side	Nelson et al. (2013) [63]

Table 8.2 Existing social media guidelines: a summary of the common tenets

1. Providers should utilize all available privacy settings to protect personal information, but should recognize that these settings may not be infallible

2. Every effort must be made to maintain patient confidentiality online, while maintaining awareness of unique challenges the online setting may provide

3. Online searches for patient information should only be done in the interest of furthering patient care, and preferably with the patient's knowledge and consent

4. Providers should consider keeping personal and professional information in separate accounts

5. Providers should consider conducting routine searches for their own information to maintain awareness of available content and their online images

6. Providers should take care to maintain the same professional boundaries online as they would in face-to-face relationships

7. Providers and patients should establish clear expectations about online communication, to include expected response time and protocols for planned absences

8. When unavailable, providers should arrange coverage for established online communications much as they would for their phone, pager, etc.

9. Providers should educate patients regarding the potential risks of connecting via social media and consider establishing a contract before entering such a relationship

10. Providers should establish clear protocols for managing emergencies that might arise in the course of a social media relationship

11. Many guidelines explicitly recommend against directly friending a patient online

American Psychiatric Association are available for mental health professionals on managing ethical concerns and avoiding ethical violations.

Overall, the social media guidelines have several things in common (Table 8.2). These fall into four categories: (1) Follow standard privacy and confidentiality practices for health and personal (i.e., including provider) information; (2) maintain "good" boundaries (e.g., don't "Friend" patients) and be aware of what information is out there about you (e.g., search self once-in-a-while); (3) establish clear expectations about online communication (modes, protocols, absences, emergencies); and (4) discuss all of the above with the patient as part of the informed consent process (e.g., reasons for additional searches). The modern psychiatrist can take advantage of, but also be cautious with, the use of social media by patients. All ages are using social media for the variety of applications, sense of being heard, self-help (social networking; CHSN), and other health complaints (e.g., suicidal ideation) [74].

8.5 Discussion

The evidence bases on patient-centered care, traditional models of care and eMH – when coupled with the long running tenets of good clinical care in the field of medicine – are a relatively decent platform for the clinician to approach new service and technological developments. In-person and eMH clinical guidelines focus on quality, affordable, and timely care in a variety of settings. Adult guidelines are the most mature, but child and adolescent guidelines are not far behind. A wide range of patients can be served, assessments can be carried out, and the technology/plant can be adjusted. Since the scope of practice in child and adolescent psychiatry involves children, adolescents, parents, and other family members, the complexity of care appears higher – more sources of data, more boundaries to attend to, a broader inter-disciplinary team membership, and a variety of additional treatments.

The consumer movement on new technologies and ways of communicating with others (text, e-mail, Twitter, Facebook) – led by adolescents and young adults – compounds the complexity of care issue described above. For those treating only adults or geriatric patients, though, this learning curve can help clinicians. Significant adjustments for use of social media include the privacy and confidentiality of health and personal information, maintaining "good" interpersonal/clinical boundaries, being aware of what information is out there about you, and clearly discussing expectations about online communication as part of the informed consent process.

The evidence base will grow rapidly and many areas need development. First, tiering of evidence would be desirable particularly in areas related to child and adolescent-specific assessments and treatments. Second, qualitative studies may be more important in this era due to the complexity involved with social media than quantitative measures. Third, we must ask "good" questions to continue apprising ourselves of developments as social media, Facebook, and texting will impact a patient's illness, interpersonal communication, and relationships with healthcare professionals "on the fly." Guidelines or stances by professional bodies may help, but only if they remain up-to-date and do not follow a decade behind to deal with the fear of the unknown in taking positions. Some medical associations (e.g., Canadian) support the conservative use of social media; some oppose it (e.g., American) though the US community has an array of supporters; others firmly oppose it (e.g., British) [69, 75, 76].

Future research will be required to understand the synergies between social media and evidence-based practice, as well as develop institutional policies that benefit patients, clinicians, public health practitioners, and industry alike. A combined, integrated mode of care (e.g., "hybrid") may be the new model or new standard of care [9, 51, 77].

Conclusions

Technology both facilitates and affects current evidence-based care, sometimes for the better and sometimes for the worse, and providers need to stay abreast of changes in contemporary practice. Continuing education and discussing the many issues involved with patients, families, and peers are suggested.

Acknowledgments American Telemedicine Association, Telemental Health Interest Group Department of Psychiatry & Behavioral Sciences, Keck School of Medicine at USC

References

1. Institute of Medicine. March 15, 2015. At: http://www.iom.edu/~/media/Files/Report%20 Files/2001/Crossing-the-Quality-Chasm/Quality%20Chasm%202001%20%20report%20 brief.pdf.
2. Council LS, Geffken D, Valeras AB, et al. A medical home: changing the way patients and teams relate through patient-centered care plans. Fam Syst Health. 2012;30:190–8.

3. Rosenthal TC. The medical home: growing evidence to support a new approach to primary care. J Am Board Fam Med. 2008;21(5):427–40.
4. Crabtree BF, Nutting PA, Miller WL, et al. Summary of the National Demonstration Project and recommendations for the patient-centered medical home. Ann Fam Med. 2010;8 Suppl 1:80–90.
5. Hilty DM, Ferrer D, Callahan EJ, et al. The effectiveness of telemental health: a 2013 review. Telemed J E Health. 2013;19(6):444–54.
6. Hilty DM, Yellowlees PM, Chan S, et al. Telepsychiatry: effective, evidence-based and at a tipping point in healthcare delivery. Psychiatr Clin North Am. In Press.
7. Yellowlees PM, Shore JH, Roberts L, et al. Practice guidelines for videoconferencing-based telemental health. Telemed J E Health. 2010;16(10):1074–89.
8. Yellowlees PM, Odor A, Iosif A, et al. Transcultural psychiatry made simple: asynchronous telepsychiatry as an approach to providing culturally relevant care. Telemed J E Health. 2013;19(4):1–6.
9. Myers KM, et al. Effectiveness of a telehealth service delivery model for treating attention-deficit hyperactivity disorder: results of a community-based randomized controlled trial. J Am Acad Child Adolesc Psychiatry. 2015;54(4):263–74.
10. Dossett EC, Shoemaker EZ, Nasatir-Hilty SE, et al. Integrated care for women, mothers, children and newborns: approaches and models for mental health, pediatric and prenatal care settings. J Womens Health Care. 2015;4:223.
11. Bisognano M, Cherouny PH, Gullo S. Applying a science-based method to improve perinatal care: the institute for healthcare improvement perinatal improvement community. Obstet Gynecol. 2014;124(4):810–4.
12. Tsivos ZL, Calam R, Sanders MR, et al. A pilot randomized controlled trial to evaluate the feasibility and acceptability of the Baby Triple P Positive Parenting Programme in mothers with postnataldepression.ClinChildPsycholPsychiatry.2014:1–23.DOI:10.1177/1359104514531589.
13. Davis MH, Everett A, Kathol R, et al. American Psychiatric Association ad hoc work group report on the integration of psychiatry and primary care, 2011. March 15, 2015. At: http://naapimha.org/wordpress/media/Integration-of-Psychiatry-and-Primary-Care.pdf.
14. Hilty DM, Shoemaker EZ, Myers KM, et al. Issues and steps toward a clinical guideline for telemental health for care of children and adolescents. J Child Adol Psychopharm. In Press.
15. APA Electronic Prescribing Guideline. March 15, 2015. At: http://www.psych.org/practice/managing-a-practice/electronic-prescribing.
16. DeJong SM, Benjamin S, Anzia JM, et al. Professionalism and the internet in psychiatry: what to teach and how to teach it. Acad Psychiatry. 2012;36(5):356–62.
17. PEW Research Center. Internet survey, 2013. March 15, 2015. At: http://www.pewinternet.org/~/media/Files/Reports/PIP_HealthOnline.pdf or smart phone information available at: http://www.pewinternet.org/data-trend/mobile/cell-phone-and-smartphone-ownership-demographics/.
18. Harvard Business Review Staff. How people really use mobile. Harvard Business Review. 2013;91(1):30–31.
19. Engle GL. The clinical application of the biopsychosocial model. Am J Psychiatry. 1980;137(5):535–44.
20. Greenberg M, Shergill S, Szmukler G, et al. Narratives in psychiatry. London: Jessica Kingsley Publishing; 2002.
21. Hilty DM, Srinivasan M, Xiong X, et al. Lessons from psychiatry and psychiatric education for medical learners and teachers. Int Rev Psychiatry. 2013;25:329–37.
22. Hamann J, Leucht S, Kissling W. Shared decision making in psychiatry. Acta Psychiatr Scand. 2003;107(6):403–9.
23. Friedlander MJ, Andrews L, Armstrong EG, et al. What can medical education learn from the neurobiology of learning? Acad Med. 2011;86(4):415–20.
24. Hebb DO. Distinctive features of learning in the higher animal. In: Delafresnaye JF, editor. Brain mechanisms and learning. London: Oxford University Press; 1961.
25. Kahneman D. Thinking, fast and slow. New York: Farrar, Straus and Giroux; 2012.
26. Turner JW. Telepsychiatry as a case study of presence: do you know what you are missing? J Comput Mediat Commun. 2001;6(4). doi:10.1111/j.1083-6101.2001.tb00132.x.

27. Kim T, Biocca F. Telepresence via television: two dimensions of telepresence may have different connections to memory and persuasion. J Comput Mediat Commun. 1997;3: NP. March 15, 2015. At: http://www.mindlab.org/images/d/DOC810.pdf.
28. Fussell SR, Benimoff NI. Social and cognitive processes in interpersonal communication: implications for advanced telecommunications technologies. Hum Factors. 1995;37:228–50.
29. Rutter DR. Looking and seeing: the role of visual communication in social interaction. Chichester/New York: Wiley; 1984.
30. McLaren P, Ball CJ, Summerfield AB, et al. An evaluation of the use of interactive television in an acute psychiatric service. J Telemed Telecare. 1995;1:79–85.
31. Elford R, White H, Bowering R, et al. A randomized, controlled trial of child psychiatric assessments conducted using videoconferencing. J Telemed Telecare. 2000;6:73–82.
32. Ball CJ, McLaren PM, Summerfield AB, et al. A comparison of communication modes in adult psychiatry. J Telemed Telecare. 1995;1:22–6.
33. Argyle M. Bodily communication. London: Methuen; 1975.
34. Hilty DM, Liu W, Marks SL, et al. Effectiveness of telepsychiatry: a brief review. Can Psychiat Assoc Bull. 2003;35(5):10–17.
35. Cukor P, Baer L, Willis BS, et al. Use of videophones and low-cost standard telephone lines to provide a social presence in telepsychiatry. Telemed J. 1998;4:313–21.
36. Ochsman RB, Chapanis A. The effects of 10 communication modes on the behavior of teams during co-operative problem-solving. Int J Man Mach Stud. 1974;6:579–619.
37. O'Malley C, Langston S, Anderson A, et al. Comparison of face-to-face and video-mediated interaction. Interact Comput. 1996;8:177–92.
38. Glueck D. Establishing therapeutic rapport in telemental health. In: Myers K, Turvey CL, editors. Telemental health. New York: Elsevier; 2013. p. 29–46.
39. Myers KM, Palmer NB, Geyer JR. Research in child and adolescent telemental health. Child Adolesc Psychiatr Clin N Am. 2011;20(1):155–71.
40. Rabinowitz T, Murphy KM, Amour JL, et al. Benefits of a telepsychiatry consultation service for rural nursing home residents. Telemed J E Health. 2010;16(1):34–40.
41. Hilty DM, Yellowlees PM, Cobb HC, et al. Models of telepsychiatric consultation-liaison service to rural primary care. Psychosomatics. 2006;47(2):152–7.
42. Yellowlees PM, Odor A, Patrice K, et al. PsychVACS: a system for asynchronous telepsychiatry. Telemed J E Health. 2011;17(4):299–303.
43. Hilty DM, Green J, Nasatir-Hilty SE, et al. Mental healthcare to rural and other underserved primary care settings: benefits of telepsychiatry, integrated care, stepped care and interdisciplinary team models. J Nurs Care. In Press.
44. Boyd DM, Ellison NB. Social network sites: definition, history, and scholarship. J Comput Med Commun. 2007;13(1):210–30.
45. Frankish K, Ryan C, Harris A. Psychiatry and online social media: potential, pitfalls and ethical guidelines for psychiatrists and trainees. Australas Psychiatry. 2012;20:181–7.
46. Facebook Newsroom. March 15, 2015. At: http://newsroom.fb.com/company-info.
47. Jain S. Practicing medicine in the age of Facebook. N Engl J Med. 2009;361(7):649–51.
48. Gutheil TG, Gabbard GO. The concept of boundaries in clinical practice: theoretical and risk-management dimensions. Am J Psychiatry. 1993;150(2):188–96.
49. Moubarak G, Guiot A, Benhamou Y, et al. Facebook activity of residents and fellows and its impact on the doctor-patient relationship. J Med Ethics. 2011;37(2):101–4.
50. Gabbard GO, Kassaw KA, Perez-Garcia G. Professional boundaries in the era of the internet. Acad Psychiatry. 2011;35(3):168–74.
51. Yellowlees P, Nafiz N. The psychiatrist-patient relationship of the future: anytime, anywhere? Harv Rev Psychiatry. 2010;18(2):96–102.
52. Koh S, Cattell GM, Cochran DM, et al. Psychiatrists' use of electronic communication and social media and a proposed framework for future guidelines. J Psychiatr Pract. 2013;19(3):254–63.
53. Clinton BK, Silverman BC, Brendel DH. Patient-targeted googling: the ethics of searching online for patient information. Harv Rev Psychiatry. 2010;18(2):103–12.
54. Gorrindo T, Groves JE. Web searching for information about physicians. JAMA. 2008;300(2):213–5.

55. Shore R, Halsey J, Shah K, et al. Report of the AMA council on ethical and judicial affairs: professionalism in the use of social media. J Clin Ethics. 2011;22(2):165–72.
56. MacDonald J, Sohn S, Ellis P. Privacy, professionalism and Facebook: a dilemma for young doctors. Med Educ. 2010;44(8):805–13.
57. Thompson LA, Dawson K, Ferdig R, et al. The intersection of online social networking with medical professionalism. J Gen Intern Med. 2008;23:954–7.
58. Chretien KC, Greysen SR, Chretien JP, et al. Online posting of unprofessional content by medical students. JAMA. 2009;302:1309–15.
59. Ginory A, Sabatier LM, Eth S. Addressing therapeutic boundaries in social networking. Psychiatry. 2012;75(1):40–8.
60. Greysen SR, Kind T, Chretien KC. Online professionalism and the mirror of social media. J Gen Intern Med. 2010;25(11):1227–9.
61. Myers KM, Lieberman D. Telemental health: responding to mandates for reform in primary healthcare. Telemed J E Health. 2013;19(6):438–43.
62. Shore JH, Mishkind MC, Bernard J, et al. A lexicon of assessment and outcome measures for telemental health. Telemed J E Health. 2013;3:282–92.
63. Nelson EL, Duncan AB, Lillis T. Special considerations for conducting psychotherapy via videoconferencing. In: Myers K, Turvey CL, editors. Telemental health: clinical, technical and administrative foundations for evidenced-based practice. San Francisco: Elsevier; 2013. p. 295–314.
64. Myers KM. AACAP practice parameter for telepsychiatry with children and adolescents. J Am Acad Child Adolesc Psychiatry. 2008;47(12):1468–83.
65. Brondbo H, Mathiassen B, Martinussen M, et al. Agreement on web-based diagnoses and severity of mental health problems in a Norwegian child and adolescent mental health service. Clin Pract Epidemiol Ment Health. 2012;8:16–21.
66. Glueck DA. Telepsychiatry in private practice. Child Adolesc Psychiatr Clin N Am. 2011;20(1):125–34.
67. Savin D, Glueck DA, Chardavoyne J, et al. Bridging cultures: child psychiatry via videoconferencing. Child Adolesc Psychiatr Clin N Am. 2011;20(1):125–34.
68. Farnan JM, Snyder Sulmasy L, et al. Online medical professionalism: patient and public relationships: policy statement from the American College of Physicians and the Federation of State Medical Boards. Ann Intern Med. 2013;158(8):620–7.
69. American Medical Association. Opinion 9.124 – Professionalism in the use of social media. AMA Code of Medical Ethics 2011. March 15, 2015. At: http://www.ama-assn.org/ama/pub/physician-resources/medical-ethics/code-medical-ethics/opinion9124.page?
70. Behnke S. Ethics in the age of the internet. Monit Psychol. 2008;39(7):74.
71. Grajales FJ, Sheps S, Ho K, et al. Social media: a review and tutorial of applications in medicine and health care. J Med Internet Res. 2014;16(2):e13.
72. Mitchell KJ, Ybarra M. Social networking sites: finding a balance between their risks and benefits. Arch Pediatr Adolesc Med. 2009;163(1):87–9.
73. Bishop M, Yellowlees P, Gates C, et al. Facebook goes to the doctor. ACM Press; 2011. p. 13–20.
74. Hidy B, Porch E, Reed S, et al. Social networking and mental health. In: Myers K, Turvey CL, editors. Telemental health. New York: Elsevier; 2013. p. 367–95.
75. Canadian Medical Association. Social media and Canadian physicians – issues and rules of engagement. March 15, 2015. At: http://www.cma.ca.libproxy.usc.edu/socialmedia.
76. British Medical Association. Using social media: practical and ethical guidance for doctors and medical students. [2013-10-27]. March 15, 2015. At: http://www.medschools.ac.uk/SiteCollectionDocuments/social_media_guidance_may2011.pdf.
77. Hilty DM, Yellowlees PM. Collaborative mental health services using multiple technologies – the new way to practice and a new standard of practice? J Am Acad Child Adolesc Psychiatry. 2015;54(4):245–6.
78. Barretto A, Wacker DP, Harding J, et al. Using telemedicine to conduct behavioral assessments. J Appl Behav Analysis 2006;39(3):333–40.

Part IV

New Therapies/Methods/Treatments

Davor Mucic

Web- and Internet-Based Services: Education, Support, Self-Care, and Formal Treatment Approaches

9

Davor Mucic, Donald M. Hilty, Michelle B. Parish, and Peter M. Yellowlees

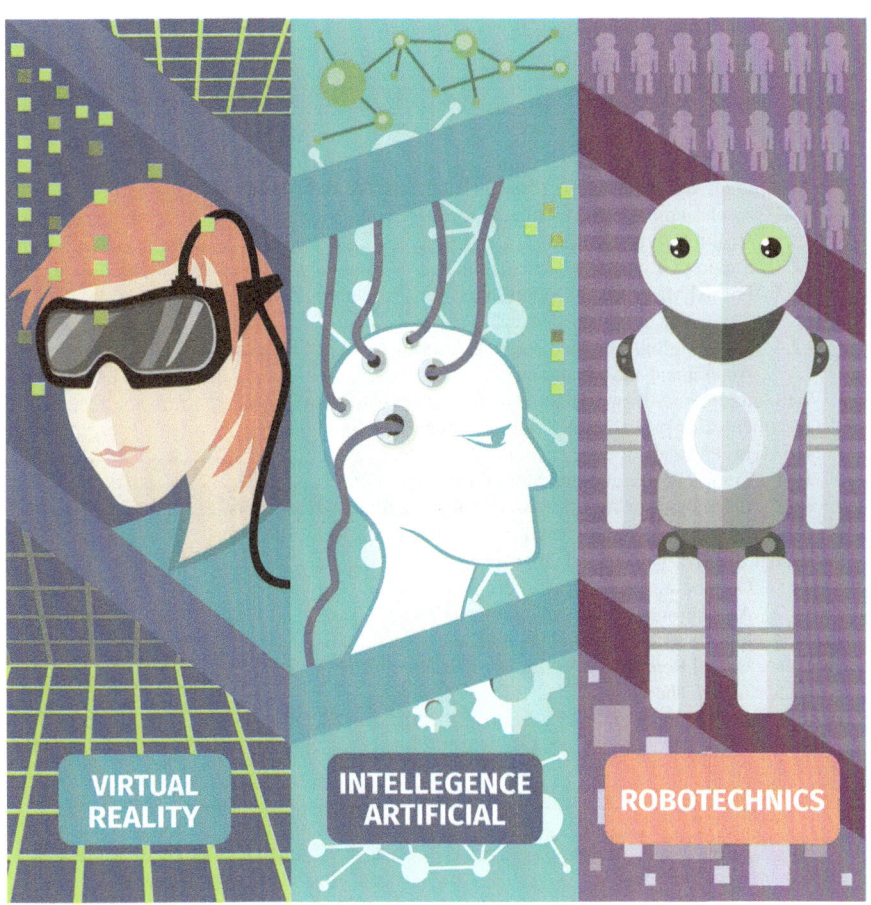

© Springer International Publishing Switzerland 2016
D. Mucic, D.M. Hilty (eds.), *e-Mental Health*,
DOI 10.1007/978-3-319-20852-7_9

D. Mucic, MD (✉)
The Little Prince Psychiatric Centre, Copenhagen, Denmark
e-mail: info@denlilleprins.org
http://www.denlilleprins.org; http://www.tv-psykiater.dk

D.M. Hilty, MD
Keck School of Medicine, University of Southern California,
Los Angeles, CA, USA
e-mail: donh031226@gmail.com

M.B. Parish, MA
UC Davis Telepsychiatry and Health Informatics, University of California, Davis School of
Medicine & Health System, 2450, 48th Street Suite 2800, Sacramento, CA 95817, USA

P.M. Yellowlees, MD, MBBS
Health Informatics Graduate Program, University of California, Davis Health System,
Sacramento, CA 95817, USA

Contents

9.1   Introduction 175
9.2   Spectrum of Web- and Internet-based Health Options for Consumers
      (and Patients and Providers) 177
      9.2.1   Health Information 177
      9.2.2   Support Groups and Participation in a "Community" 178
      9.2.3   Formal Materials or Opportunities for Consumers, Patients,
              Caregivers, and Providers 179
      9.2.4   Tools for Self-Directed Habit, Lifestyle or Illness Changes:
              Assessment and Treatment 180
9.3   Web- and Internet-Based Treatments for Patient Care: Traditional
      Treatments Easily Disseminated, Innovations/New Treatments,
      and Hybrid Models of Care 181
      9.3.1   Traditional Treatments More Easily Accessed 181
      9.3.2   Innovations or Additions to Regular Traditional Treatments 182
9.4   The Present and the Future: Innovative Treatments Used for Patients:
      Virtual Reality, Avatars, and Other Inventions 183
      9.4.1   Overview 183
      9.4.2   Asynchronous Telepsychiatry (ATP) 183
      9.4.3   Mobile Mood Diary 183
      9.4.4   Virtual Reality (VR) 184
      9.4.5   Avatar Therapy 187
Conclusion 187
References 188

Abstract

Web- and Internet-based resources are remarkably popular with the public,
patients, and providers' interventions over the last decade. Opportunities exist
for health information, support groups, formal education programs, tools for
self-directed lifestyle and illness management, obtaining advice/consultation,

and self- or provider-directed treatments (e.g., cognitive behavioral therapy or e-mental healthcare). Traditional treatments are more easily disseminated to the point-of-service. Modification of regular treatments is being developed, based on smartphone applications and applying virtual reality/avatars from games into medicine. Innovative new treatments for special populations are made possible, and hybrid models of care may be our future. Access to information, providers, that can be adjusted to patient needs and comfort, with or without clinician supervision, which creates a completely new world of opportunities. These steps empower patients to initiate, participate, and steer their care. Clinicians have to become aware of, adapt, and serve new advisory roles to patients, as we are all challenged to make the best healthcare more accessible.

9.1   Introduction

Internet-based mental health (MH) use, education, and services are on the rise by patients, general providers, and MH providers. As this is driven by consumers at large, discussions have ensued about person-centered care, knowing the whole person, or the person behind the patient [1, 2]. MH-related Internet-based services may be characterized into several categories: (1) health information via sites; (2) support groups (i.e., general or specific topic) or participation in a "community"; (3) formal educational resources; (4) tools for self-directed assessment, lifestyle change, or decision-making on the management of an illness (e.g., diabetes, depression); (5) one-time medical advice/consultation or general advice in a group led by a professional, often involving self-directed formal treatment; and (6) MH services with professionals of e-Mental Health (eMH) care – Internet-based cognitive behavioral therapy (ICBT) [3–8]. The Internet overcomes obstacles: geographic distance from services; those with special needs (i.e., autism-spectrum, sensory and motor disabilities); the housebound (i.e., physical or MH like panic disorder or phobias); and among/in particular generations (i.e., teenagers).

Thus, the Internet and World Wide Web have complemented regular MH care by adding user-friendly care options and providing greater access and customization/personalization to care. So the "content" or ranges of care are broader, and the "processes" to access services are more numerable. Patients' preferences for help-seeking, education, and treatments are becoming better known – at least to providers who evolve with practice trends and the new applications of technology. In the traditional provider-based healthcare system, providers and systems decide where, what, and how folks get care. In the person- or patient-centered system, folks just go where they want to go and access information and care. Similarly, in banking, people migrated to ATMs based on simple task completion and used tellers when necessary. Many ask, "Is it that simple for MH issues, symptoms and disorders?" Ironically, a provocative comment regarding Internet addiction and its treatment via Internet-based approaches was, "It sounds like holding AA meetings in a bar."

We approach web- and Internet-based treatments in the following context, considering information on: (1) consumer use of the spectrum of online information; (2) traditional healthcare service trends; (3) innovations by programs that had to move forward to meet their patients' needs or to overcome obstacles (i.e., rural, military) and illness-specific factors (e.g., e-treatment or communication for those with posttraumatic stress disorder (PTSD); and finally (4) quasi-experimental methodologies that have initial, good application to clinical populations, usually from the field of MH informatics (i.e., virtual reality, avatars, biosensors, other).

MH providers must meet the challenges and requirements that are emerging to fulfill the care-related requests brought about by this wave of consumer preferences and technology. With the informal and self-directed service use increasing, one question is, "If the person or patient is in care, should this be overseen by a professional, and if so, how?" In addition, "Can we assume the person or patient will plug in and get where they need to go or find the best service for them?" It may be better for patients to use regular therapy, while others would benefit from the quasi-experimental virtual reality (VR) for socialization, dealing with fears, exposure to symptoms, and to "try on" different personalities or behavioral styles. MH providers, while curious, also contend with pre-existing pathologies or seemingly new pathologies related to the Internet (e.g., addiction, group suicide, cyberbullying), disruptions of development, and high profile community events (e.g., disasters or tragedies portrayed in the media).

We will paint a picture of what MH professionals are doing, what seems to work, and some of the possibilities for helping patients in this chapter. We realize that while we seek options that are robust, standardized, or evidence-based, we also have to attend to trends, pilots, and things that don't work. With the exception of extremes, we consider that the content and process of care by technology is probably not inherently good or bad – those value judgments are important, but may have more to do with how technology is used, what it is used for, and whether health promotion is the ultimate outcome. The reader will learn about the pros and cons of:

1. The spectrum of web- and Internet-based health options for consumers (and patients), including health information, support groups, formal education programs, tools for self-directed lifestyle and illness management, options advice/consultation, and self- or provider-directed treatments (e.g., ICBT or eMH)
2. Web- and Internet-based treatments for patient care, including traditional treatments more easily disseminated, innovations/new treatments used in special populations, and hybrid models of care
3. The present and the future of web- and Internet-based quasi-experimental treatments with that of initial, good application to clinical populations, usually from the field of MH informatics (e.g., VR, avatar therapy).

9.2   Spectrum of Web- and Internet-based Health Options for Consumers (and Patients and Providers)

Certain basic rules of healthcare shape this discussion – that is, how we approach low-cost and readily accessible health resources vs. high-cost care (e.g., synchronous eMH). First, in any actual doctor/patient consultation, we know that across specialties about 80 % of all consultations/visits for any doctor are generally straightforward [9]. The 80/20 rule, then, is a concept that essentially means about 20 % of the patients use about 80 % of resources in seeing doctors. This 80/20 phenomenon means that in healthcare we really need to concentrate on the simple transactions to be efficient and to free up the most highly trained professionals to undertake the more complicated transactions. Second, the complementarity principle simply states that computers do well what humans do badly, and vice versa; we should avoid duplication. Third, it may be easier to redesign a system before putting in a new technology, rather than trying to match a technology to a currently inefficient system.

It is certain that the Internet is an important and influential source of information for consumers, as according to a 2008 survey, about 80 % of Americans rely on the Internet to find health information in order to make their healthcare decisions [10]. Globally, Africa, the Middle East, and Latin America are the fastest growing populations in terms of Internet usage [11]. In the United States, Internet use has grown dramatically over the past decade, with a jump from 44 % of the population [12]. eMH, especially telepsychiatry, is the one of the best-known areas [13]. Online health information varies in quality and readability [14–16], but it has been made very popular by enhancing coping strategies, empowerment, and self-efficacy for patients, caregivers, and providers [17]. Users report reduced feelings of anxiety and isolation, enhanced connectedness in the doctor-patient relationship, and ability to make decisions on health-related behaviors [18–20].

Social networking has been defined as "web-based services that allow individuals to (1) construct a public or semi-public profile within a bounded system, (2) articulate a list of other users with whom they share a connection, and (3) view and traverse their list of connections and those made by others within the system." [21] While it may be part of the many categories below, it is covered more in other chapters, except for directly targeted patient programs.

9.2.1   Health Information

Who are these users of the Internet [11, 12]? Most are female (86 % vs. 73 % of men) looking for information on diseases or medical problems, treatments or procedures, doctors or other health professionals, hospitals or other medical facilities, food safety or recalls, drug safety or recalls, and pregnancy and childbirth. Caregivers (a term used for adults who provide unpaid care to a parent, child, friend, or other loved ones) have access to the Internet at a high rate (79 %) and of those, 88 % look online for health information. Education affects the use of Internet: 89 % of those with a college degree vs. 70 % with a high school degree vs. 38 % with lesser degree. Income is a predictor: 95 % of adults with household income $75,000+ vs. 57 % with household income less than $30,000.

Health promotion strategies are typically at free-standing web-sites [22] and the impact of these has been reviewed [23]. Many patients migrate to sites like PatientsLikeMe (http://www.patientslikeme.com/), a consumer-driven site where individuals log on to connect with others in the community who are experiencing similar medical issues. Some options like role-playing game "Second Life" described below, which when used as an educational tool, may improve understanding of psychotic symptoms (i.e., auditory- and/or visual hallucinations [24]. For some patients this is ideal: those with anxiety (e.g., phobias or panic disorder), trauma (e.g., military personnel with PTSD), geographic obstacles (i.e., rural or otherwise long travel), poor access to care (e.g., waiting time), or who dislike local services (e.g., seen as ineffective or of limited quality).

Young people with developmental challenges may have limited access to MH services. Web and social media are changing not only communication patterns especially for them, but also the way they are looking for help, sharing experiences, and learning new behaviors. Children and adolescents comfortable with and reinforced by Internet-based chats and groups may express ideas of self-harm, negative affective states, or pessimistic cognitions of other peers [25, 26] – all of this is good, if it duplicates telling others who will respond or help them; it is more concerning, though, if it is posted and not seen.

Common prejudice is that psychotic patients are not eligible for remote consultations and for the use of technology, due to stimulus overflow and inability to deal with the abundance of information, difficulties with concentration, lack of energy, paranoia, and fear of symptom provocation. However, they succeed in using the Internet as a source of information related to their illness as well as for medication issues (e.g., to check medication side effects in the hope of finding better medication) [27–29]. Systems have been tested to provide symptom and mood regulation, medication adherence, social support, and sleep hygiene on a smartphone platform [30, 31], and sensors may predict mood or schizophrenia relapse with personalized early warning signs – such as isolation, movement inactivity, and unusual behavior [32].

Schizotypal personality disorder patients have been found to be especially likely to use the Internet, with a particular interest in social interaction on the Web [33].

9.2.2 Support Groups and Participation in a "Community"

Most support groups provide support for consumers and patients on the subject of health-related behaviors. Internet-mediated support groups can include specialized groups for individuals with disabilities or unique modes of experience [34]. Web-based support to individuals with stigmatizing or rare illness is extremely important as such groups are often socially isolated and so social networking Websites represent a tool to build community [35]. Such support is particularly suitable and well accepted by stigmatized patients who appreciate the anonymity and easy access, enabling exchange of experiences as well as flow of information [36]. They may contribute to increase knowledge, change attitudes, and alter behavior. Many programs use a peer-to-peer forum to ask questions, tell stories, and share positive ideas; others include a healthcare provider.

Social networking sites may provide a stress buffering resource for those serving in the military who experienced adverse life events [37]. In military populations, the fear of stigma among other concern reduces treatment-seeking for MH issues [32, 38]. Technology-based approaches may increase MH care access for this population. One study found that 33 % of soldiers who reported that they were not willing to talk to a counselor in person were willing to utilize at least one technology-based platform for mental healthcare [39]. Similarly, the appraised soldiers preferred using the iPhone over paper or computer due to its interface, portability, and convenience [40].

For ethnic minorities, there is more than one meaning to the use of the Internet. For the Aboriginal communities in Canada, it may represent a support medium through which the members communicate the indigenous language and cultural traditions [41, 42]. The Internet became a medium for meetings between the generations in order to share and preserve traditional knowledge – indeed, this worked better than past processes to some degree.

Caregivers' tool may benefit by the use of telecommunication technology. A review of Internet-based interventions for medical and MH disorders showed that approximately two-thirds of open or randomized controlled trials significantly reduced stress and improved quality of life in terms of specific measured outcomes [17]. Family caregivers located in rural areas found e-health support to be beneficial in comparison with conventional caregiver support [43]. The interventions range from interactive communities to bulletin board therapy groups [17].

9.2.3 Formal Materials or Opportunities for Consumers, Patients, Caregivers, and Providers

Many consumers, patients, caregivers, and providers are seeking more than health information from Websites, bulletin boards, webcasts, discussion boards, and chat rooms. They need or want more robust, structured programs (e.g., online classes, learning modules, videos, skills training). Providers often shoot for professional education courses. Caregivers feel a need to know clinical tips, self-help coping strategies, and tips on advocacy – a review of Internet-based interventions for medical and MH disorders showed that approximately two-thirds of initiatives reduced stress and improved quality of life; some of these were of open or randomized controlled trials that measured outcomes [17]. Patient populations included mental health (dementia, schizophrenia, anorexia) and medical (older adults/aging, heart transplant, traumatic brain injury, hip fracture, cancer, stroke). Caregivers' outcomes improved with satisfactory and comfortable support services delivered by cell phones [44].

Young people may benefit from web-based information, and online screening, assessment and treatment. Child and adolescent patients have been targeted over the last decade at schools, free-standing promotions in malls, at home via TV, and at primary care or MH specialist settings. A series of Internet interventions have been developed to provide broad MH promotion in children and adolescents: Kindertelefoon (www.kindertelefoon.nl), YooMagazine (www.Yoomagazine.net), Ciao, ReachOut (www.reach-out.org), and Walkalong (www.walkalong.ca).

9.2.4 Tools for Self-Directed Habit, Lifestyle or Illness Changes: Assessment and Treatment

These tools typically target good habits/health promotion, disease prevention, and informal management of symptoms or problems. Techniques might include use of a diary, a questionnaire, or a survey to provoke reflection or "stepping back" to re-evaluate one's assumptions in a conclusion. Exercise and substance (i.e., alcohol) logs are popular. Mood assessments like MoodyMe (https://itunes.apple.com/us/app/moody-me-mood-diary-tracker/id411567371?mt=8) are commonly used, as are those that map behavior patterns across time, including triggers, diet, sleep, and other related factors. Provision of stress reduction care with a mobile phone app is increasing because of a large number of potential users and economical impacts on community [45].

Mobile apps have been adjusted to the needs of patient groups, regardless of language, for example those for self-help for anxiety disorders, MH well-being and stress reduction. One example is "Fear Fighter," a computer-guided self-exposure approach to treat phobia/panic developed at the end of last century [46]. Exposure therapy is effective for phobia/panic, but qualified and trained therapist resources are scarce. Both patients and clinicians achieve benefits by having better access, saving time, and enhancing healthcare efficiency [47]. The app also enables the patient to get necessary guidance/assistance whenever and wherever he/she needs it.

The range of initiatives for support caregivers includes hotlines for consultation on key decisions (i.e., decision support), psychosocial treatments like CBT (individual or group), problem solving training, and coaching for positive parenting skills. Caregivers (and consumers) may benefit from Internet- or application-based assessment questionnaires to self-diagnose and self-refer (e.g., patient health questionnaire for depression, hospital anxiety, and depression scale). A study on public social networking accounts of college students found that 25 % of college students exhibited depressive symptoms based upon the Diagnostic and Statistical Manual of Mental Disorders (DSM) criteria, and 2.5 % met the DSM criteria for major depressive disorder. Online reinforcement from their friends may have made them more likely to discuss their depressive symptoms publicly via social networking sites [48].

Support and self-help programs allow users to ask questions to health professionals while remaining anonymous. Self-help programs are designed to offer relevant treatment approaches, typically without guidance from the therapist. Such self-help interventions without therapist guidance are especially attractive for the users that are stigmatized (e.g., severe mentally ill or individuals with drinking problem) [49].

Combined efforts by the Telemedicine and Advanced Technology Research Center, the Military Operational Medicine Research Program, United States Army Medical Research and Materiel Command, the National Center for Telehealth and Technology, and the Department of Veterans Affairs have helped in releasing apps for the general public in dedicated app stores [50]. One is called PTSD Coach [51]. It is designed to help veterans learn about and manage symptoms that commonly occur after trauma. While such apps are not designed to act as a substitute for treatment, this technology may become an important tool for managing and even initially detecting PTSD symptoms. They are used in many ways to support MH intervention including: symptom assessment, illness-specific education, treatment resource location, and tracking of treatment progress [52].

Some of the above options, while not considered "care," involve some oversight by providers for health (e.g., diabetes) and MH (e.g., depression). This usually involves bulletin boards with occasional comments or steering by professionals. For example, in an asynchronous chat group for education, the provider can use customized bursts (e.g., sending a paper to read or a video to watch) based on the discussion to provide information, correct misunderstood concepts, and know how to use a self-report measure. For one-time medical advice/consultation or general advice in a group led by a professional, sometimes the "best" outcome is a supportive referral to see a professional when things are not very simple or too many concurrent problems are at-hand.

9.3 Web- and Internet-Based Treatments for Patient Care: Traditional Treatments Easily Disseminated, Innovations/New Treatments, and Hybrid Models of Care

9.3.1 Traditional Treatments More Easily Accessed

Rapid eye movements are part of the Eye Movement Desensitization and Reprocessing approach, typically used for treatment of a patient suffering from an acute stress disorder. However, relevant experts are not easily found, which is why a videoconference-mediated treatment has been tested with promising results [53].

eMH has contributed to development of "remote speech therapy," a Swedish innovation since 2010 and now well-established in rural areas of Finland and Scotland as well [54]. The aim of the project was to reduce therapists' travel time while enabling patients in rural communities to have better access to speech and language therapy services. School children living in remote communities got the opportunity to receive therapy sessions in their schools whereas the services of a speech therapist could be received at the healthcare center.

9.3.2 Innovations or Additions to Regular Traditional Treatments

The least structured of these options is patient–doctor correspondence integrated with clinical care and the electronic health record. As the Internet increases the level of knowledge and amount of information regarding specific illness, it becomes easier for the users to talk to their doctor regarding their specific conditions and potential treatment options [20]. Schizophrenic patients especially perceive the shift in hierarchy to a more equal relationship. In this respect, a specific advantage for patients with psychosis is not having to face another person, but still being able to gain information and interact with others without feeling devalued or unsafe [27].

One promising area in this approach is supporting patients in improving attendance to treatment, which is as important as motivational work prior to conducting treatment. Psychiatric treatments fail to produce intended outcomes when patients miss their appointments; about 50 % of patients actively engage in recommended treatment regimens [55]. The reasons for non-engagement include stigma and absence of insight (denial). Each of these aspects may be influenced via direct or remote provision of education, motivation and support to enhance attendance (i.e., treatment readiness), recognition of treatment benefits, collaboration with care providers – all together, a positive psychiatric treatment history is more likely [56]. Recent patient-centered strategies to increase patient compliance are simple mail, telephone, or SMS reminders that have shown to be an effective way to support patient attendance to follow-up appointments [57, 58].

Higher intensity interventions include synchronous eMH (covered in other chapters) and Internet-based CBT (ICBT), used most often for patients with depression and anxiety. Online MH interventions are as effective as traditional in-person therapy for disorders such as depression and anxiety (e.g., CBT for panic disorder and agoraphobia) [59–63]; effect sizes and recovery rates were comparable. Based on a 30-month follow-up study for treatment of social phobia, the long-term effects of in-person delivered CBT was comparable to ICBT [61]. ICBT appears to be effective, not surprisingly, when delivered in clinical practice by a qualified therapist [64, 65]. More specifically, Internet-based CT combined with monitoring by text messages (mobile cognitive therapy, mCT), and minimal therapist support (e-mail and telephone), is an effective approach towards prevention of relapse in depression [63].

Once again, the military may be in the lead for providing Internet-based care options, with foci of remote screening and assessment, post-deployment adjustment, suicide prevention and management, and delivery of training/education [66]. Many personnel prefer to receive care at home – particularly those with anxiety, PTSD, and phobia – in addition to those who prefer to avoid the stigma of entering a mental health facility [67]. A randomized trial of home-based eMH, i.e., telepsychiatry treatment for depression, was equal or better than office-based care [68].

9.4 The Present and the Future: Innovative Treatments Used for Patients: Virtual Reality, Avatars, and Other Inventions

9.4.1 Overview

MH informatics gives us both an overview of novel assessment and treatment options, and a vision of the future. Technically, eMH is within this scope, but the field extends much further. Since MH assessment methods are time consuming and highly subjective, various automated MH assessment methods have been developed to improve efficiency as well as to provide more objective assessments [69]. Image and behavior analysis included facial expressions and gestures. Biosignals, such as skin conductance, EEG, EMG, and EGA measurements, have been used to monitor various physiological and psychological conditions. Language pattern and specifically discriminant word analyses are used in schizophrenia [70], while acoustic analysis is used for depression [71]. Online decision support is also common.

"Mental health care will soon involve clinicians logging onto online social networks: checking patients' online activity, evaluating patients' moods, administering surveys and determining if additional appointments are needed, adjusting medications, reviewing video of a significant event or issue uploaded by a patient, or even running software algorithms or other diagnostic tools to evaluate a patients mental state though the language and information shared over social networking?" [72]. This picture of MH treatment may seem a bit farfetched, but as online patient-provider interaction increases and the popularity of social networks increases, it may happen or be relevant.

9.4.2 Asynchronous Telepsychiatry (ATP)

ATP to primary care is feasible, valid, and reliable in English and Spanish-speaking patients in primary care [73]. Similar methods are used in radiology, dermatology, ophthalmology, cardiology, and pathology. One ATP model uses a basic questionnaire for screening by the provider of the patient, video capture of that interview, and uploading of patient histories for a remote psychiatrist for review in a HIPAA-adherent manner [74]. Diagnosis and treatment recommendations are made and PCPs implement care successfully about 80 % of the time and the model is cost-effective [75, 76].

9.4.3 Mobile Mood Diary

This application is similar to the paper daily diary, but on a smartphone platform. Employing CBT relies mainly on writing down daily activities, charting their moods and energy levels. Patients used to bring their recorded paper daily diary to discuss with the therapist on their weekly therapy sessions; some forgot or stop doing their CBT for whatever reason. A new application, especially for teenagers, is texting and typing on their smartphones. Psychiatrists find mobile mood diary greatly beneficial since they can look into graphs illustrating the patient's mood swings throughout the day [77].

9.4.4 Virtual Reality (VR)

VR is usually defined as computer-simulated environment that can simulate physical presence in places in the real world or imagined worlds. VR is the concept of being virtually, but not physically at a specific place, and a number of VR platforms have been developed in the past 20 years, mostly for games. VR can recreate sensory experiences, which include virtual taste, sight, smell, sound, and touch. Many companies have also developed VR platforms for entertainment, marketing, flight simulation, medical education, and other fields. In practice, it is currently very difficult to create a high-fidelity VR experience, because of technical limitations on processing power, image resolution, and communication bandwidth.

The virtual characters (avatar, virtual agent) as well as virtual environments have been developed in order to practice dynamic and real-life social interactions in a safe environment [78]. The virtual character (avatar) is the graphical representation of the user or the user's alter ego in 3D form. People are known to psychologically identify with virtual representations that do not necessarily reflect their actual appearances [79]. Thus, in virtual worlds, people can explore different versions of their self and become someone else [80]. Moreover, the appearance of avatars can cause behavioral and attitudinal shifts that might positively influence current treatment or motivate individuals who were reluctant to that due to lack of insight or stigma [81–84]. However, when participating in violent games, avatars personalize risk by simulating harm to digital representations with which people directly identify; this may contribute to behavioral change into the physical world [85].

Virtual environments are either single user virtual environments (SVEs) or collaborative virtual environments (CVEs). In an SVE, a single user explores the virtual environment, and responses from the environment or a virtual agent (avatar) must be preprogrammed. In a CVE, more than one user may inhabit the virtual environment at the same time (e.g., patient and the therapist or trainer) and can interact with each other in real-time via avatars. Users control their avatars independently and can communicate directly with each other, even when physically located in different places, through speech, movement, and gesture in the virtual space [20, 86–89]. CVEs have been used to examine and investigate the ability *to recognize* emotions [90], and also teaching students how *to manifest* their emotions and *understand* the emotions of other people [91]. One of the leading and most popular Internet-based VR applications is Second Life.

Second Life (http://secondlife.com/) allows providers and patients (represented by electronic virtual figures or avatars) to log on and meet on virtual "islands" or "clouds" (which are "private" virtual locations within the site) that can depict a variety of scenes including a virtual therapy office) [74]. It is open to the public and can be accessed free of charge. Fees are charged to purchase virtual "land" or server space and to build fantasy environments (i.e., stores, museums, or even go on a date). Virtual characters and environments represent a valuable tool for the supportive therapies and the training of social skills and non-verbal decoding (e.g., high-functioning autism), as they provide a safe, repeatable, and diversifiable learning environment [92].

In daily life, ordinary mentally healthy individuals as well as people with various MH conditions participate in Internet-mediated electronic games. The use of the software controls that change the avatar's features (i.e., the height and weight, color of skin, eyes, and hair, width of the nose, and other markers of racial identity) can have an immediate effect on the participant's sense of physical embodiment. Many participants strive for an accurate mirroring of their bodily appearance off-screen but some explore radical alterations of self [93]. These choices and the degree to which an individual feels actually present in the virtual environment may be related to MH and well-being [94]. It has been reported that participants in online role-playing games who created an avatar reflecting the "ideal self" reported greater perceived interactivity in the virtual world than those who created a replica avatar mirroring the actual self [95].

Another type of a VR platform is a fully immersive system, which uses software systems that give the user a full immersion into the VR environment. This can take place in a virtual cave, which could be a six-walled room with multiple projectors transmitting images on these walls. Some systems require a specific visual aid such as 3D glasses while others can be used with only the naked eye. A similar concept of fully immersive VR environment is the use of specific glasses that has the 3D screen inside the device. These immersive technologies are relatively costly which makes it less accessible to many providers and patients for treatment.

A review of VR reports that it has been used in the treatment of many MH conditions [74], including eating disorders, autism spectrum disorders, stress management, pain management, and diagnosis and treatment of neurological conditions such as stroke. As autism spectrum disorders are characterized by impairments in communication and reciprocal interaction [87], socio-communicative deficits are manifested via problems with spontaneously producing, understanding, and responding to non-verbal cues. Autistic individuals do not spontaneously attend to social information, and are thus less able to intuitively interact in social context [96].

One of the most effective and widely used applications in MH is VR exposure therapy (VRET), used in the treatment of phobia and trauma-related disorders like PTSD. VRET involves the use of VR applications, in conjunction with therapy, to expose patients to visual and other sensory material that represent a feared object or situation or a traumatic event. VREt allows for attenuation of the anxiety that reinforces phobia or trauma-related symptoms by providing exposure to the feared stimuli in a safe environment. VREt allows for prolonged exposure to the feared stimuli, a vital component of effective exposure therapy, and therefore it has been applied to treat phobias (e.g., social, fear of heights and flying, claustrophobia, and fear of spiders). One new approach to treat social phobia using VR incorporates transformations of the self-appearance via dissimilar avatar in order to restructure patients' distorted self-image in combination with exposure. A dissimilar virtual self provides anonymity, which reduces inhibition and anxiety and facilitates self-expression. Following this approach, a new technique is developed in order to treat social phobia using VR but based on modification of self-appearance. With this tool, therapists can help patients understand their phobia from a different perspective and work on correcting their self-image and improving their confidence in social situations.

Guidelines specific to patient-provider communication or care provision or conducting therapy in online virtual environments available are as follows[74]:

1. Patients who are only receiving generic educational information on an open VR environment can be anonymous, and should not be tracked in any way. Any providers on that island should be fully identified, and should have named or numbered avatars that clearly identify who they are, and that link to published biographies.
2. Patients who wish to move to a secure VR environment for some form of virtual therapy, whether this is individual counseling or cognitive behavioral therapy should be treated in accordance with the following protocols ensuring high practice standards, and legal and ethical processes:
   (a) All patients should undergo an in-person or telemedicine assessment to evaluate patient safety and appropriateness for treatment with this modality, establish care, confirm their diagnosis, create a treatment plan, and discuss consent. This is particularly important in a potential emergency situation where therapists have to know the physical location of a patient, as per telemedicine guidelines, in order to call for help.
   (b) All patients should then sign a written consent form if required in the state in which they reside (which can be done electronically), be trained in how to use the virtual environment, be given a tour of the private island, and receive a copy of their diagnostic assessment and treatment plan.
   (c) HIPAA compliance of the virtual environment must be documented, verified, and ensured prior to patient contact.
   (d) If patients and providers are federal employees, they can be treated in the virtual environment from any state by any provider. If the patient or the provider is not a federal employee, the treating provider must be licensed to practice in the state from which the patient logs in.
   (e) All providers will have fully authenticated avatars using their real names, and will have biographies published that link their professional identities to their avatars for patients to read.
   (f) Patients and providers will then schedule sessions on the private island for either counseling or cognitive behavioral therapy, or a combination of both.
   (g) Any major changes to the treatment plan, such as altered medications, should require an in-person telemedicine consultation.
   (h) Either the provider or the patient may at any time either cease therapy, or request a telemedicine or in-person consultation to review progress.

9.4.5   Avatar Therapy

As mentioned above, it was only a question of time when computerized technology combined with the Internet will be used in order to help in treatment of severe mental health conditions. Avatar therapy is a novel therapy based on a computer program developed within last few years by clinicians from University College in London. This approach has a potential to significantly reduce the frequency and intensity of the voices, their omnipotence, and malevolence [97]. The treatment would have a schizophrenic patient select an avatar on a computer and create a virtual representation of the scary voices that previously existed solely in his/her imagination. The system then synchronizes the avatar's lips with its speech, enabling a therapist to speak to the patient through the avatar in real time. The therapist encourages the patient to oppose the voice and gradually teaches them to take control of their hallucinations.

Within this approach the clinician plays two roles, one as a supportive therapist and the other one as the persecutory avatar. As the session proceeds, the two roles merge and avatar successively agrees to stop disturbing the patient and instead begins to make helpful suggestions in order to boost the patient's self-confidence. In accordance to this, the expression on avatar's face may be altered from menacing to neutral or even friendly smiling.

Each therapy session lasts 30 min, and afterwards, the patient is given MP3 recordings of their session, so that they can listen on a music player or computer when an auditory hallucination strikes again. Significant reduction in depressive symptoms was detected at the 3-month follow-up; increased quality of life, likewise, was due to reduction in symptoms.

More research is needed in this area, with randomized trails, reliability/validity studies, and provider training.

Conclusion

Web- and Internet-based resources are remarkably popular with the public, patients, and providers' interventions over the last decade. Opportunities exist for health information, support groups, formal education programs, tools for self-directed lifestyle, and illness management, obtaining advice/consultation, and self- or provider-directed treatments (e.g., ICBT or eMH). Traditional treatments are more easily disseminated to the point-of-service. Modification of regular treatments is in process – smartphone applications and importing of VR/avatar from games into medicine, and innovations/new treatments for special populations are rolling out new possibilities; hybrid models of care that combine in-person and the Internet care may be our future.

Patients are empowered by increased access to information, providers, and exposures – in ways that can be adjusted to patient needs and comfort, with or without clinician supervision. These steps help patients initiate, participate, and steer their care. Clinicians have to become aware of, adapt to, and use sound clinical judgment. They serve new advisory roles to patients, as we are all challenged to keep the best of MH care, yet make it more accessible. While the psychoanalytic notion that "the therapist is an empty slate" on which the patient is writing his/her own life-story is still true for some treatments, we now have a patient able to create his "virtual self" in form of avatar and interact within virtual environments in order to deal with social anxiety, recognize and express emotions, and deal with stress through titrated exposures to heal past traumas. Even those with severe MH conditions appear to benefit.

However, potential disadvantages are waiting around the corner. Because of the increase in our use of technology and computer programs utilizing avatars, spending so much time in a virtual world (e.g., Second life), a "contrast effect" is likely to occur [98, 99]. When participants are presented with attractive avatars and a world much better than the real one, the risk for massive "emigration" into virtual realities is likely to increase. Other problems persist, regarding the quality of information on Internet, its reliability, and confusion when sites are in conflict. Privacy and confidentiality concerns will continue to some degree. Patients' attitudes toward clinicians and MH care may shift, for the better or for the worse. It is critical that providers increase their awareness and understanding of web-based options to understand patients' concerns (e.g., events related to networking, interactions with others), to incorporate low-intensity but user-friendly approaches (e.g., health prevention strategies), and to offer new treatment approaches.

References

1. Miles A, Mezzich J. The care of the patient and the soul of the clinic: person-centered medicine as an emergent model of modern clinical practice. Int J Pers Centered Med. 2011;1(2):207–22.
2. Ekman I, Swedberg K, Taft C, et al. Person-centered care—ready for prime time. Eur J Cardiovasc Nurs. 2011;10(4):248–51.
3. Celio AA, Winzelberg AJ, Wilfley DE, et al. Reducing risk factors for eating disorders: comparison of an Internet- and a classroom-delivered psychoeducational program. J Consult Clin Psychol. 2000;68(4):650–7.
4. Ritterband LM, Thorndike F. Internet interventions or patient education web sites? J Med Internet Res. 2006;8(3):e18.
5. Christensen H, Griffiths K, Groves C, et al. Free range users and one hit wonders: community users of an Internet-based cognitive behaviour therapy program. Aust N Z J Psychiatry. 2006;40(1):9–62.
6. Clarke G, Eubanks D, Reid E, et al. Overcoming Depression on the Internet (ODIN) (2): a randomized trial of a self-help depression skills program with reminders. J Med Internet Res. 2005;7(2):e16.
7. Andersson G, Carlbring P, Holmstrom A, et al. Internet-based self-help with therapist feedback and in vivo group exposure for social phobia: a randomized controlled trial. J Consult Clin Psychol. 2006;74(4):677–86.
8. Ljotsson B, Lundin C, Mitsell K, et al. Remote treatment of bulimia nervosa and binge eating disorder: a randomized trial of Internet-assisted cognitive behavioural therapy. Behav Res Ther. 2007;45(4):649–61.
9. Maghazil A, Yellowlees PM. Novel approaches to clinical care in mental health: from asynchronous telepsychiatry to virtual reality. In: Lech M, Song I, Yellowlees PM, et al., editors. Mental health informatics. Heidelberg: Springer; 2014.
10. Elkin, N. How America searches: health and wellness, 2008. 7 Mar 2015. At: http://www.icrossing.com/sites/default/files/how-america-searches-health-and-wellness.pdf.
11. Internet World Stats. Internet users in the world-distribution by world regions, 2011. 28 Feb 2015. At: http://www.internetworldstats.com/stats.htm.
12. Internet World Stats. United States of America: internet usage and broadband usage report, 2011. 28 Feb 2015. At: http://www.internetworldstats.com/am/us.htm.

13. Morahan-Martin JM. How Internet users find, evaluate, and use online health information: a cross-cultural review. Cyberpsychol Behav. 2004;7(5):497–510.
14. Ferreira-Lay P, Miller S. The quality of Internet information on depression for lay people. Psychiatr Bull. 2008;32:170–3.
15. Kalk NJ, Pothier DD. Patient information on schizophrenia on the Internet. Psychiatr Bull. 2008;32:409–11.
16. Nemoto K, Tachikawa H, Sodeyama N, et al. Quality of Internet information referring to mental health and mental disorders in Japan. Psychiatry Clin Neurosci. 2007;61(3):243–8.
17. Hu C, Kung S, Rummans TA, et al. Reducing caregiver stress with internet-based interventions: a systematic review of open-label and randomized controlled trials. J Am Med Inform Assoc. 2014. doi:10.1136/amiajnl-2014-002817.
18. Andersson G, Bergström J, Carlbring P, et al. The use of the Internet in the treatment of anxiety disorders. Curr Opin Psychiatry. 2005;18(1):73–7.
19. Erwin BA, Turk CL, Heimberg RG, et al. The Internet: home to a severe population of individuals with social anxiety disorder? J Anxiety Disord. 2004;18(5):629–46.
20. Murray E, Lo B, Pollack L, et al. The impact of health information on the Internet on the physician-patient relationship: patient perceptions. Arch Intern Med. 2003;163(14):1727–34.
21. Boyd DM, Ellison NB. Social network sites: definition, history, and scholarship. J Comput Mediated Commun. 2007;13(1):210–30.
22. Siemer PC. Telemental health and web-based applications in children and adolescents. Child Adolesc Psychiatr Clin N Am. 2011;20(1):135–53.
23. Laranjo L, Arguel A, Neves AL, et al. The influence of social networking sites on health behavior change: a systematic review and meta-analysis. J Am Med Inform Assoc. 2015;22(1):243–56.
24. Yellowlees PM, Cook JN. Education about hallucinations using an Internet virtual reality system: a qualitative survey. Acad Psychiatry. 2006;30(6):534–9.
25. Griffiths KM, Calear AL, Banfield M. Systematic review on Internet Support Groups (ISGs) and depression (2): what is known about depression ISGs? J Med Internet Res. 2009;11(3):e41. doi:10.2196/jmir.1303.
26. Griffiths KM, Calear AL, Banfield M. Systematic review on Internet Support Groups (ISGs) and depression (1): do ISGs reduce depressive symptoms? J Med Internet Res. 2009;11(3):e40. doi:10.2196/jmir.1270.
27. Schrank B, Sibitz I, Unger A, et al. How use patients with schizophrenia the Internet: qualitative study. J Med Internet Res. 2010;12(5):e70. doi:10.2196/jmir.1550.
28. Koivunen M, Välimäki M, Pitkänen A, et al. A preliminary usability evaluation of Web-based portal application for patients with schizophrenia. J Psychiatr Ment Health Nurs. 2007;14(5):462–9.
29. Ahmed M. Computer-facilitated dialogue with patients who have schizophrenia. Psychiatr Serv. 2002;53(1):99–100.
30. Ben-Zeev D, Kaiser SM, Brenner CJ, et al. Development and usability testing of FOCUS: a smartphone system for self-management of schizophrenia. Psychiatr Rehabil J. 2013;36(4):289–96. PMID: 24015913.
31. Ben-Zeev D, Brenner CJ, Begale M, et al. Feasibility, acceptability, and preliminary efficacy of a smartphone intervention for schizophrenia. Schizophr Bull. 2014;40(6):1244–53.
32. Ben-Zeev D, Corrigan PW, Britt TW, et al. Stigma of mental illness and service use in the military. J Ment Health. 2012;21(3):264–73.
33. Mittal VA, Tessner KD, McMillan AL, et al. Elevated social Internet use and schizotypal personality disorder in adolescents. Schizophr Res. 2007;94(1-3):50–7.
34. Antze P. On the pragmatics of empathy in the neurodiversity movement. In: Lambek M, editor. Ordinary ethics. New York: Fordham University Press; 2010. p. 310–27.
35. Gowen K, Deschaine M, Gruttadara D, et al. Young adults with mental health conditions and social networking websites: seeking tools to build community. Psychiatr Rehab J. 2012;35(3):245–50.
36. Berger M, Wagner TH, Baker LC. Internet use and stigmatized illness. Soc Sci Med. 2005;61(8):1821–7.

37. Lewandowski J, Rosenberg BD, Jordan Parks M, et al. The effect of informal social support: face-to-face versus computer-mediated communication. Comput Hum Behav. 2011;27(5):1806–14.
38. Pietrzak R, Johnson D, Goldstein M, et al. Perceived stigma and barriers to mental health care utilization among OEF-OIF veterans. Psychiatr Serv. 2009;60(8):1118–22.
39. Wilson JA, Onorati K, Mishkind M, et al. Soldier attitudes about technology-based approaches to mental health care. Cyber Psychol Behav. 2008;11(6):767–9.
40. Bush NE, Skopp N, Smolenski D, et al. Behavioral screening measures delivered with a smartphone app: psychometric properties and user preference. J Nerv Ment Dis. 2013;201(11):991–5.
41. Alexander CJ, Adamson A, Daborn G, et al. Inuit cyberspace: the struggle for access for Inuit Qaujimajatuqangit. J Can Stud. 2009;43(2):220–49.
42. Adelson N, Olding M. Narrating aboriginality on-line: digital storytelling, identity and healing. J Commun Inf. 2013;9(2):85–90.
43. Blusi M, Dalin R, Jong M, et al. The benefits of e-health support for older family caregivers in rural areas. J Telemed Telecare. 2014;20(2):63–9.
44. Chi NC, Demiris G. A systematic review of telehealth tools and interventions to support family caregivers. J Telemed Telecare. 2015;21(1):37–44.
45. Luxton D, Hansen RN, Stanfill K, et al. Mobile app self-care versus in-office care for stress reduction: a cost minimization analysis. J Telemed Telecare. 2014;20(8):431–5.
46. Shaw SC, Marks IM, Toole S. Lessons from pilot tests of computer self help for agora/claustrophobia and panic. MD Comput. 1999;16:44–8.
47. Kenwright M, Liness S, Marks I, et al. Reducing demands on clinicians by offering computer-aided self-help for phobia/panic Feasibility study. Br J Psychiatry. 2001;179(5):456–9.
48. Moreno MA, Jelenchick LA, Egan KG, et al. Feeling bad on Facebook: depression disclosures by college students on a social networking site. Depress Anxiety. 2011;28(6):447–55.
49. Riper H, Kramer J, Smit F, et al. Web-based self-help for problem drinkers: a pragmatic randomized trial. Addiction. 2008;103(2):218–27.
50. US Department of Veterans Affairs. Department of Veterans Affairs (VA) mobile health fact sheet final [Internet]. Department of Veterans Affairs, 2013. 28 Feb 2015. At: https://mobile-health.va.gov/sites/default/files/files/VAMobileHealthFactSheet.pdf.
51. National Center for Telehealth and Technology. PTSD coach [Internet]. PTSD Coach|t2health, 2013. 28 Feb 2015. At: http://www.t2.health.mil/apps/ptsd-coach.
52. Luxton DD, McCann RA, Bush NE, et al. mHealth for mental health: integrating smartphone technology in behavioral healthcare. Prof Psychol Res Pract. 2011;42(6):505–12.
53. Todder D, Kaplan Z. Rapid eye movements for acute stress disorder using video conference communication. Tel e-Health. 2007;13(4):461–4.
54. Wakeling M, Heaney D. Competitive health services in sparsely populated areas – eHealth applications across the urban-rural dimension. Report on Scotland pilots, 2011. 28 Feb 2015. At https://www.ehealthservices.eu.
55. Agyapong VI, Rogers C, Machale S, et al. Factors predicting adherence with psychiatric follow-up appointments for patients assessed by the liaison psychiatric team in the emergency department. Int J Psychiatry Med. 2010;40:217–28.
56. Gonzalez J, Williams JW, Noël PH, et al. Adherence to mental health treatment in a primary care clinic. J Am Board Fam Pract. 2005;18:87–96.
57. Zanjani F, et al. Management of psychiatric appointments by telephone. J Telemed Telecare. 2015;21(1):61–3.
58. Kunigiri G, Gajebasia N, Sallah D. Improving attendance in psychiatric outpatient clinics by using reminders. J Telemed Telecare. 2014;20(8):464–7.
59. Amstadter AB, Broman-Fulks J, Zinzow H, Ruggiero KJ, Cercone J. Internet-based interventions for traumatic stress-related mental health problems: a review and suggestion for future research. Clin Psychol Rev. 2009;29(5):410–20.
60. Carlbring P, Ekselius L, Andersson G. Treatment of panic disorder via the Internet: a randomized trial of CBT vs applied relaxation. J Behav Ther Exp Psychiatry. 2003;34(2):129–40.

61. Carlbring P, Nordgren LB, Furmark T, et al. Long-term outcome of Internet-delivered cognitive-behavioural therapy for social phobia: a 30-month follow-up. Behav Res Ther. 2009;47(10):848–50.
62. Kiropoulos LA, Klein B, Austin DW, et al. Is internet-based CBT for panic disorder and agoraphobia as effective as face-to-face CBT? J Anxiety Disord. 2008;22(8):1273–84.
63. Kok G, Bockting C, Berger H, et al. Mobile cognitive therapy: adherence and acceptability of an online intervention in remitted recurrently depressed patients. Int Intervent. 2014;1(2):65–73.
64. Andersson G, Hedman E. Effectiveness of guided Internet-based cognitive behavior therapy in regular clinical settings. Verhaltenstherapie. 2013;23(3):140–8.
65. Andersson G, Hesser H, Veilord A, et al. Randomised controlled non-inferiority trial with 3-year follow-up of Internet-delivered versus face-to-face group cognitive behavioural therapy for depression. J Affect Disord. 2013;151(3):986–94.
66. Doarn CR, Shore J, Ferguson S, et al. Challenges, solutions, and best practices in telemental health service delivery across the pacific rim – a summary. Telemed J E Health. 2012;18(8):654–60.
67. Shore JH, Aldag M, McVeigh FL, et al. Review of mobile health technology for military mental health. Mil Med. 2014;179(8):865–78.
68. Luxton DD, Pruitt LD, O'Brien K, et al. Design and methodology of a randomized clinical trial of home-based telemental health treatment for U.S. military personnel and veterans with depression. Contemp Clin Trials. 2014;38(1):134–44.
69. Diederich J, Song I. Mental health informatics: current approaches. In: Lech M, Song I, Yellowlees PM, et al., editors. Mental health informatics. Heidelberg: Springer; 2014.
70. Diederich J, Al-Ajmi A, Yellowlees P. Ex-ray: data mining and mental health. Appl Soft Comput J. 2007;7(3):923–8.
71. France DJ, Shiavi RG. Acoustical properties of speech as indicators of depression and suicidal risk. IEEE Trans Biomed Eng. 2000;47(7):829–37.
72. Parish MB, Yellowlees PM. The rise of person-centered health care and the influence of health informatics and social network applications on mental health care. In: Lech M, Song I, Yellowlees PM, et al., editors. Mental health informatics. Heidelberg: Springer; 2014.
73. Yellowlees PM, Odor A, Patrice K, et al. Transcultural psychiatry made simple: asynchronous telepsychiatry as an approach to providing culturally relevant care. Telemed J E Health. 2013;19(4):1–6.
74. Yellowlees PM, Holloway KM, Parish MB. Therapy in virtual environments—clinical and ethical issues. Telemed J E Health. 2012;18(7):558–64.
75. Yellowlees PM, Odor A, Patrice K, et al. PsychVACS: a system for asynchronous telepsychiatry. Telemed J E Health. 2011;17(4):299–303.
76. Butler TN, Yellowlees P. Cost analysis of store-and-forward telepsychiatry as a consultation model for primary care. Telemed J E Health. 2012;18(1):74–7.
77. Trudeau M. Mental health apps: like a "therapist in your pocket". NPR mental health, 2010. 28 Feb 2015. At: http://www.npr.org/templates/story/story.php?storyId=127081326.
78. Krämer NC. Nonverbal communication. In: Hartel CR, Blascovich J, editors. Human behavior in military contexts. Washington, DC: The National Academies Press; 2008. p. 150–88.
79. Kim J. Two routes leading to conformity intention in computer-mediated groups: matching versus mismatching virtual representations. J Comput Mediat Commun. 2011;16:271–87.
80. Turkle S. Life on the screen: identity in the age of the internet. New York: Simon & Schuster; 1995.
81. Yee N, Bailenson JN. The proteus effect: the effect of transformed self-representation on behavior. Hum Commun Res. 2007;33:271–90.
82. Yee N, Bailenson JN. The difference between being and seeing: the relative contribution of self perception and priming to behavioral changes via digital self-representation. Media Psychol. 2009;2:195–209.
83. Groom V, Bailenson JN, Nass C. The influence of racial embodiment on racial bias in immersive virtual environments. Soc Infl. 2009;4:1–18.

84. Peck T, Seinfeld S, Aglioti M, et al. Putting yourself in the skin of a black avatar reduces implicit racial bias. Conscious Cogn. 2013;22:779–87.
85. Parks P, Cruz R, Ahn SJ. Don't hurt my avatar: the use and potential of digital self- representation in risk communication. Int J Robots Educ Art. 2014;4(2):11–20.
86. Schroeder R. Social Interaction in virtual environments: key issues, common themes, and a framework for research. In: Schroeder R, editor. The social life of avatars. New York: Springer; 2002. p. 1–18.
87. Bellani M, Fornasari L, Chittaro L, et al. Virtual reality in autism: state of the art. Epidemiol Psychiatr Sci. 2011;20:235–8.
88. Millen L, Cobb S, Patel H. Participatory design approach with children with autism. Int J Disabil Hum Dev. 2011;10:289–94.
89. Parsons S, Cobb S. Who chooses what I need? Child voice and user-involvement in the development of learning technologies for children with autism. In: EPSRC Observatory for Responsible Innovation in ICT, 2013. 28 Feb 2015. At: http://torrii.responsible-innovation.org.uk/resource-detail/1445.
90. Fabri M, Moore DJ. Emotionally expressive avatars for chatting, learning and therapeutic intervention. In: Jacko JA, editor. Human-computer interaction. HCI intelligent multimodal interaction environments lecture notes in computer science. Berlin: Springer; 2007. p. 275–85.
91. Cheng Y, Ye J. Exploring the social competence of students with autism spectrum conditions in a collaborative virtual learning environment – the pilot study. Comput Educ. 2010;54:1068–77.
92. Georgescu AL, Kuzmanovic B, Roth D, et al. The use of virtual characters to assess and train non-verbal communication in high-functioning autism. Front Hum Neurosci. 2014;8:807.
93. Bloustien GF, Wood D. Face, authenticity, transformations and aesthetic in second life. Body Soc. 2013;19(1):52–81.
94. Boye SM. The virtual self: exploring the influence of virtual worlds on self-concept and psychological well-being: a qualitative study, 2014. 28 Feb 2015. At: http://essay.utwente.nl/64770/1/Boye%2C%20S.M.%20-%20s1099337%20%28verslag%29.pdf.
95. Seung AJ. Avatars mirroring the actual self versus projecting the ideal self: the effects of self-priming on interactivity and immersion in an exergame. Wii fit CyberPsychol Behav. 2009;12(6):761–5.
96. Klin A, Jones W, Schultz R, et al. The enactive mind, or from actions to cognition: lessons from autism. Philos Philos Trans R Soc Lond B Biol Sci. 2003;358(1430):345–60.
97. Leff J, Williams G, Huckvale M, et al. Avatar therapy for persecutory auditory hallucinations: what is and how does it work? Psychosis. 2014;6(2):166–76.
98. Kenrick TD, Gutierres SE. Contrast effects and judgments of physical attractiveness: when beauty becomes a social problem. J Pers Soc Psychol. 1980;38(1):131–40.
99. Leding JK. The contrast effect with avatars. Comput I Hum Behav. 2015;44:118–23.

Cognitive Behavioural Therapy and Cognitive Bias Modification in Internet-Based Interventions for Mood, Anxiety and Substance Use Disorders

Matthijs Blankers, Elske Salemink, and Reinout W. Wiers

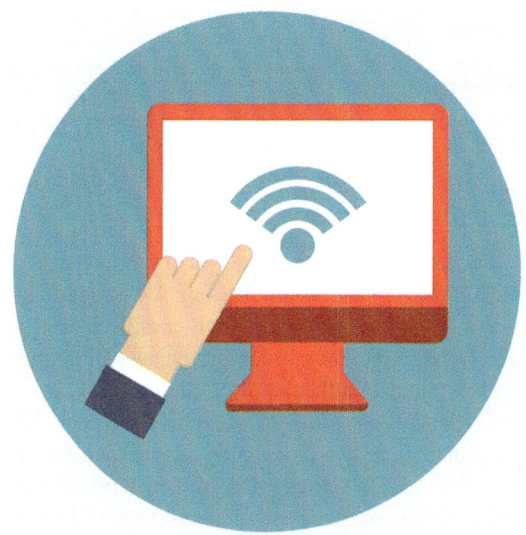

M. Blankers, PhD (✉)
Arkin Mental Health Care, Department of Research, PO Box 75848,
Amsterdam, 1070 AV, The Netherlands

Trimbos-institute, Netherlands Institute of Mental Health and Addiction,
Department of Drug Monitoring, Utrecht, The Netherlands

Academic Medical Centre, Department of Psychiatry, Amsterdam, The Netherlands
e-mail: mblankers@trimbos.nl

E. Salemink, PhD • R.W. Wiers, PhD
Addiction Development and Psychopathology (ADAPT)-Lab, Department of Psychology,
University of Amsterdam, Amsterdam, The Netherlands

© Springer International Publishing Switzerland 2016
D. Mucic, D.M. Hilty (eds.), *e-Mental Health*,
DOI 10.1007/978-3-319-20852-7_10

Contents

10.1 Introduction 194
10.2 Theoretical Background of Computerized CBT 196
    10.2.1 Background of CBT 196
    10.2.2 Background of Computerized CBT 197
10.3 Effectiveness of Computerized CBT 198
    10.3.1 Mood Disorders 198
    10.3.2 Anxiety Disorders 199
    10.3.3 Substance Use Disorders 200
10.4 Practical Applications of Computerized CBT 202
10.5 Theoretical Underpinning of Cognitive Bias Modification 202
    10.5.1 Attentional Bias 202
    10.5.2 Interpretive Bias 204
    10.5.3 Action Tendency Bias 205
10.6 Effectiveness of Cognitive Bias Modification 207
    10.6.1 Depression and Anxiety Disorders 207
    10.6.2 Substance Use Disorders 208
10.7 Practical Applications of CBM 208
10.8 Discussion and Conclusions 209
References 209

Abstract

In this chapter, the theoretical background of (computerized) cognitive behavioural therapy (CBT/c-CBT) is presented, along with cognitive bias modification (CBM), a novel set of interventions in which cognitive processes involved in a disorder are directly targeted. Next, the effectiveness of computerized CBT and CBM for common mental health disorders (depression, anxiety disorders and substance use disorders) is evaluated based on recent meta-analyses. Based on the reviewed literature, there is a reasonably strong evidence base for the effectiveness of computerized CBT interventions for depression, anxiety and substance use disorders. The evidence base for stand-alone CBM interventions is not very strong as research findings are heterogeneous – some studies report positive findings whereas others do not. The evidence base for CBM as an adjunct to computerized CBT interventions is accumulating with positive findings regarding the effectiveness. Therefore, it is concluded that based on the currently available evidence, CBM could be a useful add-on to computerized CBT in the clinical treatment of common mental health disorders.

10.1 Introduction

The past 10 years have witnessed a huge growth in the utilization of the Internet to disseminate e-mental health interventions for common mental disorders such as mood disorders, harmful alcohol use and anxiety disorders. Nowadays, a large variety of services and interventions are available, ranging from information provision, screening with tailored advice and unguided self-help modules to multisession guided Internet-based psychotherapy interventions. The advantages are evident: Internet services are ubiquitously accessible, at any time, and costs are low. The possibility of using the services anonymously can be attractive for users as well, especially in case of stigmatized disorders (e.g. substance use disorders, SUDs). Internet services and interventions might therefore contribute to narrow the treatment gap: the relative large proportion of untreated persons with mental health disorders within a given population. For example, less than 10 % of all persons with an alcohol use disorder are in treatment in Europe [1], while the economic costs of SUDs including alcohol use are among the highest of all mental and brain problems in Europe [2].

From this perspective, it is somewhat surprising that the implementation of Internet services has not been disseminated more widely yet, in particular in regions with suboptimal access to mental health facilities. This cannot be caused by a lack evidence on the effectiveness of Internet interventions for common mental disorders. The development and implementation of Internet interventions has been accompanied by many randomized clinical trials (RCTs) and other research projects. The evidence for the effectiveness and cost-effectiveness of many interventions has been demonstrated in recent reviews and meta-analyses [3–7] – although effects are often of modest size. Still, given the high prevalence of common mental disorders, the potential economic gains are enormous [4].

Many of the tested and implemented e-mental health interventions for common mental disorders are based on cognitive behavioural therapy (CBT) [8]. CBT has primarily been developed as a method to treat depression by Aaron Beck in the 1960s, while he was a psychiatrist at the University of Pennsylvania [9]. Since then, CBT has established itself as the therapeutic underpinning of many psychotherapy interventions and protocols, and more recently (computerized) CBT has become one of the standard therapeutic orientations for Internet interventions. In general, we have mainly seen a process of assimilation in the developmental trajectory from traditional face-to-face interventions for common mental disorders to technology- and Internet-enabled interventions in the last decade. In analogy to Piaget's theory of cognitive development [10], new technology is currently incorporated in already existing cognitive schemas, without changing the overall schemas of treatment. In terms of Internet interventions, digital technology is often used to deliver the traditional, previously existing CBT intervention content that has already been delivered for years or even decades to address a variety of disorders. What this field may profit from, in the same analogy from cognitive development, would be accommodation. This would be a process of incorporating new developments by altering existing cognitive schemas in order to fit in these new developments. In terms of Internet interventions, this would encompass that the content of the interventions itself is enhanced, to optimally utilize technology. The guiding question should be: "What kinds of new interventions are now possible if we use new (Internet) technology?" instead of "How can we offer existing interventions using this new technology?"

Over the past two decades many of the new findings in clinical psychology stem from neurocognitive research. Neurocognitive findings have led to a number of new, experimental treatment modalities, including technology-enabled interventions such as cognitive bias modification (CBM) as an adjunct to (computerized) CBT [11]. In CBM, a cognitive process involved in the disorder is directly targeted in an intervention. For example, in SUDs, an attentional bias and an approach-bias to substance-related stimuli have been distinguished. Both can be directly targeted in a dedicated computerized intervention, with promising first results (review: [12]). One question we address is whether the advent of technology- and Internet-based interventions proves to be an opportunity for the integration of more recent findings from (clinical) psychology into clinical practice.

In this chapter, the theoretical background of CBT and computerized CBT will first be summarized. Next, the effectiveness of computerized CBT for common mental disorders will be evaluated based on recent meta-analyses. Taking these findings into account, opportunities for accommodation of the current generation of Internet interventions will be explored. Hence, in the second part of this chapter, CBM, which is one of the promising means of accommodating CBT interventions to the technical opportunities provided by Internet technology, will be introduced. The evidence regarding the effectiveness of CBM as an adjunct to (computerized) CBT will be evaluated and advantages and disadvantages of CBM and practical applications of CBM will be discussed. Central theme of this chapter is: Will the advent of technology- and Internet-based interventions prove to be an opportunity to accommodate the clinical practice of common mental disorders to recent psychological research findings?

10.2   Theoretical Background of Computerized CBT

10.2.1 Background of CBT

CBT is a structured, short-term psychotherapy, which aims at solving current problems and in which inaccurate or unhelpful thinking is modified. The therapist tries to find ways to produce cognitive change, for example, through modifying a client's thinking and belief system, behavioural experiments or exposure, in order to produce emotional and behavioural change. CBT was initially developed for depression, but is nowadays being used for a variety of psychopathologies, including anxiety disorders, substance use disorders and eating disorders. The main constituents of a CBT intervention for depression include a focus on problem solving, behavioural activation, identifying, evaluating and responding to depressed and negative thoughts, self-perception and client's future [8].

CBT builds upon previous research in the field of psychology and is based on various theories including those by Karen Horney, Alfred Adler, George Kelly, Albert Ellis, Richard Lazarus and Albert Bandura. CBT itself is a source or predecessor for other therapeutic approaches. Those therapeutic approaches include dialectical behaviour therapy, problem-solving therapy, exposure therapy, behavioural activation and cognitive behaviour modification [8]. Many outcome studies involving CBT have been performed and published, the first one already in 1977 [13]. Nowadays, more than 500 outcome studies report evidence on the efficacy of CBT for various psychiatric disorders, psychological problems or psychological components to medical problems (e.g. pain in cancer patients). Positive results have been found in clinical settings, as well as in other settings such as community settings [14]. In more recent years, computerized CBT interventions have been shown to be effective (e.g. [15]) [8].

There are ten basic principles of CBT: [8, p. 7–11]

1. Cognitive behaviour therapy is based on an ever-evolving formulation of patients' problems and an individual conceptualization of each patient in cognitive terms.
2. Cognitive behaviour therapy requires a sound therapeutic alliance.
3. Cognitive behaviour therapy emphasizes collaboration and active participation.
4. Cognitive behaviour therapy is goal-oriented and problem-focused.
5. Cognitive behaviour therapy initially emphasizes the present.
6. Cognitive behaviour therapy is educative, aims to teach the patient to be her own therapist and emphasizes relapse prevention.
7. Cognitive behaviour therapy aims to be time limited.
8. Cognitive behaviour therapy sessions are structured.
9. Cognitive behaviour therapy teaches patients to identify, evaluate and respond to their dysfunctional thoughts and beliefs.
10. Cognitive behaviour therapy uses a variety of techniques to change thinking, mood and behaviour.

Although the basic principles apply to all patients, CBT can vary depending on the individual client, their problems or disorders, their age or life-stage, gender, intellectual level and cultural background. Also, the goals the client sets, their ability to build a strong therapeutic alliance, their motivation to bring about change and earlier therapeutic experiences shape the contents of each individual therapy [8].

10.2.2 Background of Computerized CBT

Over the past two decades, CBT has on an accumulating scale been offered using digital technology. There are several potential advantages of using computerized CBT (c-CBT) in treatment delivery. Two of the most important potential advantages are enhanced access to evidence-based psychotherapy and a reduction in therapy cost. By decreasing the amount of therapist time needed to achieve significant improvements in symptoms, a greater number of people can receive treatment by trained CBT therapists [16]. Another possible advantage of c-CBT could be that patients are reached who otherwise may not have accepted traditional therapy because of stigma or negative attitudes about treatment. The use of technology may also give patients more control and insight in the flow and progress of their therapy [16].

Yet another potential advantage of using digital technology is to teach the basic principles of CBT or to provide learning opportunities in a way that is more efficient and self-guided than would be possible in traditional therapy [16]. For example, in a recent study on drug-free patients with major depressive disorder [17] it was found that the c-CBT group showed a larger increase in CBT knowledge and a larger improvement in dysfunctional attitudes than the control group which was provided standard CBT, while the total time spent with the therapist was reduced in the c-CBT group compared to the control group. As the digital psychoeducational intervention component in the c-CBT group was designed to educate patients and develop skills through multimedia interactions and interactive exercises, this may also have led to a more consistent and engaging educational component than would typically be the case in standard therapist-led CBT [16].

However, there are also concerns regarding the acceptability and potential adverse consequences of c-CBT in comparison with therapist-led CBT. In a recent review [18], barriers to the uptake of c-CBT were systematically evaluated. The authors focused on the acceptability, accessibility and adverse consequences associated with c-CBT. Among the main results, the authors report that recruited patients have only a 38 % chance of actually starting c-CBT, with little data on why this is. When patients do start therapy, personal circumstances still negatively influence adherence in many. Though travel is eliminated by Internet-based c-CBT, time to participate in the intervention is still a limiting factor. Some additional concerns are coined regarding the accessibility to the technology – it is not known how screen readers (for partially sighted users) cope with c-CBT interventions. Also, some patients might find computerized therapy too demanding, patronizing or fast-paced and might prefer face-to-face therapy [18].

10.3 Effectiveness of Computerized CBT

Over the past decade, many RCTs on the effectiveness of various forms of c-CBT have been performed. In this section, the results with regard to the effectiveness of c-CBT for mood disorders, anxiety disorders and SUDs will briefly be reviewed.

10.3.1 Mood Disorders

There is compelling evidence that both guided (therapist or counsellor supported) and unguided Internet-based self-help efficaciously reduces (subclinical) mood disorders [3, 19–22]. Most of the research has focused on interventions to address symptoms of depression. Guided CBT Internet interventions for depression show similar effect sizes as regular face-to-face therapy [22]. In general, guided Internet interventions lead to larger reductions in symptoms than unguided interventions [21], although exceptions do exist [23, 24].

Probably the best known Internet-based CBT intervention for depression is MoodGYM. MoodGYM is an innovative, interactive Web program designed to prevent depression. It consists of five modules, an interactive game, anxiety and depression assessments, downloadable relaxation audio, a workbook and feedback assessment. MoodGYM was designed and developed by staff at the National

Institute for Mental Health Research at The Australian National University, in collaboration with researchers, mental health experts, Web and graphic designers and software engineers [25]. MoodGYM is available in Chinese, Dutch, English, Finnish and Norwegian. There is some evidence that MoodGYM is helpful for its users [26, 27]. One trial also found that the effects are still observable after 12 months [28].

Another evidence-based Internet intervention for symptoms of depression is the Dutch intervention "Kleur je leven" (Colour your life). Colour your life comprises eight modules and is based on CBT. Both a guided and an unguided version of this intervention have been shown to be effective in reducing symptoms of depression compared to an untreated waiting list [29, 30]. There is also some evidence regarding favourable cost-effectiveness of the guided version of Colour your life in comparison to a brief intervention provided by the general practitioner – although differences in effects were not found to be significant [31].

10.3.2 Anxiety Disorders

There are few systematic reviews and meta-analyses on Internet-based interventions for anxiety disorders. In their systematic review on Internet interventions for depression and anxiety, Griffiths and colleagues [32] found 16 trials in which anxiety disorders were addressed. Disorders included panic disorder, social phobia, and post-traumatic stress disorder (PTSD). Most interventions involved some level of therapist guidance, with two interventions that included face-to-face contacts. All interventions were based on CBT. Effect sizes were relatively heterogenic and ranged from 0.29 to 1.74 for participants with a diagnosed anxiety disorder. The authors concluded that guided and unguided Internet interventions for anxiety disorders are promising as self-help applications [32]. A meta-analysis by Cuijpers and colleagues [6] tested the hypothesis that Internet-based CBT for anxiety disorders is as effective as face-to-face CBT. Included studies tested Internet-based stand-alone computer, palm top or virtual reality psychotherapy interventions for adults. Addressed disorders were panic/agoraphobia, social phobia, spider phobia, flight phobia, mixed phobias, post-traumatic stress disorder and obsessive-compulsive disorder. It was found that there was no significant difference between computer-aided and face-to-face psychotherapies at post-intervention (13 studies) or at 1–3 month (three studies) or 6 month follow-ups (six studies). Drop-out rates did not significantly differ between computer-aided psychotherapy and face-to-face psychotherapy either (eight studies). The authors concluded that computer-aided psychotherapy was as effective as face-to-face psychotherapy, although a cautionary note was made regarding the results in the light of a number of methodological limitations [6]. In another review in which CBT was the dominant therapeutic tradition, Christensen and colleagues [33] concluded that recent studies have confirmed the utility of computerized interventions for anxiety. Future research should focus on identifying the active constituents of effective programmes, evaluate programmes targeted at specific populations and focus on clarifying what the optimal degree of guidance in these interventions is [19]. Two recent reviews [7, 34] report some preliminary positive results regarding the cost-effectiveness of Internet-based CBT for anxiety disorders, although the amount of evidence is rather limited.

10.3.3 Substance Use Disorders

Most of the research on Internet-based CBT interventions for SUDs has focused on interventions to reduce alcohol use or tobacco smoking. Based on a recent meta-analysis of RCTs [4], both guided and unguided CBT Internet interventions for problem drinking can be considered effective. Most of the RCTs have tested the effectiveness of unguided alcohol Internet interventions. Many of the studies indicate a small positive effect of unguided Internet-based interventions in comparison to waitlisted participants or information-only control condition [4]. There is at least one study however that fails to find evidence for effectiveness [35]. With regard to Internet-based therapy interventions addressing alcohol use, fewer studies have been performed, although the available studies show positive effects. Effect sizes of guided Internet interventions tend to be larger than unguided Internet interventions for problem drinkers [36–38], although this is not always found [4]. There are some studies on the cost-effectiveness of Internet-based CBT interventions for problem drinking. One study tested the effect of c-CBT as adjunct to a CBT in a RCT, and reported support for the cost-effectiveness of a therapist-guided Internet-based CBT intervention in comparison with the same intervention offered as self-help, without guidance [39], against a conventional cost per quality-adjusted life year (€15.000 and up) (see Fig. 10.1 for a schematic impression of the therapeutic elements of the intervention). Another study [40] used a modelling approach to present the public health cost and effects of wide implementation of Internet-based alcohol interventions in the Netherlands. The interventions on which the effects in this study were based use CBT techniques. It was found that the cost-effectiveness of the health care system to address alcohol use disorders would improve after further implementation of Internet-based alcohol interventions [40].

For smoking cessation, a number of Internet interventions have been developed and tested in RCTs. CBT and associated intervention approaches (e.g. acceptance and commitment therapy [41]) are together with techniques stemming from motivational interviewing the dominant therapeutic approach [5]. Two meta-analyses [42, 43] and a Cochrane review [5] indicate positive results of guided and unguided Internet interventions for smoking cessation in comparison to waiting list controls or minimal information-based interventions, although a substantial minority of the studies fails to find an effect, and the effect sizes of those studies that do find an effect are small. Some authors [43] conclude that only Internet interventions aiming at tobacco smokers who are motivated to quit tend to show positive results. A recent cost-effectiveness review on computer and other electronic aids for smoking cessation [44] indicates that making electronic support available to smokers actively seeking to quit is highly likely to be cost-effective. This is true if the computer intervention is delivered alongside brief advice as well as in combination with more intensive counselling [44].

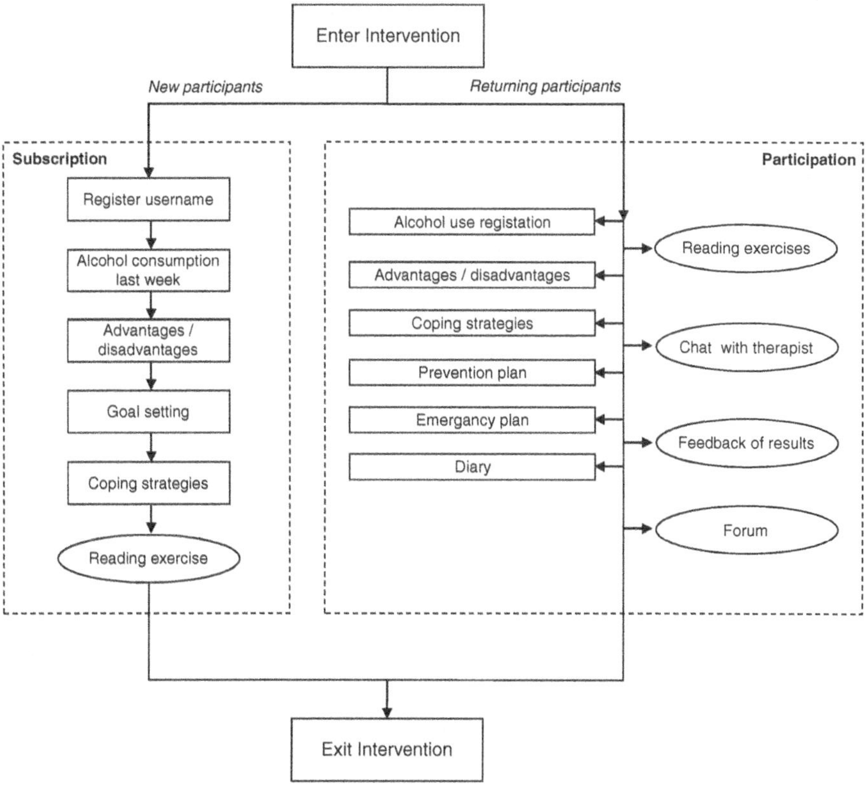

Fig. 10.1 Schematic representation of a CBT-based Alcohol Internet Intervention. Note. Figure 10.1 presents the different modules and exercises of CBT-based Alcohol Internet Intervention (see [39]). During the subscription procedure, the participant is first asked to report his or her alcohol use in the last week. Next, the advantages and disadvantages of drinking and moderation are reviewed. Then a personal goal is set: to moderate alcohol use, or to abstain from drinking. After the personal drinking goals are set, attention is focused on how this goal can be achieved. To conclude the subscription procedure, a reading exercise is provided on how to cope with alcohol craving. Only after subscription is completed, participants can enter the "participant area". Here, the six main treatment modules, four reading exercises and a result feedback page are available. In the therapist-led version of the intervention, a chat module is available for the participant and the therapist to have one-on-one chat therapy contact. A forum provides opportunities for peer-support or for reading previous posts of fellow intervention participants

For substances other than alcohol and tobacco the amount of research is limited. A German RCT on the unguided Internet-intervention "Quit the Shit"-intervention aimed at reducing cannabis use resulted in a significant decrease in use, three months after randomization [45]. In a recent RCT performed in Switzerland on unguided Internet-based CBT to address cocaine use found no difference between intervention and control group, 6 weeks after randomization [46]. However, both studies suffered from a relatively large number of participants who discontinued their participation in the study.

10.4   Practical Applications of Computerized CBT

All in all, after consideration of the advantages and disadvantages of (Internet-based) c-CBT, the British National Institute of Health and Clinical Excellence (NICE) has recommended a selection of e-mental health interventions for the delivery of c-CBT accessed via a referral from a general practitioner (GP). Three of the recommended interventions address depression (Beating the Blues, COPE and Overcoming Depression), one addresses panic/phobia (FearFighter) and one addresses obsessive-compulsive disorder (OCFighter) [47]. One of the considerations that have led to this decision is that the availability of c-CBT programmes permits increased treatment flexibility, especially for individuals who do not wish to interact with a therapist face-to-face. According to NICE, c-CBT can also be used to support therapist sessions. c-CBT may also be of benefit to individuals with, for example, agoraphobia or social phobias as it can be delivered at home. A minimal amount of therapist time is necessary for the c-CBT interventions that can be conducted at home, and the therapy has 24-h availability for the individual to access the interventions at his or her convenience [47].

10.5   Theoretical Underpinning of Cognitive Bias Modification

Positive effects have been reported regarding Internet-based CBT interventions, although further accommodation to what is possible when using computer technology would be desirable. A promising development in this regard could be to supplement c-CBT with CBM. In the following sections, the theoretical underpinning and the effectiveness and possibilities of interventions based on CBM (specifically attentional bias modification, interpretive bias modification and action tendency bias modification) will therefore be discussed. Cognitive theories argue that biases in information processing (attentional bias, interpretive bias and action tendency bias) play a crucial role in psychopathology [48, 49]. CBM started from the perspective of investigating the causal status of these cognitive processes in relation to a disorder.

10.5.1 Attentional Bias

In their seminal first study, MacLeod and colleagues [50] selected students with a medium anxiety level, and randomly assigned them to one of two conditions: one in which their attention was trained towards threatening stimuli, and one in which their attention was trained away from threatening stimuli. They did this by modifying an assessment instrument (visual probe test). In the original test, the probe to which the participant reacts (e.g. an arrow pointing up or down) appears equally often in the location of a threat stimulus and by a neutral stimulus. The attentional bias (AB) is then calculated by subtracting the reaction time on threat trials from the reaction time to non-threat trials. In a modification or training version of the task, a contingency is introduced, with the probe appearing more often on the location occupied by the threat stimulus (to induce a bias), or more often on the location occupied by the neutral stimulus (to reduce a bias) (See Fig. 10.2 for an example in the field of alcohol use). Results across two studies indicated that the attentional

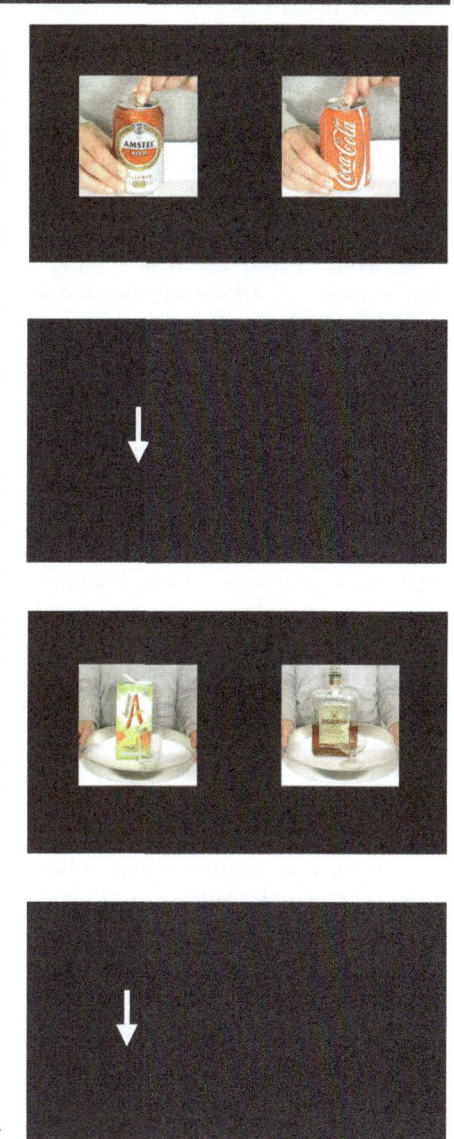

ATTENTIONAL BIAS ASSESSMENT AND TRAINING

An alcoholic and soft drink picture are simultaneously presented on screen.

An arrow appears on the location of one of the pictures. The participant needs to indicate as quickly and accurately as possible whether the arrow points up or down.

Whena correct answer is given, the next trial starts.

In the assessment version, the arrow appears equally often on the location of the alcohol and soft drink picture. In the training version, the arrow appears (almost) always on the location of the soft drink picture.

Fig. 10.2 Attentional bias assessment and training

bias modification had been successful, as assessed with different stimuli in the same task (close generalization), and further generalization was found in a subsequent stress inducing task, with participants in the attend threat condition showing greater distress than participants in the attend neutral condition [50]. Subsequent research in this domain investigated clinical applications, typically with multiple training sessions, with recent successful studies in clinically anxious patient groups [51, 52], and in unselected and targeted prevention (respectively [53]; [54]). However, it should be noted that after initial successes, many recent large Internet-studies on retraining attentional bias in patients with anxiety disorders or SUDs were less successful.

While studies examining attentional retraining in the field of anxiety have proliferated, testing the effects of this training in depression has lagged behind. One of the first studies revealed that multiple sessions of attentional retraining in dysphoric students resulted in small improvements in symptoms in students with mild depressive symptoms, but increased depressive symptoms in students with moderate to severe symptoms (Experiment 1; [55]). In a sample of depressed in- and outpatients (Experiment 2; [55]) the attentional retraining was unsuccessful in changing attentional bias and depressive symptoms. The findings in mildly depressed students were replicated [56]; there was a stronger decrease in depressive symptoms in individuals who had received the training, and these effects were mediated by change in attentional bias. Generally, effects in anxiety have been stronger than in depression. A recent meta-analysis evaluating the clinical effectiveness of attentional retraining in anxiety and depression [57] also indicated that observed effects on symptoms were mainly driven by studies on anxiety. Subsequent research applied the same logic of attentional retraining in SUDs, with initial studies testing the effect of a single session attentional bias manipulation (see Fig. 10.2). The effects of single session training across studies and substances (alcohol, smoking) can be summarized as follows: like a threat-related attentional bias, a substance-related attentional bias can be manipulated in both directions [58], but the effects do not generalize to untrained stimuli, nor to behaviour [59–61].

10.5.2 Interpretive Bias

In a similar vein, another cognitive bias was addressed in manipulation studies: an interpretation bias. Mathews and Mackintosh [62] developed a scenario-based training to modify interpretations. Participants read ambiguous social scenarios, for which half of the participants were required to generate emotionally positive outcomes, and the remaining half negative outcomes. The scenarios were three lines of text in length and remained ambiguous in terms of their emotional meaning until the final word of the text. This last word was a word fragment, the completion of which produced either a positive or negative disambiguation of the scenario. Because there was only one possible meaningful solution for each fragment, participants were forced to disambiguate the fragment in either a benign or a threatening way. Their studies with mid-range anxious students revealed that the training is capable of changing interpretations and subsequently affecting self-reported anxiety. These effects have been replicated [63] and extended to anxious populations [64–66]. Importantly, it has been shown that effects on trait anxiety were mediated by change in interpretations [67]. Note that while these effects on interpretations are consistently found, effects on emotions have been more mixed (for a review see [68]). Meta-analyses have indicated that mental imagery might increase training effects [69]. In the context of depression, interpretation retraining has been used in a more imagery-based format, where positive scenarios were presented auditorily (e.g. [70]). Several studies have shown positive effects on mood in healthy adults [71] and depressive symptoms in clinical populations [70, 72], while there is some evidence that SUDs are associated with substance-related interpretive bias [73, 74], and initial attempts are made to apply this technique in SUDs [75].

10.5.3 Action Tendency Bias

In the field of SUDs, however, a third cognitive bias was addressed–an action tendency to approach disorder-related stimuli. This bias has been observed with different instruments, for different substances, including alcohol [76, 77], cannabis use [78, 79] and cigarette smoking [80]. Applying the same logic as developed in attentional retraining, Wiers and colleagues developed a training version of the alcohol approach avoidance task [81]. This task started with an equal contingency. Half of the alcohol pictures and half of the non-alcohol pictures were to be responded to by pulling a joystick towards themselves, the other half were to be pushed away. Participants react to a feature of the stimulus unrelated to the contents, for example, the format or a little tilt left or right (see Fig. 10.3). Without notification, the contingencies changed, so that half of the (socially drinking) students were pulling most of the alcohol pictures (approach alcohol condition), and the other half were pushing most of the alcohol pictures (avoid alcohol condition). This brief intervention resulted in generalized effects, both to untrained pictures in the same task and to a different test of associations using words rather than pictures (the alcohol approach/ avoidance Implicit Association Test –IAT, see [82]). Moreover, those heavier drinking students whose approach-bias was successfully retrained towards avoidance drank less beer in a subsequent taste test than those heavier drinking students trained towards approaching beer [81].

In a first clinical application of this approach-bias retraining paradigm [83], 214 alcohol dependent patients were randomly assigned to one of two experimental conditions, in which they were trained to avoid alcohol (with or without explicit instruction, which did not differ for the results), or to one of two control conditions, in which they received no training or sham training (which also did not differ for the results). Four sessions of training preceded regular inpatient treatment, primarily CBT. In the experimental conditions only, patients' approach-bias changed into an avoidance bias for alcohol. This effect generalized to untrained pictures in the task used and to an IAT, in which alcohol and soft drink words were categorized with approach and avoidance words. Patients in the experimental conditions showed better treatment outcomes a year later (13 % less relapse), which was significant after controlling for gender. The clinical effect was not significantly related to either the

ACTION TENDENCY ASSESSMENT AND TRAINING

An alcoholic or softdrink
picture is presented on
screen; slightly tilted to the
left or right.

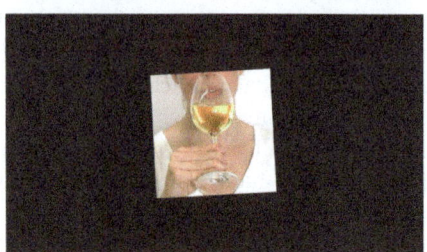

Participants need to respond,
as quickly and accurately as
possible, to the orientation of
the picture. Pictures tilted to
the left should be pushed
(and the picture shrinks in
size), pictures tiled to the
right should be pulled (and
the picture increases in size)

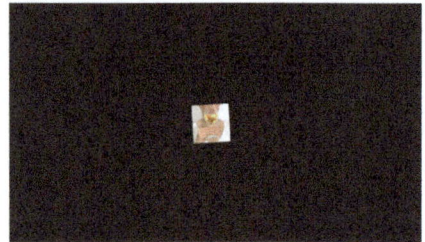

When the correct response is
given, the next trial starts.

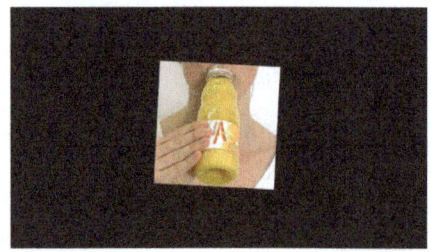

In the assessment version,
alcoholic and softdrink
pictures are equally often
presented in the push and
pull format. In the training
version, all alcoholic pictures
are presented in the push
format, and all softdrink
pictures in the pull format.

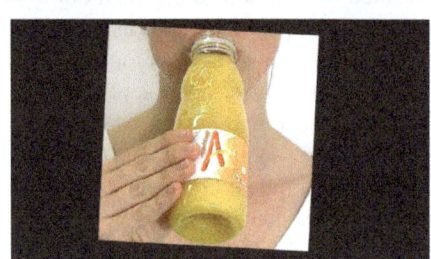

Fig. 10.3 Alcohol approach avoidance task

change of bias as assessed with the AAT or with the IAT, although further analyses
did confirm mediation by a subset of responses in the approach/avoid IAT [84]. In a
recent replication study [11], 509 alcohol-dependent patients received either 12 sessions of approach-bias retraining or no training (sham training was left out because

no difference was found between sham training and no training in [83]). Clinical effects 1 year after treatment discharge were again found (now 9 % less relapse), and in this study mediation and moderation were both found: the effect on clinical outcome was mediated by a change in the approach-bias for alcohol, and the strongest training-effect was found for participants with the strongest approach-bias for alcohol, who received the training. While these effects of CBM as adjunct to clinical CBT treatment are promising, a recent online-only study found no differential effects of CBM (attentional retraining or approach-bias retraining) as compared with placebo training; participants in all conditions reduced their drinking [85]. This suggests that a combination with CBT is necessary to obtain differential effects [12, 85]. For that reason, the combination of online CBT and CBM appears promising and is currently being tested in an RCT [86]. Recently, researchers have started investigating the potential of action tendency training in the field of anxiety with some initial promising results with respect to contamination fear [87] and social phobia [88, 89].

10.6   Effectiveness of Cognitive Bias Modification

10.6.1 Depression and Anxiety Disorders

In contrast to CBM in addiction where the added value of CBM on top of CBT has often been investigated, anxiety-related CBM has most often been applied as a stand-alone intervention. Two studies have examined the effectiveness of combining attentional retraining with CBT and results suggested that attentional retraining does not improve treatment outcome [90, 91] (but see [92] for augmentation effects in anxious children). However, in both studies, attentional retraining failed to modify attentional bias with attentional retraining. This is an important point. While it has been argued that attentional retraining is unsuccessful in the domain of anxiety [93], further analyses of results indicated that, in line with the theoretical rationale of CBM, those studies in which the bias was successfully changed almost invariably also demonstrated clinical effects, while the studies in which the bias was not successfully changed did not [94].

A recent meta-analysis revealed small effect sizes for CBM in anxiety and depression, with often non-significant effects when outliers were excluded [95]. Note, however, that CBM's effectiveness was moderated by several factors. CBM targeting interpretations was more successful than CBM targeting attentional bias (see also [96]). CBM significantly affected anxiety and depression in subclinical samples, but not in clinical samples [95]. However, that latter finding is inconsistent with another recent meta-analysis specifically directed at the clinical efficacy of attentional retraining [97], which provides support for attentional retraining as a novel evidence-based treatment for anxiety disorders. Both meta-analyses revealed that "location of training" significantly moderated its effectiveness; training was more effective in the lab [95] or in the clinic [97] compared to home-based training. As home-based training is often accomplished online, these data suggest that it might be a challenge to successfully use CBM online.

10.6.2 Substance Use Disorders

There are no meta-analyses on CBM in addiction yet. However, as summarized above and in a recent review [12], the findings so far can be summarized as follows: studies of a single session of CBM have generally not yielded good results; while the bias could be trained, effects did not generalize to untrained stimuli or to behaviour (with some exceptions: [81, 98, 99]). In clinical samples, CBM has been added to CBT for alcohol use disorders in three studies [81, 83, 100], all of which found improved clinical outcomes for patients to whom CBM was given on top of CBT, in comparison with patients who did not receive CBM or received a placebo/sham control version. However, when used as a Web-based stand-alone intervention, CBM did not reduce alcohol use and problems more than the placebo-training variety [85]. Note that a different type of training over the Internet, working memory training, did show some differential effects in reducing alcohol use and problems, in a subgroup of participants with strong automatically activated positive associations with alcohol (moderated mediation [101]), and the same intervention also showed promise in a clinical sample of stimulant use disorder patients [102]. However, this type of training is much longer (typically 25 sessions vs. CBM 4–12 sessions) and more tedious, which limits its applicability. Hence, the picture so far is that CBM is a useful add-on to CBT in the clinical treatment of SUD, with improved clinical outcomes. However, there is no evidence so far that it can work as a stand-alone intervention, and should rather be seen as a useful add-on to regular CBT.

10.7   Practical Applications of CBM

One advantage of CBM is that it may be particularly helpful for patients for whom CBT alone is not sufficient, because they have trouble acting on their higher-order goals (to remain abstinent), in the face of temptations. Indeed, there is a literature in non-SUD adolescents that in those individuals with relatively poor executive control, automatically activated cognitive processes are a more important predictor of substance use and problems than in adolescents with well-developed executive control functions [103–106]. This would suggest that CBM is especially useful for participants with relatively weak executive control functions (for an indication in anxiety, see [107]). However, this was not confirmed in the recent large trial [11], while better results were found for older participants (which could have suppressed the effects of executive control, the measure used was also not optimal). Second, adding CBM would seem especially useful for those with a strong bias (moderation). This has been confirmed in a large study [11], but it should be noted that the reliability of the measures is relatively poor, permitting no prediction yet at the individual level. Perhaps new variance-based scoring algorithms (cf., [108]) might increase the usefulness of matching patients to targeted CBM on their pretest bias scores.

Regarding disadvantages, one important caveat to the usefulness of CBM as an add-on to (online) CBT is that many patients regard the training as boring and useless, especially attentional retraining using varieties of the visual probe test [109].

One way out is to increase motivation to train by providing information on the effects of automatically triggered processes in a motivational interviewing style, thus increasing motivation to train (see [110]). Another way is to develop more engaging playful varieties of training (e.g. [53, 111]) and/or to introduce game elements (review: [112]). However, while this may increase motivation to train, we believe it is also essential to link the training to further treatment goals, as activated in CBT.

10.8   Discussion and Conclusions

In this chapter, the theoretical background and effectiveness of clinical applications of c-CBT and CBM have been discussed. Based on the reviewed literature, there is a reasonably strong evidence base for the effectiveness of c-CBT interventions for depression, anxiety and substance use disorders. Evidence regarding the cost-effectiveness is accumulating. The evidence base for stand-alone CBM interventions is not very strong as research findings are heterogeneous. The evidence base for CBM as an adjunct to c-CBT interventions is accumulating with (in general) positive findings regarding the effectiveness, in alcohol use disorders. Recently, studies have evaluated the delivery of CBT and CBM interventions using mobile devices such as smart phones and tablets. Two recent reviews on mobile apps for the delivery of health interventions including depression, anxiety disorders and SUDs concluded that the evidence regarding those interventions is not yet strong [113, 114]. Among the therapeutic orientations present in the evaluated mobile interventions was CBT. Also CBM could be administered using mobile devices based on at least two recently published studies on reducing social anxiety [115] and smoking cessation [116]. In both studies the bias was successfully changed, but no effects on behaviour could be reported. This was not surprising in the study on smoking, as these were smokers who did not intend to quit. Another promising future development is the optimization of the integration of CBM with c-CBT. To what extent can CBM and c-CBT create the synergy needed to interfere with dominant action tendencies in an emotional situation (e.g. negative mood, desire)? All in all, attempts at answering this question will lead to advancement in the delivery of mental health interventions and progress in the accommodation of depression, anxiety and SUDs to the possibilities of computer technology. Based on the currently available evidence, CBM is an interesting tool to study further as an add-on to c-CBT in the treatment of common mental health disorders.

References

1. Rehm J, Shield KD, Rehm MX, Gmel G, Frick U. Modelling the impact of alcohol dependence on mortality burden and the effect of available treatment interventions in the European Union. Eur Neuropsychopharmacol. 2013;23:89–97.
2. Effertz T, Mann K. The burden and cost of disorders of the brain in Europe with the inclusion of harmful alcohol use and nicotine addiction. Eur Neuropsychopharmacol. 2013;23(7):742–8.

3. Andrews G, Cuijpers P, Craske MG, McEvoy P, Titov N. Computer therapy for the anxiety and depressive disorders is effective, acceptable and practical health care: a meta-analysis. PLoS One. 2010;5(10):e13196.
4. Riper H, Blankers M, Hadiwijaya H, Cunningham J, Clarke S, Wiers R, Ebert D, Cuijpers P. Effectiveness of guided and unguided low-intensity internet interventions for adult alcohol misuse: a meta-analysis. PLoS One. 2014;9(6):e99912.
5. Civljak M, Stead LF, Hartmann-Boyce J, Sheikh A, Car J. Internet-based interventions for smoking cessation. Cochrane Database Syst Rev. 2013;(7):CD007078.
6. Cuijpers P, Marks IM, van Straten A, Cavanagh K, Gega L, Andersson G. Computer-aided psychotherapy for anxiety disorders: a meta-analytic review. Cogn Behav Ther. 2009;38(2):66–82.
7. Hedman E, Ljótsson B, Lindefors N. Cognitive behavior therapy via the Internet: a systematic review of applications, clinical efficacy and cost-effectiveness. Expert Rev Pharmacoecon Outcomes Res. 2012;12(6):745–64.
8. Beck JS. Cognitive behavior therapy: basics and beyond. 2nd ed. New York: The Guilford Press; 2011.
9. Beck Institute. History of cognitive therapy. Accessed: 6 Feb 2015. URL: https://archive.today/MkHiX.
10. Piaget J, Cook MT. The origins of intelligence in children. New York: International University Press; 1952.
11. Eberl C, Wiers RW, Pawelczack S, Rinck M, Becker ES, Lindenmeyer J. Approach bias modification in alcohol dependence: do clinical effects replicate and for whom does it work best? Dev Cogn Neurosci. 2013;4:38–51.
12. Wiers RW, Gladwin TE, Hofmann W, Salemink E, Ridderinkhof KR. Cognitive bias modification and cognitive control training in addiction and related psychopathology mechanisms, clinical perspectives, and ways forward. Clin Psychol Sci. 2013;1(2):192–212.
13. Rush AJ, Beck AT, Kovacs M, Hollon SD. Comparative efficacy of cognitive therapy and pharmacotherapy in the treatment of depressed outpatients. Cogn Ther Res. 1977;1(1):7–37.
14. Stirman SW, Buchhofer R, McLaulin JB, Evans AC, Beck AT. The Beck initiative: a public academic collaborative partnership to implement cognitive therapy in a community behavioral health system. Psychiatr Serv. 2009;60:1302–4.
15. Khanna MS, Kendall PC. Computer-assisted cognitive behavioral therapy for child anxiety: results of a randomized clinical trial. J Consult Clin Psychol. 2010;78(5):737–45.
16. Spurgeon JA, Wright JH. Computer-assisted cognitive-behavioral therapy. Curr Psychiatry Rep. 2010;12(6):547–52.
17. Wright JH, Wright AS, Albano AM, et al. Computer-assisted cognitive therapy for depression: maintaining efficacy while reducing therapist time. Am J Psychiatry. 2005;162:1158–64.
18. Waller R, Gilbody S. Barriers to the uptake of computerized cognitive behavioural therapy: a systematic review of the quantitative and qualitative evidence. Psychol Med. 2009;39(5):705–12.
19. Blankers M, Donker T, Riper H. E-mental health in Nederland [E-mental health in the Netherlands]. De Psychol. 2013;48:12–23.
20. Johansson R, Sjöberg E, Sjögren M, Johnsson E, Carlbring P, Andersson T, Rousseau A, Andersson G. Tailored vs. standardized internet-based cognitive behavior therapy for depression and comorbid symptoms: a randomized controlled trial. PLoS One. 2012;7(5):e36905.
21. Spek V, Cuijpers P, Nyklícek I, Riper H, Keyzer J, Pop V. Internet-based cognitive behaviour therapy for symptoms of depression and anxiety: a meta-analysis. Psychol Med. 2007;37(3):319–28.
22. Cuijpers P, Donker T, van Straten A, Li J, Andersson G. Is guided self-help as effective as face-to-face psychotherapy for depression and anxiety disorders? A systematic review and meta-analysis of comparative outcome studies. Psychol Med. 2010;40(12):1943–57.
23. Farrer L, Christensen H, Griffiths KM, Mackinnon A. Internet-based CBT for depression with and without telephone tracking in a national helpline: randomised controlled trial. PLoS One. 2011;6(11):e28099.

24. Furmark T, Carlbring P, Hedman E, Sonnenstein A, Clevberger P, Bohman B, Eriksson A, Hållén A, Frykman M, Holmström A, Sparthan E, Tillfors M, Ihrfelt EN, Spak M, Eriksson A, Ekselius L, Andersson G. Guided and unguided self-help for social anxiety disorder: randomised controlled trial. Br J Psychiatry. 2009;195(5):440–7.
25. National Institute for Mental Health Research. MoodGYM website, 2014. URL: https://moodgym.anu.edu.au.
26. Christensen H, Griffiths KM, Jorm AF. Delivering interventions for depression by using the internet: randomised controlled trial. BMJ. 2004;328(7434):265.
27. Lintvedt OK, Griffiths KM, Sørensen K, Østvik AR, Wang CE, Eisemann M, Waterloo K. Evaluating the effectiveness and efficacy of unguided internet-based self-help intervention for the prevention of depression: a randomized controlled trial. Clin Psychol Psychother. 2013;20(1):10–27.
28. Mackinnon A, Griffiths KM, Christensen H. Comparative randomised trial of online cognitive-behavioural therapy and an information website for depression: 12-month outcomes. Br J Psychiatry. 2008;192(2):130–4.
29. Spek V, Nyklíček I, Smits N, Cuijpers P, Riper H, Keyzer J, Pop V. Internet-based cognitive behavioural therapy for subthreshold depression in people over 50 years old: a randomized controlled clinical trial. Psychol Med. 2007;37(12):1797–806.
30. Warmerdam L, van Straten A, Twisk J, Riper H, Cuijpers P. Internet-based treatment for adults with depressive symptoms: randomized controlled trial. J Med Internet Res. 2008;10(4):e44.
31. Gerhards SA, de Graaf LE, Jacobs LE, Severens JL, Huibers MJ, Arntz A, Riper H, Widdershoven G, Metsemakers JF, Evers SM. Economic evaluation of online computerised cognitive-behavioural therapy without support for depression in primary care: randomised trial. Br J Psychiatry. 2010;196(4):310–8.
32. Griffiths KM, Farrer L, Christensen H. The efficacy of internet interventions for depression and anxiety disorders: a review of randomised controlled trials. Med J Aust. 2010;192(11 Suppl):S4–11.
33. Christensen H, Batterham P, Calear A. Online interventions for anxiety disorders. Curr Opin Psychiatry. 2014;27(1):7–13.
34. Arnberg FK, Linton SJ, Hultcrantz M, Heintz E, Jonsson U. Internet-delivered psychological treatments for mood and anxiety disorders: a systematic review of their efficacy, safety, and cost-effectiveness. PLoS One. 2014;9(5):e98118.
35. Wallace P, Murray E, McCambridge J, Khadjesari Z, White IR, Thompson SG, Kalaitzaki E, Godfrey C, Linke S. On-line randomized controlled trial of an internet based psychologically enhanced intervention for people with hazardous alcohol consumption. PLoS One. 2011;6(3):e14740.
36. Blankers M, Koeter MW, Schippers GM. Internet therapy versus internet self-help versus no treatment for problematic alcohol use: a randomized controlled trial. J Consult Clin Psychol. 2011;79(3):330–41.
37. Cunningham JA. Comparison of two internet-based interventions for problem drinkers: randomized controlled trial. J Med Internet Res. 2012;14(4):e107.
38. Postel MG, de Haan HA, ter Huurne ED, Becker ES, de Jong CA. Effectiveness of a web-based intervention for problem drinkers and reasons for dropout: randomized controlled trial. J Med Internet Res. 2010;12(4):e68.
39. Blankers M, Nabitz U, Smit F, Koeter MW, Schippers GM. Economic evaluation of internet-based interventions for harmful alcohol use alongside a pragmatic randomized controlled trial. J Med Internet Res. 2012;14(5):e134.
40. Smit F, Lokkerbol J, Riper H, Majo MC, Boon B, Blankers M. Modeling the cost-effectiveness of health care systems for alcohol use disorders: how implementation of eHealth interventions improves cost-effectiveness. J Med Internet Res. 2011;13(e56).
41. Bricker J, Wyszynski C, Comstock B, Heffner JL. Pilot randomized controlled trial of web-based acceptance and commitment therapy for smoking cessation. Nicotine Tob Res. 2013;15(10):1756–64.

42. Rooke S, Thorsteinsson E, Karpin A, Copeland J, Allsop D. Computer-delivered interventions for alcohol and tobacco use: a meta-analysis. Addiction. 2010;105(8):1381–90.
43. Shahab L, McEwen A. Online support for smoking cessation: a systematic review of the literature. Addiction. 2009;104(11):1792–804.
44. Chen YF, Madan J, Welton N, Yahaya I, Aveyard P, Bauld L, Wang D, Fry-Smith A, Munafò MR. Effectiveness and cost-effectiveness of computer and other electronic aids for smoking cessation: a systematic review and network meta-analysis. Health Technol Assess. 2012;16(38):1–205, iii–v.
45. Tossmann HP, Jonas B, Tensil MD, Lang P, Strüber E. A controlled trial of an internet-based intervention program for cannabis users. Cyberpsychol Behav Soc Netw. 2011;14(11):673–9.
46. Schaub M, Sullivan R, Haug S, Stark L. Web-based cognitive behavioral self-help intervention to reduce cocaine consumption in problematic cocaine users: randomized controlled trial. J Med Internet Res. 2012;14(6):e166.
47. National Institute for Health and Clinical Excellence. Computerised cognitive behaviour therapy for depression and anxiety: review of technology appraisal 51. Updated 2013. London: National Institute for Health and Clinical Excellence; 2006.
48. Mathews A, Mackintosh B. A cognitive model of selective processing in anxiety. Cogn Ther Res. 1998;22(6):539–60.
49. Wiers RW, Bartholow BD, van den Wildenberg E, Thush C, Engels RC, Sher KJ, Grenard J, Ames SL, Stacy AW. Automatic and controlled processes and the development of addictive behaviors in adolescents: a review and a model. Pharmacol Biochem Behav. 2007;86(2):263–83.
50. MacLeod C, Rutherford E, Campbell L, Ebsworthy G, Holker L. Selective attention and emotional vulnerability: assessing the causal basis of their association through the experimental manipulation of attentional bias. J Abnorm Psychol. 2002;111(1):107–23.
51. Amir N, Beard C, Burns M, Bomyea J. Attention modification program in individuals with generalized anxiety disorder. J Abnorm Psychol. 2009;118(1):28–33.
52. Schmidt NB, Richey JA, Buckner JD, Timpano KR. Attention training for generalized social anxiety disorder. J Abnorm Psychol. 2009;118(1):5–14.
53. De Voogd EL, Wiers RW, Prins PJ, Salemink E. Visual search attentional bias modification reduced social phobia in adolescents. J Behav Ther Exp Psychiatry. 2014;45(2):252–9.
54. See J, MacLeod C, Bridle R. The reduction of anxiety vulnerability through the modification of attentional bias: a real-world study using a home-based cognitive bias modification procedure. J Abnorm Psychol. 2009;118(1):65–75.
55. Baert S, De Raedt R, Schacht R, Koster EH. Attentional bias training in depression: therapeutic effects depend on depression severity. J Behav Ther Exp Psychiatry. 2010;41(3):265–74.
56. Wells TT, Beevers CG. Biased attention and dysphoria: manipulating selective attention reduces subsequent depressive symptoms. Cogn Emot. 2010;24(4):719–28.
57. Mogoaşe C, David D, Koster EH. Clinical efficacy of attentional bias modification procedures: an updated meta-analysis. J Clin Psychol. 2014;70(12):1133–57.
58. Field M, Eastwood B. Experimental manipulation of attentional bias increases the motivation to drink alcohol. Psychopharmacology (Berl). 2005;183(3):350–7.
59. Field M, Duka T, Eastwood B, Child R, Santarcangelo M, Gayton M. Experimental manipulation of attentional biases in heavy drinkers: do the effects generalise? Psychopharmacology (Berl). 2007;192(4):593–608.
60. Attwood AS, O'Sullivan H, Leonards U, Mackintosh B, Munafò MR. Attentional bias training and cue reactivity in cigarette smokers. Addiction. 2008;103(11):1875–82.
61. Schoenmakers T, Wiers RW, Jones BT, Bruce G, Jansen AT. Attentional re-training decreases attentional bias in heavy drinkers without generalization. Addiction. 2007;102(3):399–405.
62. Mathews A, Mackintosh B. Induced emotional interpretation bias and anxiety. J Abnorm Psychol. 2000;109(4):602–15.
63. Salemink E, van den Hout M, Kindt M. Trained interpretive bias: validity and effects on anxiety. J Behav Ther Exp Psychiatry. 2007;38(2):212–24.

64. Mathews A, Ridgeway V, Cook E, Yiend J. Inducing a benign interpretational bias reduces trait anxiety. J Behav Ther Exp Psychiatry. 2007;38(2):225–36.
65. Salemink E, van den Hout M, Kindt M. Effects of positive interpretive bias modification in highly anxious individuals. J Anxiety Disord. 2009;23(5):676–83.
66. Steinman SA, Teachman BA. Modifying interpretations among individuals high in anxiety sensitivity. J Anxiety Disord. 2010;24(1):71–8.
67. Salemink E, van den Hout M, Kindt M. How does cognitive bias modification affect anxiety? Mediation analyses and experimental data. Behav Cogn Psychother. 2010;38(1):59–66.
68. Lau JY. Cognitive bias modification of interpretations: a viable treatment for child and adolescent anxiety? Behav Res Ther. 2013;51(10):614–22.
69. Menne-Lothmann C, Viechtbauer W, Höhn P, Kasanova Z, Haller SP, Drukker M, van Os J, Wichers M, Lau JY. How to boost positive interpretations? A meta-analysis of the effectiveness of cognitive bias modification for interpretation. PLoS One. 2014;9(6):e100925.
70. Blackwell SE, Holmes EA. Modifying interpretation and imagination in clinical depression: a single case series using cognitive bias modification. Appl Cogn Psychol. 2010;24:338–50.
71. Rohrbacher H, Blackwell SE, Holmes EA, Reinecke A. Optimizing the ingredients for imagery-based interpretation bias modification for depressed mood: is self-generation more effective than imagination alone? J Affect Disord. 2014;152–154:212–8.
72. Williams AD, Blackwell SE, Mackenzie A, Holmes EA, Andrews G. Combining imagination and reason in the treatment of depression: a randomized controlled trial of internet-based cognitive-bias modification and internet-CBT for depression. J Consult Clin Psychol. 2013;81(5):793–9.
73. Salemink E, Wiers RW. Alcohol-related memory associations in positive and negative affect situations: drinking motives, working memory capacity, and prospective drinking. Psychol Addict Behav. 2014;28(1):105–13.
74. Woud ML, Fitzgerald DA, Wiers RW, Rinck M, Becker ES. 'Getting into the spirit': alcohol-related interpretation bias in heavy-drinking students. Psychol Addict Behav. 2012;26(3):627–32.
75. Woud ML, Hutschemaekers MH, Rinck M, Becker ES. The manipulation of alcohol-related interpretation biases by means of cognitive bias modification – interpretation (CBM-I). J Behav Ther Exp Psychiatry. 2015. pii: S0005-7916(15)00031-2.
76. Field M, Kiernan A, Eastwood B, Child R. Rapid approach responses to alcohol cues in heavy drinkers. J Behav Ther Exp Psychiatry. 2008;39(3):209–18.
77. Wiers RW, Rinck M, Dictus M, van den Wildenberg E. Relatively strong automatic appetitive action-tendencies in male carriers of the OPRM1 G-allele. Genes Brain Behav. 2009;8(1):101–6.
78. Cousijn J, Goudriaan AE, Wiers RW. Reaching out towards cannabis: approach-bias in heavy cannabis users predicts changes in cannabis use. Addiction. 2011;106(9):1667–74.
79. Field M, Eastwood B, Bradley BP, Mogg K. Selective processing of cannabis cues in regular cannabis users. Drug Alcohol Depend. 2006;85:75–82.
80. Wiers CE, Kühn S, Javadi AH, Korucuoglu O, Wiers RW, Walter H, Gallinat J, Bermpohl F. Automatic approach bias towards smoking cues is present in smokers but not in ex-smokers. Psychopharmacology (Berl). 2013;229(1):187–97.
81. Wiers RW, Rinck M, Kordts R, Houben K, Strack F. Retraining automatic action-tendencies to approach alcohol in hazardous drinkers. Addiction. 2010;105(2):279–87.
82. Ostafin BD, Palfai TP. Compelled to consume: the Implicit Association Test and automatic alcohol motivation. Psychol Addict Behav. 2006;20(3):322–7.
83. Wiers RW, Eberl C, Rinck M, Becker ES, Lindenmeyer J. Retraining automatic action tendencies changes alcoholic patients' approach bias for alcohol and improves treatment outcome. Psychol Sci. 2011;22(4):490–7.
84. Gladwin TE, Rinck M, Eberl C, Becker ES, Lindenmeyer J, Wiers RW. Mediation of cognitive bias modification for alcohol addiction via stimulus-specific alcohol avoidance association. Alcohol Clin Exp Res. 2015;39(1):101–7.
85. Wiers RW, Houben K, Fadardi JS, van Beek P, Rhemtulla M, Cox WM. Alcohol cognitive bias modification training for problem drinkers over the web. Addict Behav. 2015;40:21–6.

86. van Deursen DS, Salemink E, Smit F, Kramer J, Wiers RW. Web-based cognitive bias modification for problem drinkers: protocol of a randomised controlled trial with a 2×2×2 factorial design. BMC Public Health. 2013;13:674.
87. Amir N, Kuckertz JM, Najmi S. The effect of modifying automatic action tendencies on overt avoidance behaviors. Emotion. 2013;13(3):478–84.
88. Rinck M, Telli S, Kampmann IL, Woud ML, Kerstholt M, Te Velthuis S, Wittkowski M, Becker ES. Training approach-avoidance of smiling faces affects emotional vulnerability in socially anxious individuals. Front Hum Neurosci. 2013;7:481.
89. Taylor CT, Amir N. Modifying automatic approach action tendencies in individuals with elevated social anxiety symptoms. Behav Res Ther. 2012;50(9):529–36.
90. Rapee RM, MacLeod C, Carpenter L, Gaston JE, Frei J, Peters L, Baillie AJ. Integrating cognitive bias modification into a standard cognitive behavioural treatment package for social phobia: a randomized controlled trial. Behav Res Ther. 2013;51(4–5):207–15.
91. Boettcher J, Hasselrot J, Sund E, Andersson G, Carlbring P. Combining attention training with internet-based cognitive-behavioural self-help for social anxiety: a randomised controlled trial. Cogn Behav Ther. 2014;43(1):34–48.
92. Shechner T, Rimon-Chakir A, Britton JC, Lotan D, Apter A, Bliese PD, Pine DS, Bar-Haim Y. Attention bias modification treatment augmenting effects on cognitive behavioral therapy in children with anxiety: randomized controlled trial. J Am Acad Child Adolesc Psychiatry. 2014;53(1):61–71.
93. Emmelkamp PM. Attention bias modification: the Emperor's new suit? BMC Med. 2012;10:63.
94. Clarke PJ, Notebaert L, MacLeod C. Absence of evidence or evidence of absence: reflecting on therapeutic implementations of attentional bias modification. BMC Psychiatry. 2014;14:8.
95. Cristea IA, Kok RN, Cuijpers P. Efficacy of cognitive bias modification interventions in anxiety and depression: meta-analysis. Br J Psychiatry. 2015;206(1):7–16.
96. Hallion LS, Ruscio AM. A meta-analysis of the effect of cognitive bias modification on anxiety and depression. Psychol Bull. 2011;137(6):940–58.
97. Linetzky M, Pergamin-Hight L, Pine DS, Bar-Haim Y. Quantitative evaluation of the clinical efficacy of attention bias modification treatment for anxiety disorders. Depress Anxiety. 2015;32(6):383–91.
98. Houben K, Nederkoorn C, Wiers RW, Jansen A. Resisting temptation: decreasing alcohol-related affect and drinking behavior by training response inhibition. Drug Alcohol Depend. 2011;116(1–3):132–6.
99. Houben K, Havermans RC, Nederkoorn C, Jansen A. Beer à no-go: learning to stop responding to alcohol cues reduces alcohol intake via reduced affective associations rather than increased response inhibition. Addiction. 2012;107(7):1280–7.
100. Schoenmakers TM, de Bruin M, Lux IF, Goertz AG, Van Kerkhof DH, Wiers RW. Clinical effectiveness of attentional bias modification training in abstinent alcoholic patients. Drug Alcohol Depend. 2010;109(1–3):30–6.
101. Houben K, Wiers RW, Jansen A. Getting a grip on drinking behavior: training working memory to reduce alcohol abuse. Psychol Sci. 2011;22(7):968–75.
102. Bickel WK, Yi R, Landes RD, Hill PF, Baxter C. Remember the future: working memory training decreases delay discounting among stimulant addicts. Biol Psychiatry. 2011;69(3):260–5.
103. Grenard JL, Ames SL, Wiers RW, Thush C, Sussman S, Stacy AW. Working memory capacity moderates the predictive effects of drug-related associations on substance use. Psychol Addict Behav. 2008;22(3):426–32.
104. Thush C, Wiers RW, Ames SL, Grenard JL, Sussman S, Stacy AW. Interactions between implicit and explicit cognition and working memory capacity in the prediction of alcohol use in at-risk adolescents. Drug Alcohol Depend. 2008;94(1–3):116–24.
105. Peeters M, Wiers RW, Monshouwer K, van de Schoot R, Janssen T, Vollebergh WA. Automatic processes in at-risk adolescents: the role of alcohol-approach tendencies and response inhibition in drinking behavior. Addiction. 2012;107(11):1939–46.

106. Peeters M, Monshouwer K, van de Schoot RA, Janssen T, Vollebergh WA, Wiers RW. Automatic processes and the drinking behavior in early adolescence: a prospective study. Alcohol Clin Exp Res. 2013;37(10):1737–44.
107. Salemink E, Wiers RW. Adolescent threat-related interpretive bias and its modification: the moderating role of regulatory control. Behav Res Ther. 2012;50(1):40–6.
108. Zvielli A, Bernstein A, Koster EH. Temporal dynamics of attentional bias. Clin Psychol Sci. 2014 [Epub ahead of print].
109. Beard C, Weisberg RB, Primack J. Socially anxious primary care patients' attitudes toward cognitive bias modification (CBM): a qualitative study. Behav Cogn Psychother. 2012;40(5):618–33.
110. Boffo M, Pronk T, Mannarini S, Wiers RW. Combining cognitive bias modification training with motivational support in alcohol dependent outpatients: study protocol for a randomised controlled trial. BMC Trials. 2015;16:63.
111. Notebaert L, Clarke PJ, Grafton B, MacLeod C. Validation of a novel attentional bias modification task: the future may be in the cards. Behav Res Ther. 2015;65:93–100.
112. Boendermaker WJ, Prins PJ, Wiers RW. Cognitive Bias Modification for adolescents with substance use problems – Can serious games help? J Behav Ther Exp Psychiatry. 2015. [Epub ahead of print].
113. Payne HE, Lister C, West JH, Bernhardt JM. Behavioral functionality of mobile apps in health interventions: a systematic review of the literature. JMIR Mhealth Uhealth. 2015;3(1):e20.
114. Donker T, Petrie K, Proudfoot J, Clarke J, Birch MR, Christensen H. Smartphones for smarter delivery of mental health programs: a systematic review. J Med Internet Res. 2013;15(11):e247.
115. Enock PM, Hofmann SG, McNally RJ. Attention bias modification training via smartphone to reduce social anxiety: a randomized, controlled multi-session experiment. Cogn Ther Res. 2014;38(2):200–16.
116. Kerst WF, Waters AJ. Attentional retraining administered in the field reduces smokers' attentional bias and craving. Health Psychol. 2014;33(10):1232–40.

Psychiatric Apps: Patient Self-Assessment, Communication, and Potential Treatment Interventions

Steven Chan, John B. Torous, Ladson Hinton, and Peter M. Yellowlees

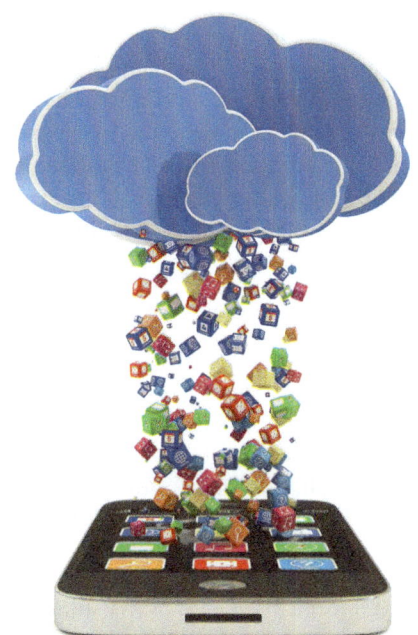

S. Chan, MD, MBA (✉) • L. Hinton, MD • P.M. Yellowlees, MD, MBBS
Department of Psychiatry, University of California,
2230 Stockton Blvd, Sacramento, CA 95817, USA
e-mail: steven@berkeley.edu; steven.chan@ucdmc.ucdavis.edu

J.B. Torous, MD
Department of Psychiatry, Harvard Longwood Psychiatry Residency
Training Program, Boston, MA, USA

© Springer International Publishing Switzerland 2016
D. Mucic, D.M. Hilty (eds.), *e-Mental Health*,
DOI 10.1007/978-3-319-20852-7_11

Contents

11.1   Introduction   218
11.2   Apps in Mental Health..   219
11.3   How Can Patients Track Their Symptoms?...   220
11.4   Keeping in Touch with Clinicians   222
11.5   How Should Clinicians Approach Current App Use by Patients?...............................   223
11.6   What Special Applications Exist for the Military?..   224
11.7   What Drawbacks and Precautions Are There?   224
Conclusion   225
References..   226

Abstract

Mobile device applications can complement traditional stages of mental health treatment, including treatment monitoring, adherence to treatment plans, psychoeducation, symptom assessment and monitoring, and clinical decision support. An increasing number of patients and clinicians have access to smartphones that can run interactive apps (applications). The advent of available wireless networks, more affordable computing, and more ubiquitous computing makes telemedicine a much more cost-effective proposition. We will provide an overview of new technologies and how they can be used in different areas of the psychiatric provider and patient's workflow.

11.1   Introduction

Technology is becoming more ingrained in health services delivery in the United States and offers a novel solution to currently unsustainable increases in healthcare spending. Increasing demand for medical services and a constrained supply of physicians and healthcare practitioners call for greater efficiency, which technology has the potential to provide. These effects also apply globally: through 2030, mental health conditions may cost the global economy $16 trillion in labor and manufacturing productivity [1]. Traditional face-to-face therapy cannot only be costly but may be insufficient alone in addressing population and global health needs. Mental health practices and innovations incorporating informatics and communication technology have been reviewed in the literature and offer the potential of greater care accessibility, reduced ongoing costs, increased personalization, and interactivity [2].

In the United States, the Affordable Care Act and Health Information Technology for Economic and Clinical Health Act's (HITECH) push to boost use of information technology and mandate use of electronic medical records, through the use of financial incentives and punishments that has created increased interest in both academic researchers and commercial sectors in technology's ability to address mental health needs.

Smartphone apps are now ubiquitous in academic medical centers, and there are numerous efforts to advance the use of such apps. Wearable computing has also seen enthusiastic uptake in the commercial space: Samsung has partnered with the University of California, San Francisco (UCSF), and has created open-reference platforms SAMI and SIMBAND [3]. Apple's HealthKit platform also has the potential to boost use of personal health records, partnering with apps, devices, academic institutions, and also the Epic electronic medical record platform [4]. The Google Glass heads-up display has seen numerous adoption and innovation in the healthcare industry [5], including in surgeries [6], emergency departments [7, 8], and even psychiatry [9].

In this chapter, we will review (1) current trends in the commercial marketplaces for mental health-related apps, (2) explore the emerging evidence base for app use in clinical care, (3) discuss how clinicians can approach app use by patients, and (4) conclude by looking at current challenges and barriers as well as potential next steps forward.

11.2 Apps in Mental Health

In mental health, however, uptake of apps has generally been slow. Behavioral health organizations were not eligible to receive any part of the $20.6 billion in financial incentives for implementing health IT. Although behavioral health organizations want to move forward in implementation, both upfront and maintenance costs have been cited as the top barrier towards implementing information technology for psychiatric hospitals, substance use services, and community mental health organizations [10]. It has also been suggested that mental health providers have also resisted adoption of technology [11].

The move towards personalized, precise assessments and interventions [12], the NIMH's recently introduced Research Domain Criteria (RDoC) [13, 14], and initiatives by the US government for the Precision Medicine [15] signal the drive towards more individualized medicine that may be based on epidemiological and consensus-driven algorithms, but driven more on informatics, laboratory medicine, and testing.

Mobile apps for psychiatry, just like telemedicine, have advantages:

- Portability—allowing for care anytime, anywhere, regardless of patient geography and transportation barriers.
- Low cost—inexpensive versus capital-intensive brick-and-mortar facilities and traditional desktop computers.
- Additional features—context-aware interventions and sensors [16] can lead to smart real-time feedback.

Mental health app demand is actually quite high. A multi-site national study of 300 patients in four US census-designated areas showed that older users were less likely to have smartphones and less willing to use them, but even across generations, a majority of respondents were willing to use apps for their mental health conditions

[17]. Similar results of smartphone usage have been shown in a large Boston urban academic outpatient mental health clinic [18]. Those with severe mental illness in a metropolitan Chicago area also used a mobile device, including cell phones, smartphones, and text messaging [19]. However, a similar study in five Tennessee community outpatient settings showed only 17 % of those who owned or shared a smartphone owned smartphones and that the most popular feature was text messaging, and downloading apps was least popular [20]. Differences in patient interest towards mental health apps have not been explored in rural versus urban settings, and the Tennessee results suggest there is still more to learn about patient attitudes and engagement.

Preliminary research suggests a need for more efficacy studies and research progress. The assessments of apps in clinical care may not follow the traditional research paradigms, and a research agenda is suggested in Chap. 6. This lack of clinical studies stands in contrast to the over 5,000 mobile device applications, including symptom tracking, cognitive behavioral therapy, and meditation applications in Apple's App Store for iOS and Google Play-enabled Android devices [21]. Though other platforms exist, such as Tizen, Android-based Fire OS, and QNX-based Blackberry OS, iOS and Android approximately equally make up 95.3 % of smartphones sold in the United States as of 2015 and thus should be the target of interventions [22].

One can categorize mental health apps within three different classifications:

- As a communication medium—for communicating with other patients, caregivers, social supports, or providers
- As an extension of traditional face-to-face clinic—augmenting psychotherapy and medical support with journaling, diaries, symptom tracking tools, and psychoeducation between appointments
- As a smart monitor—with tools that automatically predict relapse behavior or worsening affective symptoms, through sensors and data activity

11.3   How Can Patients Track Their Symptoms?

With the rise of participatory medicine and patient-centric care, patients are more empowered than ever [23]. Apps are equipping patients with new ways to self-assess, monitor, and track their symptoms. Online community groups are providing patients with the ability to share stories and even pool together symptom reporting on platforms from patient-specific sites like PatientsLikeMe to general social networking platforms such as Twitter. A 2015 meta-analysis has shown that social networking sites had a statistically significant positive effect in promoting changes in health-related behaviors [24].

Mobile apps pave the way for patients to practice self-care. As an extension of psychotherapy, symptom-gathering and monitoring apps can give patients a more interactive version of traditional paper homework, allowing them to track their activities, log their moods, and complete therapy homework [16]. *Ecological momentary assessment* (EMA) technology helps record a patient's "symptoms, affect, behavior, and cognitions close in time to experience" [25] which introduces new clinical workflow scenarios as most therapy homework is not real time and in fact delayed until the next appointment, leading to potential underreporting of symptoms [26]. Feasibility studies have demonstrated that smartphones can be used as an EMA tool [27] and have been used in research studies for psychiatry [28]. Psychometric measures such as PCL-C, PHQ-9, R-SIS, and other military population measures have been found to have internal consistencies whether recorded on smartphone, computer, or paper, but soldiers measured preferred using the iPhone over paper or computer due to its interface, portability, and convenience [29].

Mobile devices can also extend wrap-around case management services, for use in alcohol, smoking, and gambling relapses. Tobacco cessation applications have incorporated reminders, video journaling, and social networking support, such as the National Cancer Institute's QuitPal app [30] and the US Department of Veterans Affairs's Stay Quit app [31]. Smartphones have the potential to contribute to just-in-time interventions for smoking, as a large number of studies have already identified factors that contribute to smoking triggers, including the presence of other smokers, food and alcohol consumption activities, standing outside, stress, time of day, and a day of week and can thus predict antecedents of smoking [32]. A pilot study incorporating coaching and use of a smartphone's camera and Internet capabilities as a smoking cessation intervention demonstrated acceptability and feasibility [33]. This demonstrates that smartphones can be used "when and where they are needed," blending both in-person and online approaches to behavioral interventions.

These ideas have been applied towards for patients with alcohol use disorders. Researchers reported high continued use of a smartphone app that helps prevent relapses during the first four months of a study of 349 patients [34]. A publicly available app, Step Away, based on a grant from the National Institute on Alcohol Abuse and Alcoholism, provides self-help education to boost insight into the user's alcohol issue and teaching skills to manage alcohol cravings, anxiety, and moving away from a drinking lifestyle. A pilot test with 28 users with alcohol use disorder showed a reduction from 56 to 25 % of hazardous drinking behavior, with the number of drinks per day decreased by 52 % [35–37]. Unique features include alarms that occur when users are near high-risk locations (e.g., user-selected bars or liquor stores) that may trigger a relapse, a support network, and identifying pleasurable activities that can be scheduled as a substitute for alcohol.

Smartphones can also help with psychotic disorders. For instance, systems have been tested to provide symptom and mood regulation, medication adherence, social support, and sleep hygiene on a smartphone platform [38, 39]. Ambulatory self-reporting of psychotic symptoms was shown to be a feasible way of assessing psychosis for research and clinical purposes in a smartphone app tested on patients with schizophrenia [40, 41]. Integrating sensors to predict mood schizophrenia relapse with personalized early warning signs—such as isolation, movement inactivity, and unusual behavior—is being tested by Dartmouth University researchers [28, 42]. And such systems can help with side effects and physical health issues that occur as a result of serious mental illness conditions. For instance, obesity has approximately doubled the prevalence in the SMI population with schizophrenia, bipolar disorder, or major depressive disorder, compared to the general population. A study of ten participants used wearable activity monitoring devices while enrolled in a weight loss program and found that this method could help encourage such patients to lose weight, particularly with social connectivity and "friendly" competition features [43]. Inpatient psychiatric patients can also benefit from use of mobile technologies, as such devices can provide assessment of psychotic symptoms in relation to unit location, time of day, and social context, with future studies looking at integrating data with ambulatory cardiopulmonary Holter monitors [44].

Caregivers of those with schizophrenia may also play an instrumental role in smartphone app solutions for psychosis. Researchers at the University of California, San Francisco (UCSF), developed PRIME—Personalized Real-time Intervention for Motivational Enhancement—in conjunction with international design firm IDEO. The study, which is designed to be open to anyone in the United States, combines motivational interventions, goal setting, access to live coaching, and neuroplasticity-based cognitive training, based on work by researchers at UCSF and the University of California, Davis (UC Davis) [45, 46].

For depression and anxiety, a Northwestern University team built a smartphone app that employed machine learning models to predict mood, emotions, cognitive and motivational states, activities, environmental context, and social context based on 38 concurrent phone sensors' data such as ambient light, recent calls, and global positioning system coordinates. The app, Mobilyze, was shown to be feasible, with high level of satisfaction among the seven patients who used it for eight weeks [47]. Similar technology has been incorporated into the open-source Android library Purple Robot for other researchers to use [48]. The app has evolved into a suite of 13 publicly available Android apps, IntelliCare, that provide treatment education and motivational messages in an NIH clinical trial for unipolar depression and anxiety [49, 50].

Similar techniques can be used in interactive entertainment to teach self-management and behavioral awareness. Researchers in New Zealand created the immersive SPARX video game to teach cognitive behavioral therapy to adolescents who may have depression. Their randomized controlled trial found that the game clinically reduced depression and anxiety symptoms [51]. The app has been relaunched into a smartphone game, and its current commercial backers want to expand this into comorbid conditions such as cancer, diabetes, and asthma [52].

11.4 Keeping in Touch with Clinicians

An extensive body of literature research has been performed in real-time videoconferencing for mental health care as this replicates typical face-to-face psychiatric encounters and, in fact, has been shown to be as effective as face-to-face encounters [53]. This real-time videoconferencing is especially suitable for those who lack access to mental health providers in their region, those who need language or

Table 11.1 Telepsychiatry apps available on Google Play and iOS App Store

Service	Fee (as of 2/2015)	Personnel	Video	Platform
HealthLinkNow	*Not specified on Website*	Doctor or therapist	Yes	PC, Mac, mobile
American Well	$49 for a visit (10 min consultation)	MDs, therapists, nutritionists	Yes	PC, Mac, Android, iOS
1DocWay	*Not specified on Website*	Any (turnkey system)	Yes	Browser-based
Doctor on Demand	$40 for a medical visit and $50 for 25 mins with a psychologist	PhD, PsyD, LMFT	Yes	Web, Android, iOS
MDLive Breakthrough	$50 for visit (12 mins)	Doctor or therapist	Yes	Computer, Android, iOS
Cloud 9	They are selling a turnkey app	Anyone/turnkey apps	Yes	iOS, Android

cultural interpretation, those who prefer to receive care at home—particularly those with anxiety, PTSD, and phobia—and those who prefer to avoid the stigma of entering a mental health facility [54]. Telepsychiatry projects have been established, for instance, for Korean patients, with high level of acceptance and appreciation of cultural sensitivity [55].

Video mental health consults for consumers via iOS and Android devices can be performed and are provided by numerous apps (see Table 11.1). These platforms generally feature the ability to chat with a therapist over an audiovisual televideo connection.

11.5 How Should Clinicians Approach Current App Use by Patients?

Patients have thousands of apps available to them on the commercial marketplaces, and yet clinicians have little clinical evidence regarding app use in mental health and often no validated information on specific apps. Clinicians should not assume that an app that a patient is using is accurate or conforms to guidelines, as suggested by a content analysis of smoking cessation apps that noted that popular apps actually had low levels of adherence to clinical practice guidelines and evidence-based practices [56]. The vast majority of apps have not been formally evaluated as another study examining addiction recovery app reports [57]. Clinicians thus must be careful to personally assess each patient's app use to determine whether their apps appear appropriate, accurate, safe, and useful for the patient and patient's disease. In evaluating app use, clinicians must use their best judgment. Just as in routine clinical care, discussing app use with a colleague or inquiring if other clinicians have knowledge of a certain app is always a safe next step. There are also currently several Websites that offer more clinically based rating of apps, including that by the Anxiety and Depression Association of America (http://www.adaa.org/finding-help/mobile-apps) and independent, nonprofit Websites such as PsyberGuide (http://psyberguide.org/).

11.6   What Special Applications Exist for the Military?

Development of mental health apps for mobile devices has also been driven by the needs of active duty military and veterans. In the Veterans Affairs (VA) population, a majority of 188 patients anonymously surveyed and being treated for PTSD as an outpatient expressed interest in managing their symptoms with mobile devices, and 76 % had a phone or tablet capable of running apps [58]. Numerous federal agencies—the Telemedicine and Advanced Technology Research Center, the Military Operational Medicine Research Program, United States Army Medical Research and Materiel Command, the National Center for Telehealth and Technology, and the Department of Veterans Affairs—have released apps for the general public in dedicated app stores [59] and are actively conducting research studies and projects [60].

Their projects help address a range of issues, including anger and stress, mild cognitive impairment, suicidal ideation, and traumatic brain injury. Post-traumatic stress disorder (PTSD) patients through the PTSD Coach app can report their symptoms directly into their electronic medical record (EMR) [61]; qualitative analyses of a sample of users found that veterans considered the app useful for managing acute distress, acute PTSD symptoms, and issues with sleeping [62]. The Cognitive Behavioral Therapy for Insomnia (CBT-I) Coach app can also aid in recording factors surrounding insomnia and provide psychoeducation regarding cognitive behavioral techniques [63]. The PE Coach app also provides a useful complement to prolonged exposure treatment for PTSD [64]; the app itself allows users to audio record treatment sessions, record homework exercises, review homework, and track symptoms over time [65]. Follow-up studies have shown that predictors of more favorable acceptance for such an app include age less than 40 years, smartphone ownership, and previous experience in using apps [66].

11.7   What Drawbacks and Precautions Are There?

Clinicians, developers, and patients must consider a variety of aspects that may decrease the efficacy and increase the danger of using mobile mental health applications: app and device security, network service reliability, clinical efficacy, usability, and stickiness which may hamper patient adherence. Practice guidelines for behavioral interventions have not been standardized or thoroughly researched, although literature from other disciplines—including the fields of human-computer interaction (HCI), user experience (UX) design, psychology, product design, and marketing—can lead to more effective, usable apps. Social norms may also preclude those from using such devices: even the name of an app can bring about questions.

The requirement for e-health literacy may also be a barrier to adoption, as those with mental illness generally have lower levels of literacy and education and may be susceptible to poor e-health literacy [67]. Using mobile apps and wearable devices requires technical proficiency and comfort with using electronic devices. Elderly patients may not be accustomed to charging their devices on a nightly basis, for instance, may have limited vision, or may not be accustomed to using the app interface. The affordability of such devices and apps also poses a risk to those of lower socioeconomic status and effectively price them out of technological treatment.

The commercial sphere is also rife with applications that make bold claims but may not incorporate evidence-based practices, as many mobile health apps are driven by commercial intent rather than research and science [68]. There is also emerging evidence that in some instances app use can actually be harmful as reported by one study that found use of a blood alcohol level (BAL) monitoring app can actually increase drinking in men [69]. Currently, there is a paucity of data on risks, contraindications, side effects, and adverse events related to mental health app use although this will likely be an area of intense study. As mobile mental health research and academic efforts to study such continue to increase, a clearer picture of the advantages and disadvantages of app use should emerge. There is already an established literature for the efficacy of telemedicine especially in rural areas, minority populations, and developing countries [55, 70–75], thus legitimizing tele-video smartphone apps. However, smartphone apps aim to complement all aspects of mental health care, from diagnosis and monitoring to treatment and adherence although much more clinical evidence is necessary to determine if these aims are actually being realized in a safe, ethical, secure, efficacious manner.

Conclusion

Demand for and development of mental health assessment and interventions for mobile devices—including smartphone apps—as the complexity of cases increases, demand for mental health services increases, and the supply of practitioners is constrained. We anticipate moving towards mental health services combining features of both in-person and informatics-driven diagnosis, therapy, and assessment. Though the commercial sector has driven much of the initial app development, the academic community has had increased interest in studying not only the efficacy but also developing their own tools. In November 2013, ClinicalTrials.gov featured 102 open studies involving smartphones for behavior and mental disorders; that number increased to 139 open studies in February 2015 [76]. Increasing interest with new journals, such as *JMIR Mental Health*— along with a greater emphasis in healthcare technology symposia on digital health interventions—indicates a shift towards digital health for psychiatry.

Industry experts expect telemedicine and mobile health to take up to 50 % of all healthcare transactions by 2020; 25 % of all patient encounters with healthcare professionals could be driven through mobile health channels [77]. These channels encompass new devices and sensors. Though digital health has paid more attention to physical conditions, we expect more integrated health approaches with an emphasis on comorbid behavioral health conditions. "Hybrid" practices of care will become accepted and normalized over the next decade, but for this to occur, we need continued research and high-quality studies, with greater involvement by medical professional studies to integrate such tools into clinical workflows.

Acknowledgments The authors thank the UC Davis Department of Psychiatry and Behavioral Science and the APA/SAMHSA Minority Fellows Program.

Conflicts of Interest Steven Chan serves as an associate editor for iMedicalApps.com. The remaining authors declare no conflict of interest.

References

1. Jones SP, Patel V, Saxena S, Radcliffe N, Ali Al-Marri S, Darzi A. How Google's "ten Things We Know To Be True" could guide the development of mental health mobile apps. Health Aff Proj Hope. 2014;33(9):1603–11.
2. Lal S, Adair CE. E-mental health: a rapid review of the literature. Psychiatr Serv Wash DC. 2014;65(1):24–32.
3. Mottl J. Samsung debuts open Simband platform to drive digital health initiative [Internet]. FierceMobileHealthcare. 2014 [cited 15 Feb 2015]; Available from: http://www.fiercemobilehealthcare.com/story/samsung-debuts-open-simband-platform-drive-digital-health-initiative/2014-05-31.
4. Farr C. Exclusive: Apple's health tech takes early lead among top hospitals [Internet]. Reuters. 2015 [cited 15 Feb 2015]; Available from: http://www.reuters.com/article/2015/02/05/us-apple-hospitals-exclusive-idUSKBN0L90G920150205.
5. Metz C. Sorry, but Google glass isn't anywhere close to dead [Internet]. Wired. 2015 [cited 15 Feb 2015]; Available from: http://www.wired.com/2015/02/sorry-google-glass-isnt-anywhere-close-dead/.
6. Muensterer OJ, Lacher M, Zoeller C, Bronstein M, Kübler J. Google Glass in pediatric surgery: an exploratory study. Int J Surg Lond Engl. 2014;12(4):281–9.
7. Rojahn SY. Why some doctors like Google glass so much [Internet]. Wired. 2014; Available from: http://www.technologyreview.com/news/526836/why-some-doctors-like-google-glass-so-much/.
8. Borchers C. Google Glass moves into the hospital at Beth Israel [Internet]. Boston Globe. 2014 [cited 15 Feb 2015]; Available from: http://www.bostonglobe.com/business/2014/06/14/google-glass-moves-into-hospital-beth-israel-deaconess/VQNGKK9842vbRIzlM2201J/story.html.
9. Shu C. Startup brain power uses Google glass to develop apps for kids with autism [Internet]. TechCrunch. 2014 [cited 15 Feb 2015]; Available from: http://techcrunch.com/2014/12/23/brain-power/.
10. Rosenberg L. HIT: time to end behavioral health discrimination. J Behav Health Serv Res. 2012;39(4):336–8.
11. Ben-Zeev D. How I, stopped fearing technology-based interventions. Psychiatr Serv Wash DC. 2014;65(10):1183.
12. Steinhubl SR. Can mobile health technologies transform health care? JAMA [Internet] 2013 [cited 24 Nov 2013]; Available from: http://jama.jamanetwork.com/article.aspx? doi=10.1001/jama.2013.281078.
13. Morris SE, Cuthbert BN. Research domain criteria: cognitive systems, neural circuits, and dimensions of behavior. Dialogues Clin Neurosci. 2012;14(1):29–37.
14. Cuthbert BN, Insel TR. Toward the future of psychiatric diagnosis: the seven pillars of RDoC. BMC Med. 2013;11:126.
15. Collins FS, Varmus H. A new initiative on precision medicine. N Engl J Med. 2015;372:793–5.
16. Harrison V, Proudfoot J, Wee PP, Parker G, Pavlovic DH, Manicavasagar V. Mobile mental health: review of the emerging field and proof of concept study. J Ment Health Abingdon Engl. 2011;20(6):509–24.
17. Torous J, Chan RS, Yee-Marie Tan S, et al. Patient smartphone ownership and interest in mobile apps to monitor symptoms of mental health conditions: a survey in four geographically distinct psychiatric clinics. JMIR Ment Health. 2014;1(1):e5.

18. Torous J, Friedman R, Keshvan M. Smartphone ownership and interest in mobile applications to monitor symptoms of mental health conditions. JMIR Ment Health. 2014;2(1):e2.
19. Ben-Zeev D, Davis KE, Kaiser S, Krzsos I, Drake RE. Mobile technologies among people with serious mental illness: opportunities for future services. Adm Policy Ment Health. 2013;40(4):340–3.
20. Campbell B, Caine K, Connelly K, Doub T, Bragg A. Cell phone ownership and use among mental health outpatients in the USA. Pers Ubiquitous Comput. 2015;19(2):367–78.
21. Chan S, Torous J, Hinton L, Yellowlees P. Mobile tele-mental health: increasing applications and a move to hybrid models of care. Healthcare. 2014;2(2):220–33.
22. Leswing K. Android and iOS are nearly tied for U.S. smartphone market share [Internet]. Gigaom. 2015 [cited 15 Feb 2015]; Available from: https://gigaom.com/2015/02/04/android-and-ios-are-nearly-tied-for-u-s-smartphone-market-share/.
23. DeBronkart D. From patient centred to people powered: autonomy on the rise. BMJ. 2015;350:h148.
24. Laranjo L, Arguel A, Neves AL, et al. The influence of social networking sites on health behavior change: a systematic review and meta-analysis. J Am Med Inform Assoc JAMIA. 2015;22(1):243–56.
25. Moskowitz DS, Young SN. Ecological momentary assessment: what it is and why it is a method of the future in clinical psychopharmacology. J Psychiatry Neurosci JPN. 2006;31(1):13–20.
26. Torous J, Staples P, Shanahan M, et al. Utilizing a custom application on personal smartphones to assess PHQ-9 depressive symptoms in patients with major depressive disorder. JMIR Ment Health. 2015;2(1):e8.
27. Runyan JD, Steenbergh TA, Bainbridge C, Daugherty DA, Oke L, Fry BN. A smartphone ecological momentary assessment/intervention "app" for collecting real-time data and promoting self-awareness. PLoS One. 2013;8(8):e71325.
28. Ben-Zeev D. A new paradigm for illness monitoring and relapse prevention in schizophrenia [Internet]. ClinicalTrials.gov. 2013 [cited 12 Dec 2013]; Available from: http://clinicaltrials.gov/ct2/show/NCT01952041.
29. Bush NE, Skopp N, Smolenski D, Crumpton R, Fairall J. Behavioral screening measures delivered with a smartphone app: psychometric properties and user preference. J Nerv Ment Dis. 2013;201(11):991–5.
30. Pulverman R, Yellowlees PM. Smart devices and a future of hybrid tobacco cessation programs. Telemed J E-Health. 2014;20(3):241–5.
31. US Department of Veterans Affairs. Mobile app: stay quit coach [Internet]. PTSD Natl. Cent. PTSD. 2013 [cited 15 Dec 2013]; Available from: http://www.ptsd.va.gov/public/pages/stay-quit_coach_app.asp.
32. McClernon FJ, Roy Choudhury R. I am your smartphone, and I know you are about to smoke: the application of mobile sensing and computing approaches to smoking research and treatment. Nicotine Tob Res Off J Soc Res Nicotine Tob. 2013;15(10):1651–4.
33. Hertzberg JS, Carpenter VL, Kirby AC, et al. Mobile contingency management as an adjunctive smoking cessation treatment for smokers with posttraumatic stress disorder. Nicotine Tob Res. 2013;15(11):1934–8.
34. McTavish FM, Chih M-Y, Shah D, Gustafson DH. How patients recovering from alcoholism use a smartphone intervention. J Dual Diagn. 2012;8(4):294–304.
35. Dulin PL, Gonzalez VM, Campbell K. Results of a pilot test of a self-administered smartphone-based treatment system for alcohol use disorders: usability and early outcomes. Subst Abuse Off Publ Assoc Med Educ Res Subst Abuse. 2014;35(2):168–75.
36. Dulin PL, Gonzalez VM, King DK, Giroux D, Bacon S. Smartphone-based, self-administered intervention system for alcohol use disorders: theory and empirical evidence basis. Alcohol Treat Q. 2013;31(3):321–36.
37. Giroux D, Bacon S, King DK, Dulin P, Gonzalez V. Examining perceptions of a smartphone-based intervention system for alcohol use disorders. Telemed J e Health Off J Am Telemed Assoc. 2014;20(10):923–9.

38. Ben-Zeev D, Kaiser SM, Brenner CJ, Begale M, Duffecy J, Mohr DC. Development and usability testing of FOCUS: a smartphone system for self-management of schizophrenia. Psychiatr Rehabil J. 2013;36(4):289–96.
39. Ben-Zeev D, Brenner CJ, Begale M, Duffecy J, Mohr DC, Mueser KT. Feasibility, acceptability, and preliminary efficacy of a smartphone intervention for schizophrenia. Schizophr Bull. 2014;40(6):1244–53.
40. Palmier-Claus JE, Rogers A, Ainsworth J, et al. Integrating mobile-phone based assessment for psychosis into people's everyday lives and clinical care: a qualitative study. BMC Psychiatry. 2013;13:34.
41. Palmier-Claus JE, Ainsworth J, Machin M, et al. The feasibility and validity of ambulatory self-report of psychotic symptoms using a smartphone software application. BMC Psychiatry. 2012;12:172.
42. Ben-Zeev D. Mobile technologies in the study, assessment, and treatment of schizophrenia. Schizophr Bull. 2012;38(3):384–5.
43. Naslund JA, Aschbrenner KA, Barre LK, Bartels SJ. Feasibility of popular m-health technologies for activity tracking among individuals with serious mental illness. Telemed J E-Health. 2014;21(3):213–6.
44. Kimhy D, Vakhrusheva J, Liu Y, Wang Y. Use of mobile assessment technologies in inpatient psychiatric settings. Asian J Psychiatry. 2014;10:90–5.
45. DRIVE Lab. About our studies [Internet]. UCSF. [cited 15 Feb 2015]; Available from: http://drive.ucsf.edu/article/about-our-studies.
46. Fisher M, Loewy R, Carter C, et al. Neuroplasticity-based auditory training via laptop computer improves cognition in young individuals with recent onset schizophrenia. Schizophr Bull. 2015;41(1):250–8.
47. Burns MN, Begale M, Duffecy J, et al. Harnessing context sensing to develop a mobile intervention for depression. J Med Internet Res. 2011;13(3):e55.
48. Chan S. How innovation in mobile health is reshaping mental health [Internet]. iMedicalApps. 2014 [cited 25 Jan 2014]; Available from: http://www.imedicalapps.com/2014/01/mobile-mental-health-behavioral-sensor-frameworks-schizophrenia/.
49. Mohr D. Artificial intelligence in a mobile intervention for depression and anxiety (AIM) [Internet]. ClinicalTrials.gov. 2015 [cited 15 Feb 2015]; Available from: https://clinicaltrials.gov/ct2/show/NCT02176226.
50. Northwestern University Center for Behavioral Intervention Technologies. Intellicare: Mental health apps for the 21st century [Internet]. Intellicare Ment. Health Apps 21st Century. [cited 2015 Feb 15]; Available from: https://intellicare.cbits.northwestern.edu
51. Merry SN, Stasiak K, Shepherd M, Frampton C, Fleming T, Lucassen MFG. The effectiveness of SPARX, a computerised self help intervention for adolescents seeking help for depression: randomised controlled non-inferiority trial. BMJ. 2012;344:e2598.
52. Chan S. SPARX aims to use gamification to help kids manage diabetes, asthma, and other chronic conditions [Internet]. iMedicalApps. 2014 [cited 25 Jan 2014]; Available from: http://www.imedicalapps.com/2014/01/video-game-depression-anxiety-kids-diabetes-asthma-linkedwellness/.
53. Hilty DM, Ferrer DC, Parish MB, Johnston B, Callahan EJ, Yellowlees PM. The effectiveness of telemental health: a 2013 review. Telemed J e Health Off J Am Telemed Assoc. 2013;19(6):444–54.
54. Yellowlees P, Burke MM, Marks SL, Hilty DM, Shore JH. Emergency telepsychiatry. J Telemed Telecare. 2008;14(6):277–81.
55. Ye J, Shim R, Lukaszewski T, Yun K, Kim SH, Ruth G. Telepsychiatry services for Korean immigrants. Telemed J e Health Off J Am Telemed Assoc. 2012;18(10):797–802.
56. Abroms LC, Lee Westmaas J, Bontemps-Jones J, Ramani R, Mellerson J. A content analysis of popular smartphone apps for smoking cessation. Am J Prev Med. 2013;45(6):732–6.
57. Savic M, Best D, Rodda S, Lubman DI. Exploring the focus and experiences of smartphone applications for addiction recovery. J Addict Dis. 2013;32(3):310–9.
58. Erbes CR, Stinson R, Kuhn E, et al. Access, utilization, and interest in mHealth applications among veterans receiving outpatient care for PTSD. Mil Med. 2014;179(11):1218–22.

59. US Department of Veterans Affairs. Department of Veterans Affairs (VA) mobile health fact sheet final [Internet]. 2013 [cited 12 Dec 2013]; Available from: https://mobilehealth.va.gov/sites/default/files/files/VAMobileHealthFactSheet.pdf.
60. Shore JH, Aldag M, McVeigh FL, Hoover RL, Ciulla R, Fisher A. Review of mobile health technology for military mental health. Mil Med. 2014;179(8):865–78.
61. National Center for Telehealth and Technology. PTSD Coach [Internet]. PTSD Coach T2health. 2013 [cited 12 Dec 2013]; Available from: http://www.t2.health.mil/apps/ptsd-coach.
62. Kuhn E, Greene C, Hoffman J, et al. Preliminary evaluation of PTSD Coach, a smartphone app for post-traumatic stress symptoms. Mil Med. 2014;179(1):12–8.
63. US Department of Veterans Affairs. Mobile app: CBT-i coach [Internet]. PTSD Natl. Cent. PTSD. 2013 [cited 12 Dec 2013]; Available from: http://www.ptsd.va.gov/public/pages/cbti-coach-app.asp.
64. National Center for Telehealth & Technology. PE coach [Internet]. Natl. Cent. Telehealth Technol. 2013 [cited 15 Dec 2013]; Available from: http://www.t2.health.mil/apps/pe-coach.
65. Reger GM, Hoffman J, Riggs D, et al. The "PE coach" smartphone application: an innovative approach to improving implementation, fidelity, and homework adherence during prolonged exposure. Psychol Serv. 2013;10(3):342–9.
66. Kuhn E, Eftekhari A, Hoffman JE, et al. Clinician perceptions of using a smartphone app with prolonged exposure therapy. Adm Policy Ment Health. 2014;41(6):800–7.
67. Parish MB, Yellowlees P. The rise of person-centered healthcare and the influence of health informatics and social network applications on mental health care. In: Lech M, Song I, Yellowlees P, Diederich J, editors. Mental health informatics. Berlin/Heidelberg: Springer; 2014.
68. Aitken M, Gauntlett C. Patient apps for improved healthcare : from novelty to mainstream [Internet]. 2013 [cited 24 Nov 2013]; Available from: http://www.imshealth.com/deployed-files/imshealth/Global/Content/Corporate/IMS%20Health%20Institute/Reports/Patient_Apps/IIHI_Patient_Apps_Report.pdf.
69. Gajecki M, Berman AH, Sinadinovic K, Rosendahl I, Andersson C. Mobile phone brief intervention applications for risky alcohol use among university students: a randomized controlled study. Addict Sci Clin Pract. 2014;9:11.
70. Gibson K, O'Donnell S, Coulson H, Kakepetum-Schultz T. Mental health professionals' perspectives of telemental health with remote and rural First Nations communities. J Telemed Telecare. 2011;17(5):263–7.
71. Bahloul HJ, Mani N. International telepsychiatry: a review of what has been published. J Telemed Telecare. 2013;19(5):293–4.
72. Chipps J, Brysiewicz P, Mars M. Effectiveness and feasibility of telepsychiatry in resource constrained environments? A systematic review of the evidence. Afr J Psychiatry. 2012;15(4):235–43.
73. Chong J, Moreno F. Feasibility and acceptability of clinic-based telepsychiatry for low-income Hispanic primary care patients. Telemed J e Health Off J Am Telemed Assoc. 2012;18(4):297–304.
74. Grady B, Singleton M. Telepsychiatry "coverage" to a rural inpatient psychiatric unit. Telemed J e Health Off J Am Telemed Assoc. 2011;17(8):603–8.
75. Grady B. Promises and limitations of telepsychiatry in rural adult mental health care. World Psychiatry Off J World Psychiatr Assoc WPA. 2012;11(3):199–201.
76. US National Institutes of Health. Search of: smartphone|open studies – results by topic – ClinicalTrials.gov [Internet]. 2015 [cited 25 Nov 2013]; Available from: http://www.clinical-trials.gov/ct2/results/browse?term=smartphone&recr=Open&brwse=cond_cat_BXM.
77. Weinstein RS, Lopez AM, Joseph BA, et al. Telemedicine, Telehealth and mHealth applications that work: opportunities and barriers. Am J Med [Internet] 2013 [cited 25 Nov 2013]; Available from: http://linkinghub.elsevier.com/retrieve/pii/S0002934313009194.

Part V

Consequences, Limits and Risks

Davor Mucic and Donald M. Hilty

Global/Worldwide e-Mental Health: International and Futuristic Perspectives of Telepsychiatry and the Future

12

Peter M. Yellowlees, Donald M. Hilty, and Davor Mucic

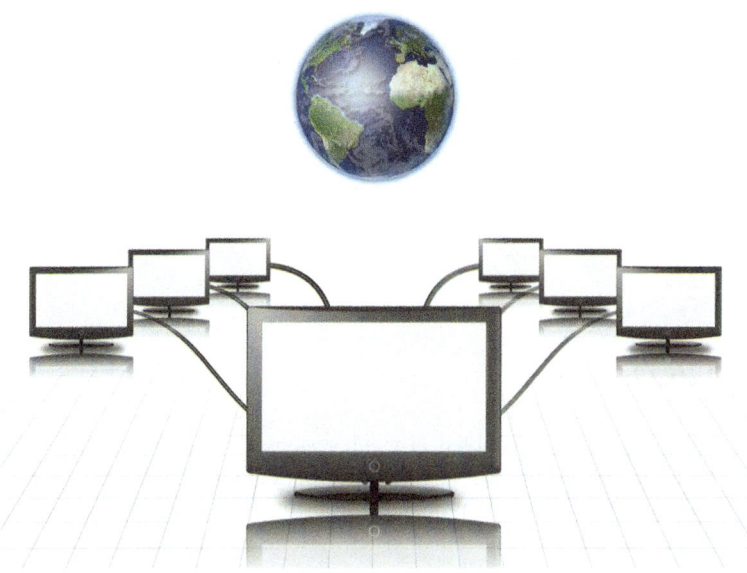

P.M. Yellowlees, MD, MBBS
Health Informatics Graduate Program, University of California, Davis Health System,
Sacramento, CA, USA

D.M. Hilty, MD (✉)
Keck School of Medicine, University of Southern California, Los Angeles,
CA, USA
e-mail: donh031226@gmail.com

D. Mucic, MD
The Little Prince Psychiatric Centre, Copenhagen, Denmark
e-mail: info@denlilleprins.org
http://www.denlilleprins.org; http://www.tv-psykiater.dk

© Springer International Publishing Switzerland 2016
D. Mucic, D.M. Hilty (eds.), *e-Mental Health*,
DOI 10.1007/978-3-319-20852-7_12

Contents

12.1   Introduction 234
12.2   Impact on the Doctor-Patient Relationship 236
12.3   Patient Advocacy and Virtual Reality in the Present and Future 239
         12.3.1   VR Systems: Future Directions 241
12.4   Hybrid Care Models Through the Use of Multiple Technologies 243
12.5   Applying Technology to Underserved Populations: Cross-cultural
         eMH and Trends in International Care 244
Conclusions 247
References 248

Abstract

Telemedicine and Internet-enabled clinical systems are already widely available and are starting to have an impact on the doctor-patient relationship and will increasingly do this more in future. Research shows that online MH interventions are as effective as traditional face-to-face therapy for disorders such as depression and anxiety. We explore the impact of technology on the doctor-patient relationship as new technologies and clinical processes are applied to patient care (e.g., virtual patient advocates). In the future, we will likely change clinical processes, add models of care (e.g., hybrids), better apply new technologies to the underserved (e.g., cross-cultural populations), and have even newer technologies to size up.

12.1   Introduction

Telemedicine and Internet-enabled clinical systems are already widely available and are starting to have an impact on the doctor-patient relationship and will increasingly do this more in future. Telemedicine consultations are now so common that they are undertaken on broadband Internet systems run in the cloud almost routinely, and professionals from all areas in mental health (MH) (from psychiatrists, psychologists, marriage and family therapists to career counselors) can now deliver e-therapy. Yellowlees and Nafiz [1] have described how MH resources and services available to patients at home or in the community may be provided through a multitude of Internet devices, ranging from computers to iPhones, including:

- Online/video/telephone-based patient support groups and Websites for health information
- Telepsychiatry consultations and e-mail/phone/instant messaging with physicians and other providers from fixed and mobile locations
- Multimedia educational materials developed by patients and providers for both patient and provider education
- Scheduling systems, personal electronic health records, and tools for self-directed decision support and chronic disease management

Commercial Websites offering telepsychiatry services such as Healthlinknow. com not only offer information for both professionals and clients on how telepsychiatry works but also services like MH consultations for clients in larger cities and smaller remote communities, prisons, and clinics. Online cognitive behavior therapy (CBT) programs, such as fearfighter.com and "beating the blues" offer computer-aided CBT (CCBT) for a fraction of the cost of a traditional face-to-face therapy. Fearfighter is a Website designed to treat panic and phobia with multistep interventions and has full outcome measurement tracking and patient support in the form of e-mail interactions, secure messaging, and telephone interactions (fearfighter.com).

It is estimated that 70 % of Americans own smartphones and 50 % of adults have used their phone to look up health or medical information. There are numerous mood-tracking applications for cell phones now. These apps are generally either free or cost just a few dollars (generally $2–$10) and allow users to track their quality and amount of sleep, stress and mood behavioral triggers, general health, and most importantly their mood (ranging from depression, anxiety, stress, post-traumatic stress, brain injury, and many more). There are reminder alarms if you forget to check in and notepad features that allow users to journal each day. The T2 Mood Tracker (developed by the National Center for Telehealth and Technology) is a good example and allows users to pick and choose which symptoms apply to them as well as tracking their symptoms.

The following are sample comments by users of the T2 Mood Tracker application [1]:

> I have adult ADD, depression and GAD. The reminder feature is very helpful or I wouldn't remember to use it consistently. I like that I can track each of my issues separately, which helps me to notice which issues are giving me more trouble. This makes me feel a lot less anxious in itself, since part of the problem with managing mental issues is knowing which ones are the root symptoms, and which are symptoms of the root cause not being addressed.

This tool (T2 Mood Tracker) provides the tracking and journaling that so many psychologists and other MH providers encourage clients to use in order to really monitor their functioning. If used regularly, this app could be phenomenal in helping individuals to learn control over their own mind and body.

Developed by universities and experts in the field, there are also free self-help Websites for those seeking alleviation from symptoms of mental disorders. MoodGYM is an innovative, interactive Web program designed by researchers at the Centre for Mental Health Research at the Australian National University and is designed for the treatment of depression and anxiety [2]. Using flash diagrams and online exercises, MoodGYM teaches CBT to its 400,000 plus users – a proven treatment for depression as well as relaxation and meditation techniques. Research trials have shown that MoodGYM significantly reduces depression symptoms for its users, and the benefits have been shown to last for up to 12 months when compared to control groups [3, 4].

Research shows that online MH interventions are as effective as traditional face-to-face therapy for disorders such as depression and anxiety. For example, treatment outcomes are comparable with both face-to-face and online CBT in alleviating symptoms of panic disorder and agoraphobia. Based on a 30-month follow-up study for treatment of social phobia, research showed that the long-term effects of face-to-face delivered CBT was comparable to Internet-based treatment. In regard to depression, research shows that both CBT and psychoeducation obtained online can reduce symptoms of depression.

Telepsychiatry consultations are now well established with guidelines existing for both adult and child psychiatry and have been demonstrated to be diagnostically valid and show substantial patient satisfaction [5, 6]. Details of the evidence base for telepsychiatry and the telepsychiatry literature are provided elsewhere in this book.

This chapter will help the reader review trends in international e-mental healthcare: (1) the best of what is being done now with new technologies, (2) the application of new technologies to patient care (e.g., virtual patient advocates), and (3) how we will move forward with changes in clinical processes, models of care (e.g., hybrids), applying new developments to the underserved (e.g., cross-cultural populations), and sizing up even newer technologies over the next decade or two.

12.2 Impact on the Doctor-Patient Relationship

It has been described how on a typical day a military psychologist might provide an hour of therapy to a patient struggling with anxiety in Guam, another hour to a client in Japan experiencing post-traumatic stress disorder, and a third hour to a soldier in his home state of Hawaii who might be dealing with depression [1]. All of this therapy is provided from an office at Tripler Army Medical Center in Honolulu, but only one of the sessions is done face-to-face.

The doctor-patient relationship is central to the general practice of medicine, but it is especially important in psychiatry and other MH care fields because it plays a prominent role in the therapeutic process. In his book *The Doctor, His Patient and the Illness*, Balint described the doctor-patient relationship as a process involving three stages: the collection of symptoms from the patient (including the physical and mental state exams), a diagnostic evaluation, and seeking mutual agreement on a management plan.

Psychiatrists have been described as having three potential roles in the doctor-patient relationship – that of authority, facilitator, or partner. In the authority role, the psychiatrist makes all the decisions for the patient – this role is becoming less common although some patients still prefer to be told what to do and not to have major input into the decision-making process. In the facilitator role, the psychiatrist guides his or her patients to appropriate information that will help the patient make informed treatment choices. Finally, in the partner role, the psychiatrist assists with research into therapeutic options and information analysis but the patient is often the primary researcher. Ultimately, in the partner role, the patient makes their own decisions and this is often described as patient-focused care.

With the advent of videoconferencing, e-mail, and instant messaging, the relationship of the doctor-patient has undoubtedly changed, however, as Andersson has written, "Emerging evidence across trials clearly suggests that the computer cannot totally replace human contact" [7]. In-person consultations will remain the core of most psychiatrist-patient relationships but the Internet is becoming a major component of most health consultations and will continue to change the way that psychiatrists and other MH professionals work. Initially, patients may have a traditional face-to-face visit but this might be followed with video visits such as online therapy and psychoeducation with in-person visits occurring as needed so that increasing numbers of patients and doctors now have what Yellowlees has described as a hybrid relationship.

With the use of e-therapy using videoconferencing, e-mail, or telephone/texting or messaging, it is vital that both practitioners and clients understand and appreciate the limited nature of this medium and practitioners need to:

- Assess if the client is suitable for online treatment, taking into consideration if the client is in immediate crisis, is engaged in active suicidal ideation or if there are other serious concerns such as domestic violence or severe drug use
- Have back-up resources in place to address urgent issues
- Educate clients and provide informed consent
- Assess the suitability of clients and work within ethical parameters

E-therapy has numerous benefits, such as the convenience of undergoing treatment in the privacy of your home versus having to drive to see a mental healthcare provider. It allows patients and practitioners to bypass time and geographical boundaries, allowing access to mental healthcare for those with limited mobility or for people who live in remote locations. And although in-person therapy is considered the gold standard, researchers are discovering that online treatments can be as effective and therapeutic but this is not to say that there are no opposing opinions and certain issues that still need addressing.

One issue with online therapy is the artificial distance created between the doctor and the client, and researchers have argued that this can have both positive and negative consequences. The clinical limitations of distance involve lack of visual and auditory cues, body language, and spontaneous clarification (if communication is via e-mail or text), which can be very important in some instances in therapy. However, with treatments of disorders that have a potential element of shame, stigma or embarrassment, such as post-traumatic stress disorder, eating disorders, or for those struggling with social anxiety, the prospect of receiving treatment from a distance can be appealing [7]. Researchers have hypothesized that online counseling may create a sense of disinhibition where clients feel more comfortable discussing sensitive topics online compared with a traditional in-person setting [8]. Dr. Fishkind, a psychiatrist based out of Texas has written:

> We've had over 60,000 patient encounters…only six have been refused to be seen via teleconferencing…when it comes to mental health issues and the difficult things you need to talk about in a crisis, a lot of patients feel it's less threatening and easier to be open and communicative via telemedicine.

In the treatment of children and adolescents, the authors have argued that in certain cases telepsychiatry might be a superior method of psychiatric assessment than face-to-face consultations [9]. They discussed five case studies, one of which is the following:

> A 15-year old girl was referred for a consultation by her primary care provider, and she agreed to individual face-to-face therapy for the first time after her first telepsychiatry consultation. Despite multiple attempts in the past, she had declined to do so. The girl stated that she felt more comfortable in front of a monitor than with "a real psychiatrist." Both the girl and her mother reported that in the past she had refused to open up. After the telepsychiatry session, an appointment with a local psychologist was secured for individual therapy. At 2-month follow up, the girl reported improvement with her energy level, sleep, and social motivation. She had been meeting with her therapist consistently every week since the initial consultation with us.

An adolescent psychiatrist who treats adolescents Virginia, was noted to say that:

> [Patients] feel great about seeing me on the television and they actually become more animated when they see me that way, especially kids with anxiety issues. They do very well with telemedicine [1].

Distance (when e-mail is utilized as a medium) also allows for a "zone of reflection," which has been described as a slowing down of the therapy process which allows both parties to pay close attention to their own thoughts and feelings while still engaged in a dialogue [10]. The author also suggested that some clients might also be more comfortable expressing themselves in writing and the process of writing itself can be therapeutic and encourage insight [10].

Numerous ethical and legal questions have been raised as the healthcare field advances increasingly towards using the Internet routinely for clinical mental healthcare, including:

* The practicalities of the use of e-mail in the doctor-patient relationship
* State licensing and credentialing concerns if therapist and client are in different states
* Confidentiality and privacy for both patients and providers
* The right of providers to not be always available to patients and to have appropriate downtime and work-life balance

In order to ensure confidentiality and privacy, practitioners need to utilize safeguards such as firewalls and password protection, but even with these precautions a misdirected e-mail to an unintended recipient increases liability exposure for the psychiatrist. A possible solution to this could be the use of encryption technology. An encrypted e-mail has an unintelligible sequence of characters that can only be unscrambled with a decryption key from the sender (the psychiatrist in this example).

Although many of the American Psychological Association ethics code apply to online therapy, such as informed consent, doing no harm, and competence to practice, Deborah Baker, JD, past director for prescriptive authority and regulatory affairs in APA's Practice Directorate has been quoted as saying "...*technology is pushing ahead at a rapid pace, psychology licensing laws have not yet caught up. All health and mental health-care professions are wrestling with many of the same issues*".

The locus of power in healthcare is shifting as we move to this future of increasing amounts of care delivered online in one form or another. Instead of the doctor having full control of the patients' needs, a consumerist model has emerged in which patients and their doctors are partners in managing the patients' care. The age of the "Industrial Age Medicine" has been replaced by the new model of the "Information Age Care" as envisioned by Ferguson and Smith. In this new information age, the relationships of healthcare practitioners and their patients are increasingly developing into collaborative partnerships as patients have more control over their healthcare needs than ever before.

The Industry Council Chairman for the American Telemedicine Association has predicted that telemedicine will continue to grow as demands for real-time remote delivery systems grow across the healthcare spectrum. The mental healthcare field needs to seize this opportunity, as this is clearly where the future of healthcare is headed.

We have described how mental healthcare is changing and moving forward in most clinical environments, certainly in Western Countries, and how it is becoming more patient-centric and consumer-focused. But what about the role of those who support patients – their families, friends, and anyone else who might be what has typically been described in the past as a patient advocate. Someone who works with patients to ensure that they receive the best possible care, understands the decisions they have to make, and frequently guides patients through our sometimes highly complicated health system.

12.3   Patient Advocacy and Virtual Reality in the Present and Future

In a future of increasingly online healthcare, the patient will require assistance in a series of novel ways. Currently such assistance is delivered by in-person patient advocates but in future these roles will be taken over or supplemented by what has been described as a virtual patient advocates (VPA) [11]. An encouraging advancement in technology, the VPA is a computerized, animated character (often referred to as an avatar) designed to integrate best practices from provider-patient communication theory. It emulates face-to-face conversation complete with non-verbal communication such as gaze, posture, and hand gestures. The authors have described a study conducted at Boston Medical Center using a VPA called the Gabby System, which showed that some of the study participants preferred talking to the VPA rather than interacting with a real person [11]. One explanation for this could be that the study demographic was comprised of young women who were "digital natives" and had never known a world without the Internet. Additional studies on how older populations of patients feel about using avatars as patient advocates are necessary because there may be less enthusiasm for this form of support amongst patients not familiar with virtual reality (VR) environments.

"Louise" is another VPA system designed as part of Boston Medical Center's Project RED, an initiative to improve and re-engineer hospital discharges while improving patient safety and reducing readmissions. Louise is designed to work with people who have limited computer skills. While it does take some initial nursing time to set up the use of this software program, it has been shown to reduce hospital utilization (readmission and emergency visits). An advantage of using a VPA is that the program avatar can potentially be accessed at the convenience of the patient from wherever he or she may be located and yet it can seem quite real, as if the patient is talking to an actual person. As Mucci has noted, "the virtual patient advocate is patient and kind, shows empathy and humor, has medical knowledge, and shows confidence. All of these things make her trustworthy to patients. They appreciate the private time they are allowed to listen and ask questions – and that they decide when they have had enough."

The same authors noted that the use of VPAs for children would be an interesting area of study. Children might find that interacting with a "virtual friend" is less threatening than dealing with an adult, especially if the avatar is also a child. Many children are accustomed to cartoon characters as well as avatars in video games so it might be a very natural transition from those characters to a VPA. The VPA could be tailored to explain things at the level of understanding that is appropriate for the child. It has been described how recent developments in clinical VR have taken the concept of the patient avatar, or VPA, one step further as is evidenced by a project developed by Rizzo et al. which they described the provider avatar [11]. The SimCoach project was developed to create virtual human support agents that can act as online guides and therapists and was designed to attract and engage military service members, veterans, and their significant others who might not be inclined to seek help from a live healthcare provider. These support agents are no longer at the level of a prop to add context or minimal faux interaction in a virtual world, they are designed to perceive and act in a 3D virtual world, engage in face-to-face spoken dialogues with real users (and other virtual humans) and in some cases, they are capable of exhibiting human-like emotional reactions. Rizzo and his team then created SimSensai which took SimCoach to the next level and added cameras and Microsoft's Kinect sensor to observe and analyze face, gesture, and vocal parameters that help the agent better react to the patient's emotional state. The virtual therapist model as developed for the SimCoach and SimSensei projects could also be applied to the patient navigator role in future and opens up a whole new style of potentially automated clinical practice, and one where machine-based translation and interpretation programs, used across different languages, could potentially open up a global market.

Another example of the expansion of the VPA role is the creation of robot caregivers [11]. Many countries have begun investing in robot development and researchers in the USA are developing robot-caregiver prototypes. These caregiving robots would be different than the ones already commonly in use to assist in surgery or deliver medications – these robots are meant to be your friend and caregiver and have the potential to be helpful in the area of MH.

As the future of healthcare delivery unfolds, reimbursement is increasingly being tied to the efficiency and quality of care, and this will incentivize the use of computer-based technologies and processes such as Virtual Patient Advocates. In some instances, however, there is no substitute for in-person delivery of patient care and support. This is where a hybrid model of the Patient Advocate role may prove useful. When accompanying a patient to provider appointments or facilitating the relationship of the patient to the healthcare provider, being physically present is important. Using fixed and mobile devices as a tool to be "virtually physically present" may allow the Patient Advocate to become more versatile and to become accessible to remotely located patients. The role of patient advocate and the form that role takes – be it in-person, digital/online, avatar, or some hybrid model of these technologies – should be expressly tied to the patient population for which the role is employed [11]. As various studies have shown, some patient populations lend themselves better to one form of this role over another. There are, however, many viable forms a patient navigator/advocate role can take and there is a place for the online/virtual patient navigator role in the future of healthcare, and especially mental healthcare, and given that the VPA already exists, it will move into the area of VR systems where therapy is already being delivered.

12.3.1 VR Systems: Future Directions

One of the applications that is being increasingly widely adopted and used for mental healthcare education and clinical purposes is VR [12]. VR is the concept of being virtually but not physically at a specific place. Some VR platforms involve three-dimensional imaging and surround audio that make the user feel like in the real world. The user can go or do certain things that in real life might be difficult or impossible. Many companies have used virtual reality for games and entertainment and it has been used in flight simulation for teaching pilots how to fly without risking equipments and lives. Recently though, VR has been used in many other professional fields. For example, businesses are using VR applications to market their products, educators are using them for teaching and for public awareness, and doctors to communicate with and treat their patients.

One of the leading more popular VR applications is Second Life (www.secondlife.com). Second Life is a VR platform that is open to the public and can be accessed free of charge. Every user is given an avatar that can be customized to reflect one's own physical appearance or character. Avatars can walk, run, or fly from one island to another. Some can go shopping, visit museums, or even go on a date. It all depends on the user's preference and liking.

Another type of a VR platform is a fully immersive system. These fully immersive software systems give the user a full immersion in the VR environment. This can take place in a virtual cave, which could be a three-, four-, five-, or six-walled room with multiple projectors transmitting images on these walls. Some systems require a specific visual aid such as three-dimensional glasses while others can be used with only the naked eye. A similar concept of fully immersive VR environment is the use of specific glasses that have the three-dimensional screen inside the device. The price of these systems has reduced remarkably in recent years and it is now possible to buy a simple 3D device that connects with a smartphone which is inserted inside it so that the phone screen becomes the screen of the 3D device, for as little as $30US. These cheap and simple systems are increasingly being used to help patients who have simple phobias of spiders or heights as discussed below.

VR systems have already been described by Maghazil and Yellowlees as playing a role in treating patients with many conditions including but not limited to eating disorders, anxiety disorders, some autism spectrum disorders, stress management, pain management, strokes, brain injury, psychiatric disability, cognitive impairment, and dysfunctions of the central nervous system. Phobias and traumas can also be treated through VR exposure therapy (VRE). VRE has been proven to treat many patients by exposing them to visual and other sensory materials that represent the patient's feared object or traumatic event as previously experienced. Many phobias including social phobias, fear of heights and flying, claustrophobia and fear of spiders have been treated with VRE, and military organizations have started utilizing VRE for treating post-traumatic stress disorders (PTSD) and other combat-related disorders. The future is bright for the continued expansion of these approaches to treatment.

Second Life is an educational tool that has been used all around the world. To observe faculty teaching health informatics to groups of students attending a seminar on a private teaching area in Second Life, go to www.youtube.com and put in the search terms "informatics" and "MHI214" and review a number of videos posted demonstrating how to teach groups of students on this platform. These films demonstrate well the wide range of avatars adapted and modified by the students and you will see Yellowlees communicating with spacemen, rabbits and highly sexualized versions of humans as part of his most unique looking student group. Many universities, colleges, libraries, and government bodies have adopted VR software for education and many instructors and educators prefer Second Life over other distant learning methods because it is more personal and provides more opportunity for creativity. Research conducted in the UK in 2007 showed that as early as that time over 80 % of United Kingdom's universities had developed teaching or learning tools in Second Life and that over 300 universities around the world were already teaching courses or performing research on this VR platform alone.

The benefits of using VR platforms for educational purposes in the medical field are obvious and it is likely that these games like environments will be increasingly popular and used in future. Health educators can target many audiences and ethnic groups to promote health awareness, and games, billboards, and videos are simple approaches that can target big audiences. Healthcare providers can also use these virtual environments to educate their patients about diseases or conditions they may acquire. Instead of flipping through a brochure or going through web pages, VR can offer important and beneficial sources of information with more appealing visual aids, especially in mobile environments.

12.4   Hybrid Care Models Through the Use of Multiple Technologies

The increasing numbers of practitioners using a hybrid approach to care, as described previously, is one of many variations on the theme of providing patient-centered care that is affordable, timely, and easy to access. An excellent example is the Seattle-based project run by Meyers and her colleagues who have employed multiple in-person and technological approaches to provide evidence-based assessment and treatment to children with ADHD living in several states in North West USA [13]. In this project, child psychiatrists both provide direct care and education online, patients see physicians, behaviorists, and psychiatrists online and in person, and the whole delivery platform for care and monitoring is online, but focused on primary care clinics, from where all therapy sessions are coordinated.

An innovative model of collaborative MH services has been implemented using multiple technologies and this is not only a new way to practice psychiatry, but is also likely to lead in many instances to lead to a new standard of practice, showing that telemedicine is versatile and will increasingly support and enable the implementation of specialized treatments where and when the patients need them. We know that most mental healthcare takes part in primary care across the world and that most patients with psychiatric disorders never see or are never evaluated by a psychiatrist; such versatile telehealth models help remedy this problem. Myers project has affirmed the contemporary view that psychiatrists may use technology to disseminate their skills (consulting, training, supervision) and develop innovative treatment programs that an interdisciplinary team (primary care providers, behavior therapists, community partners like teachers, family, care coordinators and psychiatrists) may efficiently deliver. We propose that the model of combined interventions should now become the new standard of practice in child psychiatry for treating children who have ADHD combined with other psychiatric disorders, whether the children live in rural or metropolitan areas.

One consideration is the development of a new standard of care. It has been suggested that this combination of hybrid clinical approaches as demonstrated by Myers and new collaborative research processes suggest that we should be able to move towards a new standard of care [14]. We need MH providers and others to attitudinally shift to hybrid models of in-person and technology-delivered care – many have headed that way already, including the Department of Veterans Affairs, the new younger generation of psychiatrists, and patients and families who will push us to move the e-care connection even further. We need a technology platform for care that integrates the best of stepped models of care, access to specialists, a continuum of e-service delivery options (e.g., e-mail/phone, [15]; asynchronous, [16]), interdisciplinary role definition (and cross-training), and training on shared MH models to improve our efficiency.

To accelerate the necessary attitudinal changes, the use of hybrid models of care should be taught in all psychiatric residency programs as well as within other disciplines and at medical and nursing schools. Then we will be able to work on quality improvement, sustainability, new approaches to collecting clinical outcome evidence that are not purely dependent on traditional randomized controlled trials, and the further integration of technology into daily practice to provide the context and the infrastructure for continuing discoveries in science and in psychiatry. In our own MH disciplines, we see the next steps being the further integration and implementation of algorithmically and evidence-driven care within this hybrid model and how we can learn to effectively use mobile technologies.

So, while all of this is exciting and interesting, how does it fit in with global MH services and the provision of cross-cultural internationalized care?

12.5 Applying Technology to Underserved Populations: Cross-cultural eMH and Trends in International Care

The aim of this key section is to build on the innovations described above and to understand how the issues that will impact national and international cross-cultural MH services learn how e-Mental Health (eMH) may improve the quality of care toward ethnic minorities worldwide including reducing of stigma that is very often culturally conditioned and obtain an insight into potential obstacles and suggested solutions for development of both national and international cross-cultural eMH services. While various eMH applications have been tested and developed over the last five to six decades, there are relatively few published reports describing the use of telepsychiatry in the provision of MH care to cross-cultural patients [16–19].

The term "cross-cultural telepsychiatry" covers the delivery of culturally appropriate MH care from a distance in "real time" by the use of videoconferencing i.e., "synchronous telepsychiatry" and/or "asynchronous" ("store and forward" model, where we speak about a transmission of recorded clinical-related material, i.e., assessment, psychiatric interview/consultation between referring physicians and specialist) [20]. Equal access to MH services is a human right for both domestic and immigrant population in modern communities worldwide. However, due to geographical distances and other barriers, e.g., cultural, religious and linguistic, cross-cultural patient population face difficulties in access to MH professionals in a desired way.

eMH applications offer new possibilities for reducing disparities in access to relevant mental healthcare to most vulnerable patient groups, such as refugees, migrants, and asylum seekers worldwide. It has been reported that patients who face language barriers (i.e., refugees, asylum seekers, and migrants are less likely than others to have a usual source of medical care and who frequently receive preventive services at reduced rates have an increased risk of non-adherence to medications, are less likely than others to return for follow-up appointments after visits to the emergency room, and have higher rates of hospitalization and drug complications [21]. Language barriers are also likely to affect patients' trust in their providers.

Patients who do not speak the language of respective care providers have reported feelings of being discriminated against in clinical settings, whereas communicating with health professionals in a common language is associated with increased trust and confidence [22]. Several studies have found that language barriers are associated with lower rates of patient satisfaction and poor care delivery in comparison with care received by patients who speak the language of the care provider [23, 24].

Cross-cultural patient treatment within MH care demands a high standard of communication between the patient and the care provider, since linguistic, cultural, or even racial barriers may affect patient satisfaction. Cultural differences and language difficulties result in communication gaps where important nuances are either obscured or missed. In such a situation, both patients and professionals are often exposed to the "lost-in-translation syndrome." To take account of these problems, a number of telepsychiatry services have been established to increase the quality of mental healthcare for certain ethnic minorities.

Telemedicine provides operational and logistical efficiencies that enable medical interpreters to be more readily accessible to healthcare providers and is increasingly being used in hospitals and clinics via mobile carts, tablets, or smartphones. Compared with phone interpretation, videoconferencing enables interpreters to observe and interpret non-verbal cues for the provider [25], making interpreters more available with no need to travel between consultations. Videoconferencing has been successfully deployed in numerous organizations and has led to decreased delays and increased efficiency of interpreters, with one institution reportedly saving approximately $368,000 per year [26].

The use of technology services/applications described in this book have a potential to provide efficient and cost-effective opportunities to reach individuals and groups with poor service access despite geographically distances and/or national borders. However, when it comes to remote real-time eMH consultations via videoconferencing, there are only few studies describing international, cross-border studies and none involve developing countries [27]. A consulting psychiatrist was licensed in Australia, but living in New Zealand, provided care for two patients in a facility in Australia; one of the cases was a new consultation and the other was a follow-up [28]. A six-month trial of telepsychiatry tertiary care from South London to the island of Jersey reported five teleconsultations of a single second opinion and four case reviews [29]. International eMH and tele-education for Swedish medical students about cross-cultural issues in refugees with MH problems was conducted between Sweden, the USA, and Australia. There was one real patient at the American site and one simulated patient at the Australian site, with patient interviews by experts while medical students observed by videoconference and participated in the discussion [30]. Videoconferencing provided psychoanalytic clinical care and training to psychoanalytic candidates in China by US psychoanalysts, and this involved 40 psychoanalytic and 30 psychodynamic psychotherapies [31].

The most comprehensive international eMH service in the world was established in Denmark in mid-2006 as a part of cross-cultural telepsychiatry pilot-project launched by The Little Prince Psychiatric Centre located in Copenhagen [32, 33]. Due to lack of bilingual clinicians in Denmark, psychiatrists who spoke Arabic, Polish, Kurdish, and ex-Yugoslavian languages, but were physically located in Sweden, were employed to provide care due to their cross-cultural skills. Furthermore, bilingual psychiatrists not only have the selected skills but a detailed knowledge of the MH system in Scandinavia as well as knowledge about health systems in the patients' home countries. Over a period of 18 months, 31 patients (i.e., refugees, migrants, and asylum seekers) were assessed and treated via videoconferencing by providers who spoke the patients' own language. Videoconferencing equipment connected the Swedish Department of the Little Prince Psychiatric Centre with two hospitals, one asylum seekers' center and one social institution in Denmark. The distances from the Swedish station located in Malmö to the Danish telepsychiatry stations were from 140 to 300 km. Overall, high patient satisfaction was reported and minor disadvantages of eMH were offset by the fact that the doctors and the patients linguistically and culturally matched. The use of bilingual clinicians with a similar ethnic and cultural background to their patients compensates for the distance and lack of physical presence.

Experiences from projects over the last decade – described above and in Chap. 5 – may pave the way for development of an International eMH Network within European Union (EU).

Clinical and scientific objectives and goals of such international telemental health service are to:

1. Improve the mental healthcare across national boundaries by providing psychiatric consultations between countries within EU
2. Develop international treatment teams with select skills (e.g., sign language and many foreign languages staff)
3. Provide acute psychiatric assessments at a distance
4. Establish a second opinion service and shared care service between MH professionals and general practitioners
5. Improve discharge planning by involvement of clinicians with specialized skills and expertise
6. Develop subsequent follow-up service via videoconferencing
7. Increase access to child, adult, geriatric, forensic, and deaf services specialty staff
8. Provide distance supervision and staff consultation
9. Provide psychoeducation of patients' family members
10. Improve distance learning via case conferencing and best practice demonstration across the national boundaries
11. Create a database over cross-cultural and other select skills professionals within EU

The potential outcomes of the above are many:

1. Increased access to specialized expertise (e.g., sign language and many foreign languages staff)
2. Increased speed and accuracy of diagnosis and treatment that otherwise will be provided by translators
3. Increased access to child, adult, geriatric, forensic, and deaf services specialty staff
4. Increased continuity of care and professional contact
5. Improved education of the stuff and psychoeducation of the patients and their family members
6. Increased efficiency and effectiveness through improved performance

7. Cost benefits as result of reduced staff and translator costs: travel time, staff time, decreased use of translators
8. Reduced waiting time/waiting lists for the treatment due to increased access to respective resources
9. Decrease in the number of inappropriate admissions and readmissions into the acute sector

While waiting for development of eMH services in a larger scale within EU, a MasterMind (*MA*nagement of MH di*S*orders *T*hrough advanc*E*d technology and se*R*vices – telehealth for the *MIND*) project was launched in March 2014 (ending in February 2017) [34]. Total investment of 14,000,000,00 EUR aims to result in a set of guidelines and a "toolbox" for the promotion and facilitation of implementation of a safe and effective eMH service across Europe with a primary focus on remote treatment of depression. The videoconferencing service will be used for creating a network between health professionals who can then support each other and share knowledge. Videoconferencing can be used for establishing a network from specialist to specialist, specialist to non-specialist. Furthermore, videoconferencing can be used for providing specialist treatment in areas where this service is scarce, e.g., rural areas. The aim is to provide the patients with more holistic and patient-centered care while ensuring that they have access to high-quality treatment in their immediate environment.

An alternative equally innovative, disruptive approach to providing international cross-cultural care is the use of language translation smartphone apps. These apps are potentially available any time with any patient, automatically interpreting language in speech-to-speech, text-to-speech, and speech-to-text modes. A combination of automated speech recognition (ASR, also known as text-to-speech or voice dictation) and machine translation (MT) technologies are already in use to translate Websites, generate subtitles in different languages in YouTube videos, and provide closed captions for simultaneous teleconferencing on Skype.

Google Translate is one of the more well-known apps available on Android, iOS, and the Web. ASR and MT technology vendor Nuance has been demonstrated in clinical settings [35]; others are creating non-commercial open source software [36]. Modern-day ASR and MT technologies also employ machine-learning algorithms to make interpretation more accurate over time; no longer will we see the sometimes bizarre language translations from traditional software that employs static linguistic rules.

Conclusions

We have explored the impact of technology on the doctor-patient relationship as new technologies and clinical processes are applied to patient care (e.g., virtual patient advocates). These approaches will make the relationship more flexible and productive as it occurs across time and distance, no longer restricted to the clinic office.

In the future, we will likely change clinical more processes, especially as virtual reality, synchronous, asynchronous, and mobile technologies combine, add models of care (e.g., hybrids), and better apply new technologies to the underserved (e.g., cross-cultural populations) all around the world. And on top of that we will undoubtedly have even newer technologies to size up – technologies and clinical processes that as of today have not even been dreamed of.

Aside with the development of new technological devices, we will hopefully see establishment of international services in order to exchange professional expertise as well as assess and even treat patients on distance via patients' respective mother tongue rather than via interpreters.

References

1. Yellowlees PM, Nafiz N. The psychiatrist-patient relationship of the future: anytime, anywhere? Rev Psychiatry. 2010;18(2):96–102.
2. MoodGym. 7 Mar 2015. At: https://moodgym.anu.edu.au/welcome.
3. Christensen H, Griffiths K, Groves C, et al. Free range users and one hit wonders: community users of an internet-based cognitive behaviour therapy program. Aust N Z J Psychiatry. 2006;40(1):59–62.
4. Mackinnon A, Griffiths KM, Christensen H. Comparative randomised trial of online cognitive-behavioural therapy and an information website for depression: 12-months outcomes. Br J Psychiatry. 2008;192(2):130–4.
5. Neufeld JD, Bourgeois JA, Hilty DM, et al. The e-Mental Health Consult Service: providing enhanced primary care mental health services through telemedicine. Psychosomatics. 2007;48:135–41.
6. O'Reilly R, Bishop J, Maddox K, et al. Is telepsychiatry equivalent to face to face psychiatry: results from a randomized controlled equivalence trial. Psychiatr Serv. 2007;258:836–43.
7. Andersson G, Carlbring P, Holmstrom A, et al. Internet-based self-help with therapist feedback and in vivo group exposure for social phobia: a randomized controlled trial. J Consult Clin Psychol. 2006;74(4):677–86.
8. Suler J. The psychology of cyberspace. CyberPsychology Behav. 2001;4:675–80.
9. Pakyurek M, Yellowlees PM, Hilty DM. The child and adolescent telepsychiatry consultation: can it be a more effective clinical process for certain patients than conventional practice? Tel J e-Health. 2010;16(3):289–92.
10. Suler J. Psychotherapy in cyberspace: a 5 dimensional model of online and computer-mediated psychotherapy. CyberPsychology Behav. 2000;3(2):151–60.
11. Kent S, Yellowlees PM. The virtual patient advocate. J Telemed eHealth. 2015 [Epub ahead of print].
12. Maghazil A, Yellowlees PM. Novel approaches to clinical care in mental health: from asynchronous telepsychiatry to virtual reality. In: Lech M, Song I, Yellowlees PM, et al., editors. Mental health informatics. Berlin/Heidelberg: Springer; 2014.
13. Myers KM, Vander Stoep A, Zhou C, et al. Effectiveness of a telehealth service delivery model for treating attention-deficit hyperactivity disorder: results of a community-based randomized controlled trial. J Am Acad Child Adolesc Psychiatry. 2015;54:263–74, (in press).
14. Hilty DM, Yellowlees PM. Collaborative mental health services using multiple technologies – the new way to practice and a new standard of practice? J Amer Acad Child Adol Psychiatry. 2015;54(4):245–6.
15. Hilty DM, Yellowlees PM, Cobb HC, et al. Models of telepsychiatric consultation-liaison service to rural primary care. Psychosomatics. 2006;47(2):152–7.
16. Yellowlees PM, Odor A, Burke MM, et al. A feasibility study of asynchronous telepsychiatry for psychiatric consultations. Psychiatr Serv. 2010;61(8):838–40.
17. Sherrill WW, Crew L, Mayo RM, et al. Educational and health services innovation to improve care for rural Hispanic communities in the U.S. Educ Health (Abingdon). 2005;18:356–67.
18. Shore J, Kaufmann LJ, Brooks E, et al. Review of American Indian veteran telemental health. Tel e-Health. 2012;18(2):87–94.

19. Yeung A, et al. A study of the effectiveness of telepsychiatry-based culturally sensitive collaborative treatment of depressed Chinese Americans. BMC Psychiatry. 2011;11:154.
20. Hilty DM, Ferrer DC, Parish MB, et al. The effectiveness of telemental health: a 2013 review. Telemed J E Health. 2013;19:444–54.
21. Flores G. Language barriers to health care in the United States. N Engl J Med. 2006;355:229–31.
22. Mutchler JE, Bacigalupe G, Coppin A, Gottlieb A. Language barriers surrounding medication use among older Latinos. J Cross Cult Gerontol. 2007;22:101–14.
23. Carrasquillo O, Orav EJ, Brennan TA, et al. Impact of language barriers on patient satisfaction in an emergency department. J Gen Intern Med. 1999;14:82–7.
24. Sarver J, Baker DW. Effect of language barriers on follow-up appointments after an emergency department visit. J Gen Intern Med. 2000;15:256–64.
25. Nápoles AM, Santoyo-Olsson J, Karliner LS, O'Brien H, Gregorich SE, Pérez-Stable EJ. Clinician ratings of interpreter mediated visits in underserved primary care settings with ad hoc, in-person professional, and video conferencing modes. J Health Care Poor Underserved. 2010;21(1):301–17.
26. O'Neill DD, Anthony S, Laws M. Every language now. In: Berkowitz L, McCarthy C, editors. Innovation with information technologies in healthcare. London: Springer; 2013. p. 167–77. Accessed March 7, 2015. At: http://link.springer.com/10.1007/978-1-4471-4327-7_13.
27. Jefee-Bahloul H, et al. Pilot assessment and survey of Syrian refugees' psychological stress and openness to referral for telepsychiatry (PASSPORT Study). Telemed J E Health. 2014;20(10):977–9.
28. Samuels A. International telepsychiatry: a link between New Zealand and Australia. Aust N Z J Psychiatry. 1999;33:284–6.
29. Harley J. Economic evaluation of a tertiary telepsychiatry service to an island. J Telemed Telecare. 2006;12(7):354–7.
30. Ekblad S, Manicavasagar V, Silove D, et al. The use of international videoconferencing as a strategy for teaching medical students about transcultural psychiatry. Transcult Psychiatry. 2004;41:120–9.
31. Fishkin R, Fishkin L, Leli U, et al. Psychodynamic treatment, training, and supervision using internet-based technologies. J Am Acad Psychoanal Dyn Psychiatry. 2011;39:155–68.
32. Mucic D. International telepsychiatry: a study of patient acceptability. J Telemed Telecare. 2008;14:241–3.
33. www.denlilleprins.org
34. Mastermind. 28 Feb 2015. At http://www.southdenmark.com/showcases/terapi-hjemme-i-dagligstuen.aspx/.
35. Seligman M, Dillinger M. Real-time multi-media translation for healthcare: a usability study. In: Summit MT, editor. XIII: the Thirteenth Machine Translation Summit. Asia-Pacific Association for Machine Translation (AAMT). 2011. p. 595–602. March 7, 2015. At: http://www.mt-archive.info/10/MTS-2011-Seligman.pdf.
36. Teixeira CSC. Multilingual systems, translation technology and their impact on the translator's profession. In: Neustein A, Markowitz JA, editors. Where humans meet machines. New York: Springer; 2015. p. 300–9. http://link.springer.com/10.1007/978-1-4614-6934-6.

How Does the Internet Influence the Doctor–Patient Relationship?

Mark Agius and Helen Stangeland

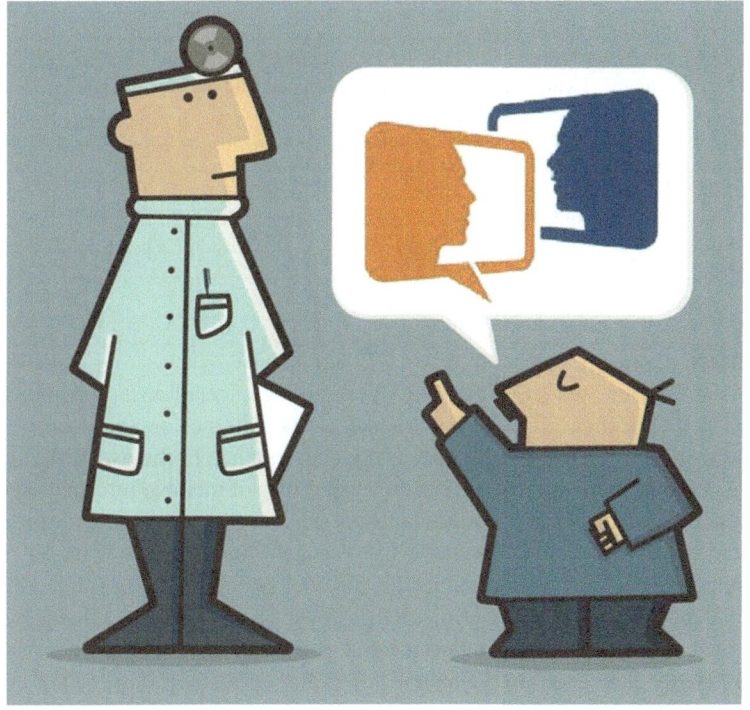

M. Agius (✉)
Department of Psychiatry University of Cambridge and Clare College Cambridge,
University Foundation Trust, Wickford, Essex, UK
e-mail: ma393@cam.ac.uk

H. Stangeland
Third Medical Faculty, Charles University Prague, Prague, Czech Republic

© Springer International Publishing Switzerland 2016
D. Mucic, D.M. Hilty (eds.), *e-Mental Health*,
DOI 10.1007/978-3-319-20852-7_13

Contents

13.1   Introduction 252
13.2   The Doctor–Patient Relationship 253
    13.2.1   Trust 253
    13.2.2   Holistic Approach 253
    13.2.3   The Standard Pathway to Care 254
    13.2.4   The Therapeutic Effect of Doctors 255
    13.2.5   The Relationship of Evidence-Based Medicine
         to the Doctor–Patient Relationship 255
    13.2.6   Consultation Analysis 255
    13.2.7   Consultation Style 257
13.3   Applying Our Knowledge About the Consultation to Telemedicine 257
13.4   Has the Doctor–Patient Relationship in Fact Been Affected by the Internet? 258
13.5   How the Internet Affects the Doctor–Patient Relationship: The Research Data 259
    13.5.1   A Better Informed Patient Equals Better Overall Health 259
    13.5.2   Disparities Between Patient Groups 259
    13.5.3   The Active Patient 260
    13.5.4   Time and Effectiveness 260
    13.5.5   Patient's Ability to Critically Review Internet Information 261
    13.5.6   Bringing Health Information from the Internet into the Doctors' Office 261
    13.5.7   Change to the Patient–Doctor Relationship 261
    13.5.8   Internet Skills and Guidance 262
13.6   Conclusions and Recommendations Going Forward 263
    13.6.1   Recommendations 263
    13.6.2   Some Possible Problems 263
Conclusion 264
References 264

Abstract

In this chapter, we consider the doctor–patient relationship as classically described. We then consider the impact of the Internet on the doctor–patient relationship in two ways. One way is the consequence of the use of the Internet for videoconferencing; the other is the availability of medical information on the Internet in various forms, so that patients are able to easily access information before or after the consultation, while various Websites may even be recommended during the consultation itself. The doctor–patient relationship continues to be central to the practice of medicine; however, the Internet influences it in a number of ways, and it is important that clinicians are aware of these so as to optimise the help given to the patient.

13.1   Introduction

Over the last few years, with the Internet becoming widely available, concerns have been raised that the doctor–patient relationship may be in some way changed or even compromised by the ease of availability of information which patients may glean from the Internet. There has been concern that by removing the position of the doctor as the sole source of medical information there will be change in the balance of the relationship between doctor and patient to the detriment of one or other party [1, 2].

The aim of this chapter is to examine these concerns, firstly by examining the nature of the doctor–patient relationship, then by examining the reasons for these concerns, subsequently by discussing the data presently available as to how the doctor–patient relationship has in fact been affected by the Internet. Finally, we shall produce some suggestions, based in fact on the literature about the relationship itself and our understanding of it as to how the use of the Internet can in fact be seen as potentially enhancing, rather than harming the doctor–patient relationship [3–5].

13.2 The Doctor–Patient Relationship

In the UK, both General Practice and Psychiatry have made the idea of the doctor–patient relationship the central tenet of medical practice [6].

The key concept of the doctor patient relationship is the consultation, which has been described by Sir James Spence as "The occasion when, in the intimacy of the consulting room, a person who is ill, or believes himself to be ill, seeks the advice of a doctor whom he trusts" [7]. It is this consultation which is the central moment in the relationship between two persons; one of whom may have a problem, but also much life experience, while the other, who also has had years of life experience and study of the art of medicine, is believed by the first to have the knowledge and skills to help find a solution [6].

13.2.1 Trust

Trust between the two persons concerned is essential to a successful outcome, but it can only be achieved by the two, doctor and patient, valuing each other as individual persons, each with their own knowledge, experiences and frailties. There is the need for each of the two to accept the other: for the doctor to accept that the patient genuinely needs help but has intellect and willingness to understand what may be offered and make appropriate choices and for the patient to understand that the doctor may indeed have the knowledge to help solve his situation, but at the same time also has his/her human frailties and weaknesses, and indeed is not infallible, though well intentioned [6].

13.2.2 Holistic Approach

However, the doctor's approach must take many considerations into account; it must be holistic. Sir James continued "Before explanation and advice can be given to a patient, three diagnoses must be made: the diagnosis of the disease, of the concept or fears of the disease in the mind of the patient and of the patient's capacity to understand the explanation" [7]. A patient's illness may take on many different aspects, depending on what the patient understands about the doctor's explanation of the disease and what the patient fears or is concerned about, and the doctor's advice must take this into account [6].

Ian McWhinney has said, "This is not a matter of rejecting the reductive (disease) theory, but enlarging its scope to overcome its limitations" [8]. The holistic approach recognises that illness is closely related to the personality and experience of the patient and that man cannot be understood in isolation from his environment. The holistic view acknowledges that every illness is different and that the physician himself is an important aspect of the healing process. The function of the doctor and his communication skills in the healing process is of great importance [9].

Brown and Freeling have stated: "The doctor's function is to understand the whole of his patient's communication so that he could assess the whole person and be able to consider the effect of any intervention in an illness on the whole life of his patient" [9].

Trust is essential. Francis Peabody as early as 1927 pointed out "Do you see what an opportunity you have? The foundation of your whole relation with the patient is laid in those first few minutes of contact. Here is a worried, lonely, suffering man, and if you begin by approaching him with sympathy, tact and consideration, you get his confidence and he becomes your patient" [9].

13.2.3 The Standard Pathway to Care

It should be remembered that patients consult doctors after a great deal of consideration on their part. Tuckett, in 1976, pointed out that, "Individuals have symptoms much of the time, and that dealing with them, particularly by self-medication, is a day-to-day activity; that individuals visit the doctor on average for only one of about ten symptoms that they suffer; that when they do go these symptoms have not necessarily got worse; that their motives for going and what they want from the doctor, may often have more to do with some change in their social circumstances than with any change in symptoms" [10].

The fact that patients tend to consider a great deal before consulting the doctor and that they usually think very hard, discuss with family and friends, even look up in books or consult pharmacists or other mental health professionals they have access to, before seeing the doctor, is the "health seeking behaviour" which has been described by Goldberg and Huxley as a "first filter" in their pathway to care [11–14]. This is very relevant to the issue of the use of the Internet by patients; the Internet is in fact one more source which the patient might use in attempting to clarify his/her thoughts and achieve some understanding of his/her situation before going to see the doctor. Hence, it is analogous to all the other sources of information the patient may have access to, even though it is a very accessible and powerful one [15, 16].

13.2.4 The Therapeutic Effect of Doctors

There is the need that both patient and doctor recognise the other as a unique person, as all human persons are indeed unique, and therefore in themselves have a value which is inestimable, because there shall never be another person like the one who is before them.

Michael Balint, in 1964, listed the doctor's tasks as "listening", "understanding" and "using" the understanding so that it should have a therapeutic effect [17]. Balint had pioneered "Balint Groups", which were in fact psychotherapeutic groups for doctors who could discuss within the group the difficulties which they encountered in relating to individual patients. This is how doctors work with patients in order to help them recover. The therapeutic effect of the doctor himself should never be underestimated. One of us [MA] was privileged in his GP training to have met a doctor who was one of the original members of the first Balint Group. This doctor always quoted Balint as repeating "Remember that the first thing a doctor prescribes to a patient is himself."

13.2.5 The Relationship of Evidence-Based Medicine to the Doctor–Patient Relationship

It is all too easy in a medical system which is dominated by evidence-based treatment algorithms which prescribe "best practice" and which are dependent on biologically developed medication to fall into the trap of treating the disease identified only by science rather than attempting to help the patient. Such a mechanistic approach, which pays little heed to the patient's needs, fails to recognise the patient as a person. It is necessary that doctors "think laterally", in order that they may identify aspects of the patient's condition apart from the primary illness which in themselves require treatment. One of us (MA) frequently recounts to students a mistake he once made as a General Practitioner, when he treated a patient with severe rheumatoid arthritis, who was severely distressed, without recognising that the patient was actually also suffering from depression secondary to her arthritic condition. As a result, important needs of the patient remained unaddressed.

13.2.6 Consultation Analysis

What we have so far argued depends very much on the concept of viewing both the doctor and the patient as unique individuals who have their own understanding, experience and knowledge which may have been gleaned from many sources, one of which is the Internet but others are books, friends and acquaintances with whom they have discussed their symptoms and which will have influenced how they each enter the consultation. It is the task of the doctor to ensure that the consultation is managed appropriately, so that both doctor and patient can understand each other, share their knowledge, apply it to a common problem, which is the one that the patient has brought, and then come up with a common solution [3–5].

Consultation analysis has developed as part of doctor's training in order to emphasise how this mutual understanding can be brought about in the consultation [18].

Roger Neighbour describes the phases of a consultation in his book "The Inner Consultation" as a five-stage mode [19]. The doctor first connects with the patient and develops rapport and empathy. He then "Summarises" with the patient their reasons for attending, including their feelings, concerns and expectations from the consultation. Having made a diagnosis, he then "hands over" or shares with the patient an agreed management plan which hands back control to the patient. He then "Safety-nets" or makes contingency plans with the patient in case the clinician is wrong or something unexpected happens. Finally, once the patient has left, the doctor "housekeeps" or takes measures to ensure the clinician stays in good shape for the next patient.

Another excellent model for the consultation is Silverman's Calgary Cambridge method of analysing consultations [20], which is now used by a large number of medical schools in the UK. This method is based on previous work by Pendleton et al. [21] and is an evidence-based approach to integration of the "tasks" of the consultation and improving skills for effective communication. Silverman divides the consultation into: Firstly initiating the session by establishing rapport and thence establishing the reasons for the patient consulting. From this develops a shared agenda between doctor and patient. Next information is gathered; the patient tells his/her story. The doctor used open-ended questions initially, only using closed questions later to get additional information. The doctor identifies verbal and non-verbal cues given by the patient. Next the doctor builds the relationship further – developing rapport, recording notes, accepting the patient's views and feelings and demonstrating empathy and support. Then the doctor provides explanation and develops a treatment plan with the patient by giving digestible, understandable information and explanation. Finally, he closes the session by summarising and clarifying the agreed plan.

The emphasis throughout is on mutuality and sharing of both the doctor's and patient's prior knowledge, fears and concerns, the doctor's acceptance of these with empathy and the development of a mutual plan between doctor and patient [18].

Some of this knowledge, as well as fears and concerns, may have been gleaned by the patient from the Internet [15, 16]. Hence, the doctor must work together with the patient to clarify, using his medical training and understanding, what the patient has understood from many sources including Internet sources to place this knowledge in the context of the patient's real situation and develop a plan together with the patient in order to best manage the situation.

During the consultation, one must accept that the doctor and patient may see the consultation as having different aims. For the doctor, the history, examination and investigation results in a differential diagnosis, while for the patient, expression of his ideas, expectations and feelings results in an understanding of the patient's beliefs and concerns by the doctor. An integration of both these viewpoints is necessary in the consultation in order that a joint plan of action can be developed [18].

13.2.7 Consultation Style

The doctor's consultation style is important. A patient-centred consultation style is less authoritarian: It encourages the patient to express their own feelings and concerns and uses open questioning, because of the doctor's interest in the psychosocial aspect of illness, before going to closed questions to clinch the diagnosis [18].

Thus, an integrated approach to information gathering, seeking to identify physical psychological and social factors, is likely to produce a better outcome [18].

Body language is important in establishing rapport and empathy. Even how the doctor sits affects how he projects himself. If the patient is across the desk and the doctor sits like a headmaster, then the consultation becomes more authoritarian, while if the patient and doctor are not separated by a desk, then the consultation is held on a more equal footing [18].

Therefore the doctor–patient relationship is very dependent on the adoption of a consultation style which leads to an open discussion between doctor and patient which leads to the sharing of information by both parties, so as to come to a common mutually agreed solution to the problem which the patient has presented for discussion, which is to be implemented by a mutually agreed plan [18]. Some but not necessarily all of this information may have been provided by the Internet [15, 16].

13.3   Applying Our Knowledge About the Consultation to Telemedicine

Up to now we have discussed the doctor–patient relationship in general terms. It should be added here that in the opinion of the present authors what has been said is equally applicable when the consultation is carried out not in a room, as is conventional, but across a televised screen, with the doctor and patient in different localities.

Hence, it is clear that even in a televised consultation the doctor and patient can use an open consultation style, including appropriate body language, which develops an appropriate rapport, and empathy and leads to the development of a mutually agreed plan. Perhaps the best evidence for this is the fact that in British Clinical Schools and General Practice training programs, the common method of training doctors in the consultation skills mentioned above is in fact the videoing of consultations [real or simulated] and their consequent analysis for the aspects of a good consultation which we have mentioned above [22–24].

Data on telepsychiatry carried out in this way is well summarised by Hilty et al. [25]; it appears that there are no major impediments to the development of the doctor–patient relationship in terms of communication and satisfaction. Hilty rightly points out that many factors affect perception of the telemedicine visit and communication by those taking part. Disclosure may be affected by the presence of others in the room, belief of being videotaped and concerns about stigma. Furthermore, patients who have not used telemedicine before may feel anxious, may be distracted by the equipment, or may be self-conscious about seeing himself/herself on a screen [25].

The free flow of the consultation may be interrupted by signal delay [26], so that a turn-taking conversation occurs rather than the free-flowing conversation indicative of a high-rapport interaction [27], and if parties speak at the same time they may perceive the other as interrupting [25]. However, no differences with the development of rapport were found in a small cohort which experienced brief signal delays [26]. Patients tend to respond in a "conservative" or "stilted" way when audio delay occurs with videoconferencing [28].

The environment of a telepsychiatry consultation is different from that of a face-to-face consultation, and as a result several cues, for example gait, are missing [29]; however, at present, it is assumed that the videoconferencing provides an appropriate physical environment for good decision-making [25]. Cukor et al. have reported that telepsychiatry enables a "social presence" to be established which enables both doctor and patient to share a virtual space, get to know one another and discuss complex issues [30].

Non-verbal communication is of great importance in establishing mutual connections and understanding. This it does through eye contact, gestures, posture, fidgeting, nods, grins, smiles, frowns and lip reading [28]. It is reported that decreased ability to detect non-verbal cues occurs during videoconferencing for patient interviews [31]. This has been described as the "cuelessness" phenomena [32]. A task-oriented focus with a depersonalised content may occur as a consequence of this during telepsychiatry consultations. It has been noted that higher levels of mutual gaze were recorded in telepsychiatry [33], which was higher than usual interpersonal interactions [34]. This may help understanding between the two participants [25]. It appears that patients have reported lower levels of anxiety in telepsychiatry during the consultation, while physicians reported increased anxiety [25]. Patients also reported some sense of not having been understood [25].

An in-person conversation takes less time than videoconferencing [35, 36].

It appears that telepsychiatry does not significantly interfere with the development of a therapeutic alliance [37]; however, we have reviewed the consequences of the use of telepsychiatry utilising the Internet here because it is important to be aware of the changes which we have discussed above when performing a diagnostic consultation over the Internet. Similarly, there is literature about delivering psychological therapy over the Internet using videoconferencing [38], and similar changes in delivering therapy will occur [39].

13.4 Has the Doctor–Patient Relationship in Fact Been Affected by the Internet?

Doctors have expressed concern that Internet access results in a more time-consuming consultation, because patients become more demanding and have more complex questions or may have misinterpreted the information they have acquired on the Internet [40].

However, rather than disrupting the doctor–patient relationship, the availability of information gleaned from the Internet appears to enhance to a degree the discussion between the patient and the doctor [1, 40–42]. Because of information gleaned from the Internet, patients appear better informed about their condition and better able therefore to help develop a jointly agreed treatment plan [40, 43].

It is nowadays a very frequent occurrence that patients seek information on the Internet before consulting the doctor, often without informing the doctor of that fact; however, fortunately, patients tend to value their doctor's opinion more highly than the information which they have found on the Internet [44]. Often, patients might also simply want the physician to explain, contextualise or just give their professional opinion about the information they bring to the consultation [4].

If the doctor has not fully explained the situation to the patient, some patients seem to consider the Internet as a low-cost extension of their doctors' guidance, seeking information that the doctor had not made clear during the consultation [42, 45, 46]. On the other hand, anxiety and lack of trust in the physician can be the drive for individuals to use the Internet [46]. Given the wide availability of the Internet, it is useful for doctors to give the patients recommended Internet sites which they can use as supplementary sources of psychoeducation for the patient to reinforce the knowledge imparted in the consultation.

13.5   How the Internet Affects the Doctor–Patient Relationship: The Research Data

We can now review in some more detail the data published so far regarding the impact of the Internet on the doctor–patient relationship.

13.5.1 A Better Informed Patient Equals Better Overall Health

Over the past several years, the Internet has given a broader access to health-related information and patients seem to use this possibility frequently [15, 16].

- It is suggested that this factor actually improves the overall health to the individual patient by "*making subsequent health-related behavioural changes*" [47]. Several patients report changing their thinking about their health after exposure to health-related information on the Internet [48, 49].
- It appears that patients seem to consider the Internet as a low-cost extension of their doctors' guidance, using it to seek information that the doctor had not made clear during the consultation [42, 45, 46]. Because of this, it would appear logical that the doctor should, during the consultation, offer some sites which he considers useful for the patient to consult.
- Internet support forums can be beneficial in giving patients psychological support [43].

13.5.2 Disparities Between Patient Groups

Socioeconomic factors can play a role regarding the propensity of patients to seek information on the Internet. Several factors are involved in lowering the threshold for searching the Internet for information. These include age, sex, education, household income and work positions. Education seems to weigh most out of these factors. In general, the younger and higher educated people, especially women, seems to educate themselves about their health [3, 4, 41, 44, 46, 47, 50–52]. However, the outcome of consultations does not seem to be changed by the use of the Internet because the patients still regarded the doctors' opinion as having the highest value [44].

The elderly have a lower tendency to seek health-associated information and tend to maintain the traditional paternalistic relationship to their physician [53]. This has a strong connection to their generally lower computer skills [53]. Still, demographic and situational variables may play an important role here as well [53].

Sometimes, anxiety and lack of trust in the physician can be the drive for individuals to use the Internet [46].

13.5.3 The Active Patient

It has been reported that the use of information which the patient has abstracted from the Internet has led to a shift from the traditional paternalistic physician–patient relationship towards a more dynamic relationship based on partnership [1, 40–42].

- The patients who discuss the health-related information they have retrieved from Internet seem to be more confident and active instead of being a passive recipient. Hence, patients who have used the Internet to seek information may feel that they have a better sense of control over their situation.
- This can especially be true for the long-term (chronic) patients who must manage their disease for a long period of time and visit the doctor more frequently than the average person. Since a chronic disease, such as diabetes, must be controlled at all times, the patient becomes more familiar with his/her body and how it responds to different treatments. These patients seem to educate themselves to a higher degree about their disease and treatment options on the Internet, and they then discuss these options with their physician [42].
- In general, the patients seem to communicate better due to their increased understanding of their situation and so they are more able to participate in the decision making regarding their treatment [40, 43].
- Often, patients might also simply want the physician to explain, contextualise or just give their professional opinion about the information they bring to the consultation [4]. This is particularly important, since there is evidence that the patients still regard the doctors' opinion as having the highest value, as compared to the Internet [44].

13.5.4 Time and Effectiveness

The informed patient can decrease the time spent in consultation with the doctor, making the diagnosing more smooth and effective [1, 16].

- Internet information can help patients evaluate the importance of their complaints before the consultation, in order to get the best use of the limited time with the doctor [4].

- The doctor might also benefit from the quick access to health-related information during consultations [52, 55].
- On the other hand, some doctors have claimed that Internet access results in a more time-consuming consultation, because patients become more demanding and have more complex questions or may have misinterpreted the information they have acquired on the Internet [40].

13.5.5 Patient's Ability to Critically Review Internet Information

Whereas there are many excellent sites on the Internet, unfortunately, the quality of the Internet information is poorly controlled, and since patients lack the theoretical knowledge, they are unable to filter and critically review the information [44]. This along with other misinterpretations can lead to unnecessary fear and anxiety for the patient [40].

- Support forums also give the opportunity for patients to exchange experiences and opinions about their disease. This is regarded as positive but it can become problematic when the forum users encourage others to demand instead of asking the physicians about their diagnosis and treatment [42].
- Although most doctors seem to be positive toward the Internet-educated patients, some doctors fear that the number of patients with more specific demands or other inappropriate requests will increase [1].

13.5.6 Bringing Health Information from the Internet into the Doctors' Office

Some patients seem to experience hesitation to discuss information from the Internet with the doctor. They do not want to offend or seem challenging towards the doctor [56]. Not all patients share information with their doctor [5].

- Patients who have checked the Internet for answers before going to the doctor may have higher anxiety levels compared with those who did not check the Internet [4, 46].
- Others do not hesitate to bring information to the doctor and feel that if they show the doctor that they have invested time, then the doctor will take their problems more seriously. Other motives include *making the most* out of the consultation, clarifying their information and developing a more equal relationship with their GP [4, 40].
- On the other hand, patients can become overconfident and give less value to their doctor's opinion [2, 40, 42]. These patients may use the health information from the Internet to verify the doctors' competence [42, 56]. This can cause some problems and damage the doctor–patient relationship if the doctor's communication skills are not adequate.

13.5.7 Change to the Patient–Doctor Relationship

The shift in roles and dynamics between the doctor and the patient has raised the question of whether access to Internet information improves or worsens the doctor–patient relationship [1, 2]. In most instances, adequate communication skills will ensure that Internet information will lead to a positive improvement of the relationship [3–5].

• As long as the doctor has the ability to listen and use good communication skills to show interest in what the patient wishes to tell, the relationship seems to improve. The feeling of being heard and taken seriously is very important for the patients and can increase trust considerably [4].
• Even though most physicians feel that the Internet might have a positive effect on their relationship to their patients [40], some doctors report that they have difficulties dealing with Internet information, either because they lack communications kills or because they are not adequately updated on what information there actually is on the Internet [57].
• If the doctor feels that his/her authority is being challenged and reacts by acting in a superior or condescending way, the relationship can worsen or possibly be destroyed [4].
• This is not so true for patient groups who are in managed care or have other disadvantages [44].
• Good communication skills seem to result in greatly improved relationships even though the doctor does not necessarily agree with the information which the patient brings.
• Faster diagnosis and better use of consultation time can also contribute to a better relationship [55].

13.5.8 Internet Skills and Guidance

Traditionally, doctors have been the only source of information for patients. The Internet has changed this dramatically and information now flows freely and in an uncontrolled way. Since patients have different predispositions to understand, evaluate and filter information, there are suggestions that health staff should keep themselves updated regarding what the patients might find on the Internet and know where to direct and guide the patients to the best sites of the web. As the Internet influences patients more and more, this would be beneficial for both the doctor and the patients [1, 2, 5, 41, 42, 44, 58].

Until now, giving Internet recommendations and guidance from doctors and other health staff has not been normal procedure for doctors and other health staff [42, 59].

The Internet can prove to be an effective tool not only for education of the patient's current disease but also for prevention. This is especially true for the younger patient group [50]. The elderly do not always have the same adequate computer skills [54] and educating them in using the Internet to make better choices regarding their health has been attempted. However, there is no documentation that educating the elderly in computer skills actually makes a difference in their usage of this information source [53].

13.6   Conclusions and Recommendations Going Forward

There is no question that the Internet is here to stay with us for the foreseeable future. While it is true that the Internet is extremely widely available, and therefore is very frequently used, there is no reason to believe that its impact on the consultation is in any way really different from the other sources of patient information (family, friends, books, articles, etc.) which have been available for much longer. These have been described earlier as the "first filter" in the patient's "pathway to care" [11–14]. Hence the model of the consultation which we have already described [19–21] should be very effective in responding to the needs of the patient, including his/her questions about what he has read on the Internet. Such a consultation model includes empathy and a patient-centred consultation style, which is less authoritarian and which encourages the patient to express their own feelings and concerns and uses open questioning before going to closed questions to clinch the diagnosis. It also includes a collaborative approach to planning interventions to which the patient contributes, now putting to good use the information he had extracted from the Internet and the questions that he had wanted to raise with the doctor. This will lead to a successful consultation [19–21]. Such a model is not "Internet specific", but the presence of information from the Internet can be used to enhance it.

13.6.1 Recommendations

Indeed, since both doctor and patient will be aware that information on the Internet is of varying quality, doctors should have available to themselves a series of useful Websites which they can refer patients to for supplementary information regarding the problem they are dealing with. There are available a number of excellent sites based in the UK, such as the NICE site, which is excellent for information on the recommended National Health Treatment Pathways for all major conditions and also sites of NGOs who advocate for and support patients with specific conditions; Parkinson's UK, British Diabetic Association, Epilepsy Society, Depression Alliance, Manic Depression Fellowship are a few among many such NGOs. There also exist sites for some specific psychotherapies such as cognitive therapies that doctors can judiciously recommend to appropriate patients. Some examples of these are "Living Life to the Full" or "Beating the Blues" [60].

Thus, doctors can, by recommending appropriate sites on the Internet to patients as part of their joint plan to solve the problem, enhance the patient's knowledge and increase the Patient's resilience.

13.6.2 Some Possible Problems

However, there may be some problems with Internet use linked with the nature of the Internet itself. All should be easily solved by the application of the consultation skills described above. Here we briefly discuss some such problems.

13.6.2.1 Discussion Boards

It is worth commenting on the issue of discussion boards, support forums and blogs. Internet support forums can be beneficial in giving patients psychological support [43]. Support forums also give the opportunity for patients to exchange experiences and opinions about their disease. However, a risk has been observed that forum users might encourage others to demand instead of asking the physicians about their diagnosis and treatment [42]. It is wise for doctors to point out to patients that blogs and support forums contain subjective information which applies to the individual writers but not necessarily to all patients or indeed to the individual viewer. Therefore, information obtained from these sources needs to be particularly discussed with health professionals to establish appropriate guidance for the individual patient.

13.6.2.2 Misleading Information on the Internet

Another issue which can arise is that of Websites which give misleading information, which could seriously affect the patient's chance of recovery. These misleading Websites are often found within the Mental Health Field. One example of such a group of Websites are the "pro-anorexia" Websites [61–64]. Dealing with information from these sites will be particularly challenging, but again, the use of the consultation skills we have described should be sufficient to overcome the difficulties.

13.6.2.3 Social Media

A comment should be made about another possible use of the Internet for consultation purposed. This is the use of Social Media such as Facebook or Twitter. The General Medical Council has recently issued guidance regarding this [65]. Essentially, the issue is that confidentiality cannot be ensured on social media sites; therefore, consultations, discussion of patient's condition and prescription cannot be carried out on these sites.

Conclusion

It is the present authors' view that appropriate training for doctors in consultation skills and the use of patient-centred consultation methods will enable doctors to consult effectively with patients who access the Internet for health care advice. The present evidence suggests that this is true, and that, on balance, access to the Internet can in fact enhance the impact of the consultation.

References

1. Moick M, Terlutter R. Physicians' motives for professional internet use and differences in attitudes toward the internet-informed patient, physician-patient communication, and prescribing behavior. Med 2 0. 2012;1(2):e2.
2. AlGhamdi KM, Moussa NA. Internet use by the public to search for health-related information. Int J Med Inform. 2012;81(6):363–73.
3. Rider T, Malik M, Chevassut T. Haematology patients and the internet – the use of on-line health information and the impact on the patient-doctor relationship. Patient Educ Couns. 2014;97(2):223–38.

4. Bowes P, Stevenson F, Ahluwalia S, Murray E. 'I need her to be a doctor': patients' experiences of presenting health information from the internet in GP consultations. Br J Gen Pract. 2012;62(604):e732–8.
5. Russ H, Giveon SM, Catarivas MG, Yaphe J. The effect of the Internet on the patient-doctor relationship from the patient's perspective: a survey from primary care. Isr Med Assoc J. 2011;13(4):220–4.
6. Agius M, Micallef C. On patient centred psychiatry. Psychiatr Danub. 2008;20(3):339–41.
7. Spence J. The purpose and practice of medicine. London: OUP; 1960.
8. McWhinney I. An introduction to family medicine. London: OUP; 1981.
9. Brown K, Freeling P. The doctor-patient relationship. Edinburgh: Churchill-Livingstone; 1976.
10. Tuckett D. An introduction to medical sociology. London: Tavistock; 1976.
11. Goldberg D. Epidemiology of mental disorders in primary care settings. Epidemiol Rev. 1995;17:182–90.
12. Goldberg D, Huxley P. Common mental disorders: a bio-social model. London: Routledge; 1991.
13. Goldberg D, Huxley P. Mental illness in the community: the pathway to psychiatric care (International Behavioural and Social Sciences Library). London: Routledge; 2001.
14. Verhaak P. :Determinants of the health-seaking Process :Goldberg and Huxley's first level and first filter. Psychol Med. 1995;25:95–104.
15. Iverson SA, Howard KB, Penney BK. Impact of internet use on health-related behaviors and the patient-physician relationship: a survey-based study and review. J Am Osteopath Assoc. 2008;108(12):699–711.
16. Wald HS, Dube CE, Anthony DC. Untangling the web—the impact of Internet use on health care and the physician-patient relationship. Patient Educ Couns. 2007;68(3):218–24.
17. Balint M. The doctor, his patient, and the illness. London: Churchill Livingstone; 1964.
18. Agius M. The medical consultation and the human person. Psychiatr Danub. 2014;26 Suppl 1:15–8.
19. Neighbour R. The inner consultation. Lancaster: MTP; 1987.
20. Silverman J, Kurtz S, Draper J. Skills for communicating with patients. 3rd ed. Oxford: Radcliffe; 2013.
21. Pendleton D, Schofield T, Tate P, Havelock P. The new consultation: developing doctor-patient communication. London: OUP; 2003.
22. Cahill P, Papageorgiou A. Video analysis of communication in paediatric consultations in primary care. Br J Gen Pract. 2007;57(544):866–71.
23. Salisbury C, et al. The content of general practice consultations: cross-sectional study based on video recordings. Br J Gen Pract. 2013;63(616):e751–9.
24. Pringle M, Stewart-Evans C. Does awareness of being video recorded affect doctors' consultation behaviour? Br J Gen Pract. 1990;40(340):455–8.
25. Hilty DM, et al. How telepsychiatry affects the doctor–patient relationship: communication, satisfaction, and additional clinically relevant issues. Primary Psychiatry. 2002;9:29–34.
26. Manning TR, Goetz ET, Street RL. Signal delay effects on rapport in telepsychiatry. CyberPsychology Behav. 2000;3:119–27.
27. Tickle-Degnen L, Rosenthal R. The nature of rapport and its nonverbal correlates. Psychol Inq. 1990;1:285–93.
28. Fussell SR, Benimoff NI. Social and cognitive processes in interpersonal communication: implications for advanced telecommunications technologies. Hum Factors. 1995;37:228–50.
29. Kim T, Biocca F. Telepresence via television: two dimensions of telepresence may have different connections to memory and persuasion. J Comput-Mediated Commun. 1997;3:NP.
30. Cukor P, Baer L, Willis BS, et al. Use of videophones and low-cost standard telephone lines to provide a social presence in telepsychiatry. Telemed J. 1998;4:313–21.
31. McLaren P, Ball CJ, Summerfield AB, Watson JP, Lipsedge M. An evaluation of the use of interactive television in an acute psychiatric service. J Telemed Telecare. 1995;1:79–85.
32. Rutter DR. Looking and seeing : the role of visual communication in social interaction. Chichester. New York: Wiley; 1984.

33. Ball CJ, McLaren PM, Summerfield AB, Lipsedge MS, Watson JP. A comparison of communication modes in adult psychiatry. J Telemed Telecare. 1995;1:22–6.
34. Argyle M. Bodily communication. London: Methuen; 1975.
35. Ochsman RB, Chapanis A. The effects of 10 communication modes on the behavior of teams during co-operative problem-solving. Int J Man-Machine Studies. 1974;6:579–619.
36. O'Malley C, Langston S, Anderson A, et al. Comparison of face-to-face and videomediated interaction. Interacting Comput. 1996;8:177–92.
37. Manchanda M, McLaren P. Cognitive behaviour therapy via interactive video. J Telemed Telecare. 1998;4:53–5.
38. Postel M, de Haan H, De Jong C. E-therapy for mental health problems: a systematic review. Telemed e-Health. 2008;14(7):707–14.
39. Nelson E, Duncan A, Lillis T. Special considerations for conducting psychotherapy over videoconferencing. In: Myers K, Turvey C, editors. Telemental health: clinical, technical, and administrative foundations for evidence-based practice. London: Elsevier Insights; 2012.
40. van Uden-Kraan CF, Drossaert CH, Taal E, Smit WM, Seydel ER, van de Laar MA. Experiences and attitudes of Dutch rheumatologists and oncologists with regard to their patients' health-related internet use. Clin Rheumatol. 2010;29(11):1229–36.
41. McMullan M. Patients using the Internet to obtain health information: how this affects the patient-health professional relationship. Patient Educ Couns. 2006;63(1–2):24–8.
42. Hewitt-Taylor J. Bond CS What e-patients want from the doctor-patient relationship: content analysis of posts on discussion boards. J Med Internet Res. 2012;14(6), e155.
43. Valero-Aguilera B, Bermúdez-Tamayo C, García-Gutiérrez JF, Jiménez-Pernett J, Vázquez-Alonso F, Suárez-Charneco A, Guerrero-Tejada R, Cózar-Olmo JM. Factors related to use of the Internet as a source of health information by urological cancer patients. Support Care Cancer. 2012;20(12):3087–94.
44. Murray E, Lo B, et al. The impact of health information on the internet on the physician-patient relationship: patient perceptions. Arch Intern Med. 2003;163(14):1727–34.
45. Armstrong N, Powell J. Patient perspectives on health advice posted on Internet discussion boards: a qualitative study. Health Expect. 2009;12(3):313–20.
46. D'Agostino TA, et al. Toward a greater understanding of breast cancer patients' decisions to discuss cancer-related internet information with their doctors: an exploratory study. Patient Educ Couns. 2012;89(1):109–15.
47. AlGhamdi KM, Almohideb MA. Internet use by dermatology outpatients to search for health information. Int J Dermatol. 2011;50(3):292–9.
48. Cooley DL, Mancuso AM, Weiss LB, Coren JS. Health-related Internet use among patients of osteopathic physicians. J Am Osteopath Assoc. 2011;111(8):473–82.
49. Marin-Torres V, et al. Internet as an information source for health in primary care patients and its influence on the physician-patient relationship. Aten Primaria. 2013;45(1):46–53.
50. Beck F, et al. Use of the internet as a health information resource among French young adults: results from a nationally representative survey. J Med Internet Res. 2014;16(5), e128.
51. Houston TK, Allison JJ. Users of internet health information: differences by health status. J Med Internet Res. 2002;4(2), E7.
52. Bernard E, et al. Internet use for information seeking in clinical practice: a cross-sectional survey among French general practitioners. Int J Med Inform. 2012;81(7):493–9.
53. Campbell RJ, Nolfi DA. Teaching elderly adults to use the internet to access health care information: before-after study. J Med Internet Res. 2005;7(2), e19.
54. Lin X, et al. Health literacy, computer skills and quality of patient-physician communication in Chinese patients with cataract. PLoS One. 2014;9(9), e107615.
55. Purcarea VL, Petrescu DG, Gheorghe IR, Petrescu CM. Optimizing the technological and informational relationship of the health care process and of the communication between physician and patient—factors that have an impact on the process of diagnosis from the physician's and the patient's perspectives. J Med Life. 2011;4(2):198–206.
56. Chiu YC. Probing, impelling, but not offending doctors: the role of the internet as an information source for patients' interactions with doctors. Qual Health Res. 2011;21(12):1658–66.

57. Jacob J. Consumer access to health care information: its effect on the physician-patient relationship. Alaska Med. 2002;44(4):75–82.
58. Tonsaker T, Bartlett G, Trpkov C. Health information on the internet: gold mine or minefield? Can Fam Physician. 2014;60(5):407–8.
59. Dominguez M, Sapina L. Pediatric cancer and the internet: exploring the gap in doctor-parents communication. J Cancer Educ. 2015;30(1):145–51.
60. Chadwick S. Some useful web resources for depression and bipolar disorder. Cutting Edge Psychiatr Pract. 2013;3:359–60.
61. Tierney S. The dangers and draw of online communication: pro-anorexia websites and their implications for users, practitioners, and researchers. Eat Disord. 2006;14(3):181–90.
62. Abbate Daga G, Gramaglia C, Pierò A, Fassino S. Eating disorders and the internet: cure and curse. Eat Weight Disord. 2006;11(2):e68–71.
63. Harshbarger JL, Ahlers-Schmidt CR, Mayans L, Mayans D, Hawkins JH. Pro-anorexia websites: what a clinician should know. Int J Eat Disord. 2009;42(4):367–70.
64. Christodoulou M. Pro-anorexia websites pose public health challenge. Lancet. 2012;379(9811):110.
65. General Medical Council Doctor's use of Social Media 25-03-2013

Pathological Use of the Internet

Vladimir Carli and Tony Durkee

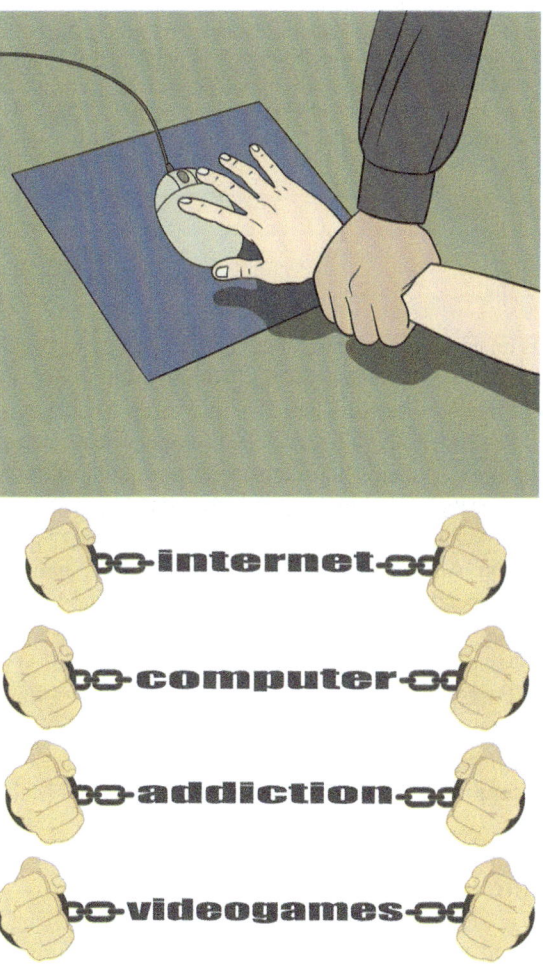

V. Carli, MD, PhD (✉) • T. Durkee, MSc
Swedish National Centre for Suicide Research and Prevention of Mental Ill-Health (NASP),
Karolinska Institutet, Granits väg 4, Stockholm 17177, Sweden
e-mail: vladimir.carli@ki.se; tony.durkee@ki.se

Contents

14.1   Introduction   270
14.2   Trends in Internet Use and Online Activities...   271
14.3   Pathological Internet Use: Diagnosis, Assessment and Aetiologic Theories...............   274
       14.3.1   Nomenclature   274
       14.3.2   Diagnostic Classification...   274
       14.3.3   Assessment   275
       14.3.4   Phenomenology of Pathological Internet Use   277
       14.3.5   Cognitive-Behavioural Model of Pathological Internet Use   278
       14.3.6   Neurobiological Conceptions of Pathological Internet Use   279
14.4   Epidemiology of Pathological Internet Use...   279
       14.4.1   Socio-Demographics of Pathological Internet Users   284
       14.4.2   Psychosocial Factors Related to Pathological Internet Use...........................   284
       14.4.3   Co-morbidity   284
       14.4.4   Suicidal Behaviours and Pathological Internet Use   285
14.5   Treatment Strategies for Pathological Internet Use...   285
Conclusion   286
References...   286

Abstract

The Internet is an extensive medium that is progressing into becoming essential in everyday life. It has opened a new realm of communication, social interactivity and education with endless possibilities for increasing proficiency and erudition. Although the Internet was initially developed for the primary purpose of facilitating research, information seeking and interpersonal communication, for some Internet users, it has become the central focal point in their daily lives. Trends show that mean hours online per week has risen exponentially during the last two decades among the general population. Among specific subgroups, however, studies have shown that some individuals spend between 20 and 80 h per week on the Internet, with some sessions lasting up to 15 h. These individuals often experience clinical depression, anxiety, social isolation and despair. This phenomenon is referred to as pathological Internet use (PIU). Given the complex nature of this condition, this chapter provides a multidimensional overview on the convergence of phenomenological, neurobiological, epidemiological and psychological aspects of PIU in order to provide a better understanding for general practitioners, clinicians and mental health professionals.

14.1   Introduction

Due to technological advances and improved accessibility to information technologies, a substantial increase in Internet usage has been observed across populations and cultures alike. Undertones of the rapid widespread use of the Internet are thought to evolve from its simplistic features, such as accessibility, affordability and anonymity [1]. Accessibility refers to the limitless content that is readily available online. The ample increase in broadband and Wi-Fi connections, along with high-tech advances in mobile phones, has led to a momentous surge in the availability of the Internet that is independent of place and time. This trend has subsequently led to its growing affordability as well. Affordability refers to the overall decline in costs for Internet subscriptions, which is likely due to the increase in Internet providers and direct competition. Anonymity refers to the concealment of both real and perceived identity. The anonymity of the Internet allows users to privately partake in online behaviours without the fear of being stigmatized. This extrapolated anonymity of the Internet provides the user with an anecdotal sense of control over the content, undertone and nature of the online experience [2]. This theory is corroborated by the work of Turkle [3], who suggested that there are two active components that captivate users to go online:

1. the pleasure of control (i.e. individuals tend to have a higher level of control in the virtual world compared to the real world) and
2. the perceived variability of identity in the simulated world (i.e. individuals are able to disguise their true identity online).

The evolution of Internet usage is paired inextricably with the escalation of its excessive use. The convergence of online socialization (addictive Internet applications) and Internet ubiquity with premorbid personality and cognitive dysfunction are major factors in the phenomenology of excessive use and subsequent Internet pathology [4]. This complex interaction is believed to occur on a continuum of biological, psychological and social underpinnings.

Based on the composite nature of this phenomenon, this chapter has three specific objectives:

1. To outline multidimensional approaches used to investigate pathological Internet use (PIU), which are required to fully understand and appreciate its complexity
2. To present a conceptual framework that converges phenomenological, neurobiological, epidemiological and psychological aspects of PIU in order to explore its underlying facets and aetiological pathways
3. To present clinicians methodological approaches to this clinical problem and potential solutions

14.2 Trends in Internet Use and Online Activities

Internet use has grown exponentially worldwide comprising to nearly 3 billion users. Statistics show that the Asian and Pacific regions account for the majority of Internet users worldwide (44.8 %), followed by Europe (21.5 %), North America (11.4 %), Latin America (7.0 %), Middle East (3.7 %) and Oceania (1.0 %) [5].

Internet user penetration levels have reached 40 % globally, with higher rates observed in developed countries (78 %) compared to developing countries (32 %). Europe has the highest penetration rate of both Internet users (73.1 %) and Internet accessibility (76.2 %) compared to the Americas (61.8 % and 54.6 %), Commonwealth of Independent States (CIS) (50.8 % and 48.2 %), Arab States (37.4 % and 33.7 %), Asia and Pacific regions (30.1 % and 32.0 %) and Africa (16.8 % and 9.4 %), respectively (see Fig. 14.1). Global trends have also shown a parallel incline in Internet usage and accessibility rates during the past 10 years (see Fig. 14.2).

Out of the total 2.8 billion estimated Internet users worldwide, 54 % (1.5 billion) are males and 46 % (1.3 billion) are females. Gender disparities between geographic regions and economic standings are noted. In developed countries, 80 % of males and 74 % of females are active Internet users compared to 33 and

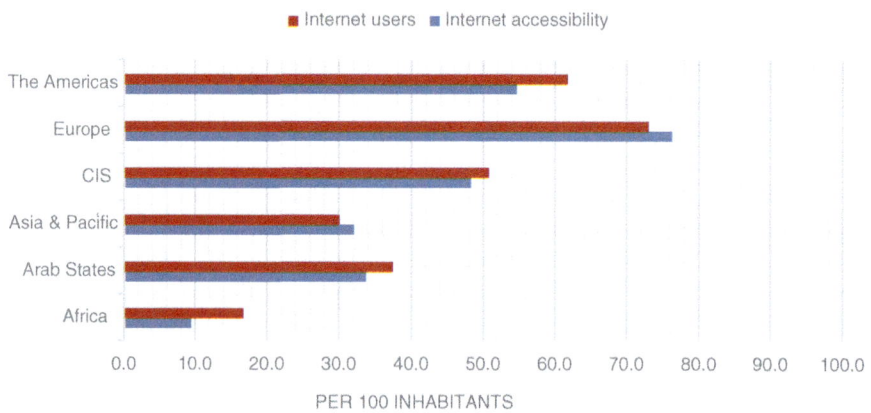

Fig. 14.1 Penetration rates of Internet users and accessibility by geographic region, 2013 (*Data source:* International Telecommunications Union (ITU) [29])

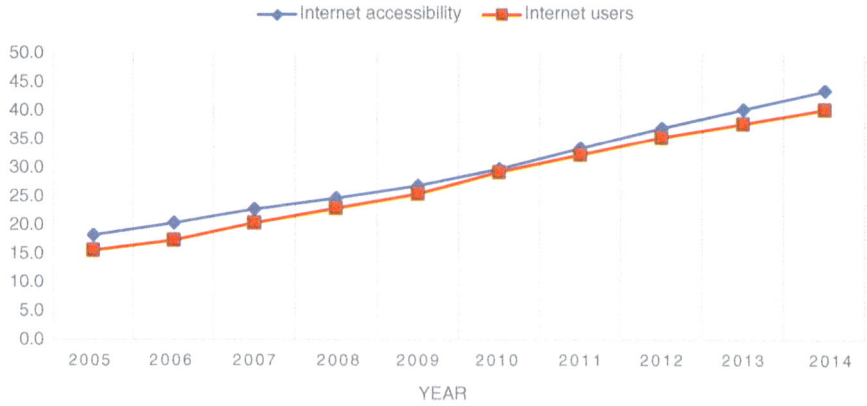

Fig. 14.2 Global trends in penetration rates of Internet users and accessibility, 2005–2014 (*Data source*: International Telecommunications Union (ITU) [29])

29 % in developing countries, respectively [6]. Similar to gender, Internet usage appears to differ by age groups. A recent report on information and communications technology (ICT)[7] showed that 100 % of respondents aged <18 years reported to use the Internet compared to those aged 19–24 years (99 %), 25–35 years (90 %), 36–45 years (91 %), 46–55 years (86 %), 56–65 years (88 %) and >66 years (65 %).

In a survey of the U.S. general population [7], 78 % of Internet users reported to go online at least once a week. Among this group, 87 % reported to check their email at least once per day, while 20 % reported to send instant messages on a daily basis. Results showed that the majority of Internet users tended to surf the Web (78 %), followed by social networking and video sharing (51 %), playing online video games (36 %), downloading or watching videos (35 %), downloading or listening to music (33 %), paying bills (29 %), listening to online radio stations (28 %), shopping online (22 %), visiting religious or spiritual sites (11 %) and gambling (4.4 %). The addictive potential of certain online activities could prove more harmful than others. In a large, cross-national study, Tsitsika and colleagues [8] reported that online gambling and social networking had the strongest correlation with PIU followed by online gaming, visiting chat rooms and Internet forums. Online activities based on social interactivity appear to have the strongest addictive potential.

Time spent online among the general population has increased substantially over the past decade. Statistics show that mean hours online per week has more than doubled from 9.4 in 2000 to 20.4 in 2012 (see Fig. 14.3). Internet use among pathological users, however, have been estimated to range from 20 to 80 h online per week, with individual sessions lasting up to 15 h per day [9]. In a recent review assessing trends among pathological Internet users [10], results showed that subjects spent an average of 4.3 h online per-day compared to 2.9 observed among the general population in the aforementioned.

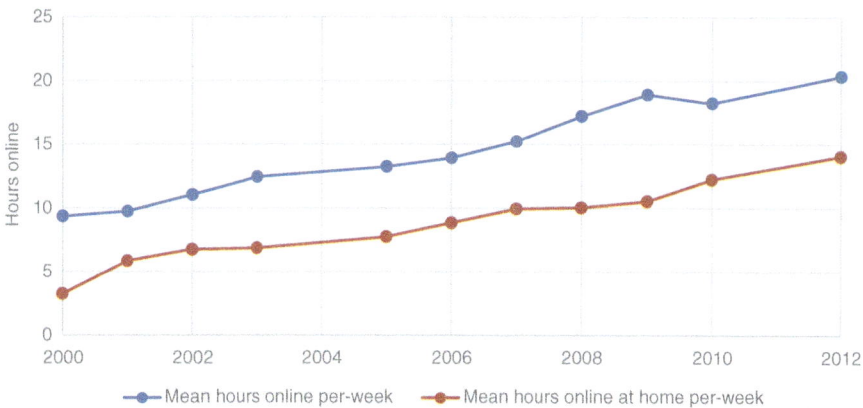

Fig. 14.3 Trends in mean hours online per-week among the general population, 2000–2012 (*Data source*: Digital future report [7])

14.3 Pathological Internet Use: Diagnosis, Assessment and Aetiologic Theories

The taxonomy of pathological Internet use still lacks specificity in many aspects. In order to conceptualize these ambiguities, there are three distinct problem areas to consider: *nomenclature, diagnostic classification* and *assessment*.

14.3.1 Nomenclature

In terms of nomenclature, a review of the scientific literature shows considerable heterogeneity between studies. There are an array of terms that have emerged in recent years to describe this phenomenon, including, but not limited to, Internet addiction, Internet addiction disorder, excessive Internet use, problematic Internet use, computer addiction, cyber addiction, net addiction, compulsive Internet use, Internet dependence, Internet overuse, Internet related disorder, Internet behaviour dependence and pathological Internet use. Despite this heterogeneity, there are some universal components that constitute a PIU definition. These constituents often involve characteristics related to the inability to control one's Internet use, excessive or poorly controlled preoccupations, urges or behaviours with marked distress and functional impairments.

14.3.2 Diagnostic Classification

The diagnostic classification of PIU is still very much ambiguous. There is currently no international consensus on the diagnostic criteria for Internet pathology. It is neither listed in the Diagnostic and Statistical Manual of Mental Disorders (DSM)-Fourth Edition nor the International Classification of Diseases (ICD) nosological systems. In the scientific literature, PIU has conceptually been modelled as an impulse-control disorder and derived from the DSM-IV diagnostic criteria of pathological gambling. It has been proposed that the diagnostic construct of pathological gambling, as a behavioural addiction, is most akin to the pathological nature of Internet use. The major challenge facing PIU, however, is its conception as an addictive disorder. Debates continue to flare as to whether PIU merits inclusion in the DSM nosological system as an official addictive disorder. In the midst of this contention, the recently published DSM-5 has integrated behavioural addiction (non-substance-related addictive disorders) as an official diagnostic category, while including Internet gaming disorder (IGD) into the appendix pending further research. The diagnostic criteria for Internet gaming disorder includes nine specific symptoms: preoccupation, withdrawal, tolerance, loss of control, continued use irrespective of problem awareness, neglect of alternative recreational activities, escapism and mood modification, deception and jeopardizing relationships or jobs. These explicit criteria have also been widely used in developing psychometric instruments for ascertaining PIU diagnoses; however, the nosological ambiguity and lack of conceptual clarity surrounding the concepts of IGD and PIU lead to questions of its validity. Despite the lack of conformity on the diagnostic classification of PIU, there is a general accord among researchers that PIU is, in fact, a legitimate condition that is strongly related to severe interpersonal social and work/vocational.

14.3.3 Assessment

There are a number of different scales and questionnaires that have been developed over the years to assess PIU (see Table 14.1). One of the earliest measures utilized in scientific-based research is the Young's Diagnostic Questionnaire (YDQ). The YDQ was developed according to the DSM-IV diagnostic criteria for pathological gambling. In the YDQ, a diagnosis is based on a pattern of Internet usage, over the past 6 months, in which results in clinical impairment or distress as indicated by the presence of the following criteria: (1) preoccupation with the Internet; (2) need for longer amounts of time online to achieve satisfaction; (3) repeated unsuccessful efforts to control, cut back, or stop Internet use; (4) restlessness, moodiness, depression, or irritability when attempting to cut down or stop Internet use; (5) staying online longer than originally intended; (6) jeopardizing or risking the loss of a significant relationship, job, or educational or career opportunity because of the Internet; (7) lying to family members, therapists, or others to conceal the extent of involvement with the Internet; and (8) using the Internet as a way of escaping from problems or of relieving a dysphoric mood. The 8-item YDQ score ranges from 0 to 8 and can be categorized as follows: adaptive users (scoring 0–2), maladaptive users (scoring 3–4) and pathological users (scoring $\geq$5). The YDQ reflects eight of the nine criteria for IGD in the DSM-5. Although the YDQ has shown to have a relatively acceptable internal consistency ($\alpha = 0.71$), there are still critiques of its validity. Beard and Wolf criticized the questionnaire for being more rigid than the assessment of pathological gambling and suggested that the first five criteria in the YDQ could be met without any loss of psychological or social functioning. They proposed that a diagnosis of PIU should include individuals endorsing the first five criteria (preoccupation, tolerance, inability to cut back, restlessness or moodiness when attempting to reduce use and spending more time online than intended) and at least one of the three latter criteria (adverse consequences, lying to conceal Internet use and use of Internet to escape from problems).

In light of these debates, Young modified the YDQ to account for severity and multifaceted aspects of Internet pathology. Referred to as the Internet Addiction Test (IAT), this 20-item measure assesses psychological dependence, compulsive use, withdrawal, daily routines, productivity, social life and feelings. IAT scores range from 29 to 100 with higher levels indicating a stronger addiction. The IAT was structured in English, and it has already been translated and psychometrically evaluated in Italian, French, German, Finnish, Chinese, Arabic and Korean. The IAT consists of a 5-point Likert scale and has shown to have high face validity, reliability and internal consistency ($\alpha = 0.88$).

Table 14.1 Psychometric instruments for measuring pathological Internet use

Study	Instrument	Description	Scale	Target	Reliability[a]
Young (1998)	Young's Diagnostic Questionnaire (YDQ)	8 items	Yes/No	Adults Adolescents	$\alpha=0.71$ [30, 31]
Young (2008)	Internet Addiction Test (IAT)	20 items	5-point Likert scale	Adults Adolescents	$\alpha=0.88$ [32, 33]
Thatcher and Goolam (2005)	Problematic Internet Use Questionnaire (PIUQ)	20 items	5-point Likert scale	Adults Adolescents	$\alpha=0.90$ [34]
Chen (2005)	Chen Internet Addiction Scale (CIAS)	26 items	4-point Likert scale	Adolescents	$\alpha=0.90$ [35]
Morahan-Martin and Schumacker (2000)	Pathological Use Scale (PUS)	13 items	Yes/No	Adults	$\alpha=0.88$ [36]
Brenner (1997)	Internet-Related Addictive Behaviour Inventory (IRABI)	32 items	Yes/No	General population	$\alpha=0.87$ [37]
Meerkerk et al. (2008)	Compulsive Internet Use Scale (CIUS)	14 items	5-point Likert scale	General population	$\alpha=0.90$ [38]
Caplan (2002)	Generalized Problematic Internet Use Scale (GPIUS)	29 items	5-point Likert scale	Adults	$\alpha=0.78-0.85$ [39]
Caplan (2010)	Generalized Problematic Internet Use Scale (GPIUS2)	15 items	8-point Likert scale	Adults Adolescents	$\alpha=0.91$ [40]
Armstrong et al. (2000)	Internet Related Problem Scale (IRPS)	20 items	10-point Likert scale	Adults	$\alpha=0.88$ [41]
Ceyhan (2007)	Problematic Internet Usage Scale (PIUS)	33 items	Vertical scale	Adults	$\alpha=0.94$ [42]
Davis et al. (2002)	Online Cognition Scale (OCS)	36 items	7-point Likert scale	Adults Adolescents	$\alpha=0.94$ [12]

[a]Cronbach's alpha coefficient

Similar to the IAT, the Chen Internet Addiction Scale (CIAS) and the Problematic Internet Use Questionnaire (PIUQ) are based on the DSM-IV criteria for impulse control disorders. The CIAS is a 26-item self-reported measure with good reliability and validity. In terms of scoring, the minimum and maximum score of the CIAS is 26 and 84, respectively. Higher scores indicate increased severity of addiction to the Internet. It has been primarily used to measure the severity of adolescent PIU in China; however, it is beginning to expand to other Asian countries. This 4-point Likert scale measure has indicated a relatively robust internal consistency ($\alpha=0.90$) and is one of the most utilized scales in Asian populations. The PIUQ is an 18-item measure with a 5-point Likert scale. Total scores range from 18 to 90 with higher scores indicating a greater addiction. Results from a validation study provided good evidence for the reliability and construct validity of the PIUQ ($\alpha=0.90$).

In contrast with the previous scales, which are based on pathological gambling, the Internet-Related Addictive Behaviour Inventory (IRABI) was constructed on the basis of the diagnostic criteria for substance abuse in the DSM-IV. This 32-item measure includes questions related to negative life consequences and side effects of PIU, such as relationship problems and time management issues. The IRABI score ranges from 1 to 32 with higher scores indicating a greater addiction. The IRABI questionnaire has illustrated a relatively good internal consistency ($\alpha=0.87$).

The most robust measures, however, appear to be based on cognitive models, namely the Generalized Problematic Internet Use Scale (GPIUS2) and Online Cognition Scale (OCS). The GPIUS2 consists of 15 items that are rated on an 8-point Likert scale. The items form five subscales, namely, preference for online social interaction, mood regulation, cognitive preoccupation, compulsive use and negative outcome. GPIUS2 has 15 items and all the items are on a scale ranging from 1 (definitely disagree) to 8 (definitely agree). The higher points scored indicate a greater addiction. The OCS is a 36-item questionnaire comprising a 7-point Likert scale. Items are based on symptoms elucidated in the scientific literature, particularly focused on cognitions rather than behaviours, and adapted from related measures of procrastination, depression, impulsivity and pathological gambling. OCS scores range from 36 to 252, with higher scores indicating higher levels of pathological Internet use. The internal consistency of both scales were highly robust at $\alpha=0.91$ and $\alpha=0.94$, respectively.

14.3.4 Phenomenology of Pathological Internet Use

The aetiological pathway and progression of PIU have been theorized using different model-based approaches. According to Griffiths [11], behavioural addictions, such as PIU, develop via biopsychosocial processes that share basic underlying mechanisms and constitute six core components:

- Salience
- Mood modification
- Tolerance
- Withdrawal symptoms
- Conflicts
- Relapse

Salience includes preoccupation with online activities on a number of levels, namely cognitive (compulsive thoughts about online activities), emotional (cravings for next online session) and behavioural (neglecting social and personal responsibilities). Mood modification occurs when individuals use the Internet to alleviate depressed moods or escape from real-life problems. Tolerance is denoted by the necessity to spend more time online in order to attain the desired effect experienced during the initial stages of the addiction. Withdraw symptoms are unpleasant feelings that arise when the individual attempts to decrease or discontinue their Internet usage; this can occur on the physiological level (shaking or tremors) and psychological level (depression or irritability). Conflicts are denoted by interpersonal conflicts (jeopardizing personal relationships) and intrapsychic conflicts (subjective feelings of losing control). Relapse denotes the unsuccessful attempts to reduce or discontinue Internet use. This approach is widely used in research on PIU and related conditions, however, other approaches have also proven effective in operationalizing the conception of Internet pathology.

14.3.5 Cognitive-Behavioural Model of Pathological Internet Use

According to Davis [12], PIU comprises two types: specific pathological Internet use and generalized pathological Internet use. Specific PIU is denoted as a content-specific addiction, such as online gambling. This form of dependency is assumed to exist even in the absence of the Internet (e.g. pathological gamblers visit casinos rather than gamble online). Generalized PIU, however, refers to Internet misuse that is independent of Internet content. This frequently involves a dependency that is based on the unique virtual milieu that only the Internet can provide, such as massively multiplayer online role-playing games (MMORPG).

Davis utilizes a diathesis-stress model to describe the causation of PIU that involves pre-existing vulnerabilities (diathesis) and life events (stressor). The respective model denotes that there are certain aetiological factors that induce addictive behaviour. These include necessary, sufficient and contributory factors. The necessary factor is a preconditioned component for the manifestation of symptoms. Sufficient factors are aetiological elements that guarantee the occurrence of symptoms, while contributory factors significantly increase the development of various symptoms, but are not necessary or sufficient for the occurrence of pathology.

According to this model, causal factors of PIU are placed on a continuum ranging from distal to proximal. Distal causes are contiguous to the onset of the dependency, while proximal causes are towards the end. Psychopathologies are considered a distal necessary cause for the manifestation of PIU symptoms, while exposure to the Internet is considered to be the stressor. It should be noted that the underlying psychopathology alone does not result in PIU symptoms, but is a basic component in the aetiology of the disorder. Depending on the level of response the users receive from their initial online experience ascertains whether they continue to use the Internet. Through a process termed operant conditioning (i.e. a type of learning in which behaviours are modified by its antecedents and consequences), the user develops a pattern of Internet use through positive and negative reinforcement.

Positive experiences then serve to condition the individual to repeat the use of online activities to achieve the same positive effect. Maladaptive cognitions are thought to be proximal causes of the disorder and are a sufficient cause for the manifestation of Internet pathology. In terms of ruminative cognition style, this model suggests that individuals are constantly thinking about online activities rather than real-life issues. These types of persons often experience PIU for longer periods of time and with more severe symptoms than those who do not adopt this cognitive style.

14.3.6 Neurobiological Conceptions of Pathological Internet Use

The neurobiological mechanisms of addiction consist of the molecular and neurochemical changes that occur in an individual during the initial phase of testing the substance or behaviour to the latter stages of a fully developed addiction. The mesolimbic dopamine system has been the principle focal point of neurobiological research in explaining the activating and positive reinforcing effects of substances and behaviours.

The dopaminergic system appears to play a central role in the neurobiological structure of PIU. In a study by Kim and colleagues [13], results showed that individuals with PIU had significantly lower levels of dopamine D2 receptors in subdivisions of the striatum. Further inquiries by Hou et al. [14] supported this finding by showing that individuals with PIU had significantly reduced levels of striatal dopamine transporter (DAT) expression. In genomics, the nicotinic acetylcholine receptor subunit alpha 4 (CHRNA4) gene has been linked with dopaminergic neurotransmission. Based on this premise, Montag and colleagues [15] investigated the liaison between the polymorphism of the CHRNA4 gene and PIU, with results denoting a positive relationship.

Neuroimaging has gained popularity in recent years within the field of addiction, based largely on its ability to measure dopaminergic function and neurochemical changes among individuals. In a recent systematic review of neuroimaging studies on PIU and Internet gaming disorder [16], results indicated that, on the neurological level, PIU and Internet gaming disorders led to neural adaptation and structural changes in the brain as a result of prolonged use, while on the molecular level, PIU was epitomized by a general deficiency in dopaminergic activity.

14.4 Epidemiology of Pathological Internet Use

Prevalence data on PIU are hampered by methodological weaknesses, primarily due to the heterogeneity of definitions and diagnostic instruments. A systematic analysis revealed that previous studies have generally adopted inconsistent definitions and diagnostic criteria, utilized sampling methods that are prone to bias and applied predominantly exploratory rather than confirmatory data analyses [17]. In view of these shortcomings, comparative analyses of PIU prevalence data should include studies that employed similar methodologies. Given the YDQ is widely operational in current research, studies using this questionnaire and endorsing the same cut-off criteria (5/8 items for a PIU diagnosis) were selected and analysed (see Table 14.2).

Table 14.2 Review of studies using comparable methodologies to measure the prevalence of pathological Internet use among adult and adolescent populations

Study	Study design	Sample size	Population	Instrument	Cut-off score	Prevalence
Adult populations						
Kheirkhah et al. (2010) [43]	Cross-sectional	$N = 1,856$	General population Mean age = 20.25, SD = 4.19 years Iran	YDQ	5/8 items on YDQ	22.8 %
Bakken et al. (2009) [44]	Cross-sectional	$N = 3,399$	General population Age range = 16–74 years Norway	YDQ	5/8 items on YDQ	1.0 %
Huang et al. (2009) [45]	Cross-sectional	$N = 4,400$	College students Mean age = 20.19, SD = 1.26 years Age range = 16–30 years China	YDQ	5/8 items on YDQ	9.5 %
Leung (2004) [46]	Cross-sectional	$N = 699$	General population Age range = 16–24 years Hong Kong	YDQ	5/8 items on YDQ	37.9 %
Adolescent populations						
Siomos et al. (2012) [47]	Cross-sectional	$N = 2,017$	Students Mean age = 15.05, SE = .05 years Age range = 12–19 years Greece	YDQ	5/8 items on YDQ	15.2 %
Siomos et al. (2008) [48]	Cross-sectional	$N = 2,200$	Students Mean age = 15.34, SD = 1.66 years Age range = 12–18 years Greece	YDQ	5/8 items on YDQ	8.2 %
Fisoun et al. (2012) [49]	Cross-sectional	$N = 1,270$	Students Mean age = 15.99, SE = .05 years Age range = 14–18 years Greece	YDQ	5/8 items on YDQ	5.3 %

Gong et al. (2009) [50]	Cross-sectional	N = 3,018	Students Mean age = 15.8, SD = 2.1 years Age range = 11–23 years China	YDQ	5/8 items on YDQ	5.0 %
Lin et al. (2009) [51]	Cross-sectional	N = 1,289	Students Mean age = 17.46, SD = 1.00 years Age range = 16–19 years Taiwan	YDQ	5/8 items on YDQ	23.4 %
Johansson and Gotestam (2004) [52]	Cross-sectional	N = 3,237	Students Mean age = 14.9 years Age range = 12–18 years Norway	YDQ	5/8 items on YDQ	1.9 %
Wang et al. (2013) [53]	Cross-sectional	N = 10,988	Students Mean age = 17.2 years Age range = 13–23 years China	YDQ	5/8 items on YDQ	7.5 %
Li et al. (2014) [54]	Cross-sectional	N = 24,013	Students Mean age range = 7.58–15.92 years China	YDQ	5/8 items on YDQ	6.3 %

Among the adult population, there were only four studies identified in the literature that assessed the prevalence of PIU using the YDQ with the predefined cut-off
criteria. The lowest rates were found among a sample of Norwegian adults ($n=3,399$)
aged 16–74 years with only 1 % of subjects meeting the criteria of addiction. On the
other end of the scale, the prevalence of PIU among a sample of young adults
($n=699$) aged 16–24 years in Hong Kong had a staggering PIU prevalence rate of
37.9 %. The remaining two studies reported a PIU prevalence rate of 9.5 % in China
and 22.8 % in Iran, respectively. Despite the homogeneity of methodologies used in
these studies, there was still a large variation of PIU prevalence observed between
countries. This could signal that there is a latent sociocultural factor that is influencing the results.

Among the adolescent population, eight studies were identified in the literature
that assessed the prevalence of PIU using the YDQ with the predefined cut-off
criteria. The sample sizes ranged from $n=1,270$ adolescents in Greece to
$n=24,013$ in China. Mean ages ranged from 7.58 years in China to 17.46 years in
Taiwan. With the exception of the high prevalence observed in Taiwan (23.4 %)
and Greece (15.2 %), the remaining prevalence rates appeared more homogenous.
Similar to the adult population, Norway had the lowest prevalence of 1.9 %. The
remaining prevalence rates were in Greece (5.3 % and 8.2 %) and China (5 6.3 %
and 7.5 %).

In a large, cross-cultural study on the prevalence of PIU in European adolescents,
results showed relatively high and diversified rates between countries [18]. The
study included a representative sample of 12,395 school-based adolescents recruited
from randomly selected schools across study sites in eleven European countries:
Austria, Estonia, France, Germany, Hungary, Ireland, Israel, Italy, Romania,
Slovenia and Spain. Using the YDQ, Internet users were categorized into three
groups: adaptive Internet users (scoring 0–2), maladaptive Internet users (scoring
3–4) and pathological Internet users (scoring >5). The prevalence rate of maladaptive and pathological Internet use for the total sample was 13.5 % and 4.4 %, respectively. Female students presented a higher rate of maladaptive Internet use (14.3 %
in females vs. 12.4 % in males), while males reported a significantly higher rates of
pathological Internet use (5.2 % in males vs. 3.8 % in females). Gender variations
for both maladaptive and pathological use were observed between countries. In
regards to maladaptive use, males had a higher prevalence than females in Estonia
and Slovenia, while in Romania, the opposite was observed. The remaining countries showed similar rates for both genders. In regards to pathological use, small
variations in prevalence rates were found between male and female adolescents in
all countries except Israel, wherein males had a twofold higher prevalence than
females. Significant country differences were found in the prevalence of both maladaptive and pathological use, with Israel denoting the highest prevalence of both
maladaptive use (18.2 %) and pathological use (11.8 %), while Italy signified the
lowest prevalence in these two groups (8.8 % and 1.2 %), respectively (see
Table 14.3).

Table 14.3 Prevalence of pathological Internet use among adolescents in Europe using Young's Diagnostic Questionnaire

Country	Sample	Adaptive use (n = 9,823)						Maladaptive use (n = 1,608)						Pathological use (n = 525)					
		Males		Females		Total		Males		Female		Total		Males		Females		Total	
	n	n	%	n	%	n	%	n	%	n	%	n	%	n	%	n	%	n	%
Austria	943	289	82.8	495	83.3	784	83.1	50	14.3	80	13.5	130	13.8	10	2.9	19	3.2	29	3.1
Estonia	1,034	392	82.5	411	73.5	803	77.7	61	12.8	115	20.6	176	17.0	22	4.6	33	5.9	55	5.3
France	1,003	281	88.4	558	81.5	839	83.7	30	9.4	108	15.8	138	13.8	7	2.2	19	2.8	26	2.6
Germany	1,438	573	83.4	588	78.5	1,161	80.7	81	11.8	127	16.9	208	14.5	33	4.8	36	4.8	69	4.8
Hungary	1,008	369	88.9	533	89.9	902	89.5	37	8.9	53	8.9	90	8.9	9	2.2	7	1.2	16	1.6
Ireland	1,067	506	87.2	417	85.6	923	86.5	47	8.1	57	11.7	104	9.8	27	4.7	13	2.7	40	3.7
Israel	951	513	68.0	153	68.1	666	70.0	142	18.8	31	15.8	173	18.2	100	13.3	12	6.1	112	11.8
Italy	1,188	341	89.7	729	90.2	1,070	90.1	33	8.7	71	8.8	104	8.8	6	1.6	8	1.0	14	1.2
Romania	1,136	303	77.3	629	84.5	932	82.0	69	17.6	83	11.2	152	13.4	20	5.1	32	4.3	52	4.6
Slovenia	1,164	288	83.5	611	74.6	899	77.2	41	11.9	156	19.1	197	16.9	16	4.6	52	6.4	68	5.8
Spain	1,024	452	85.4	392	79.2	844	82.4	58	11.0	78	15.8	136	13.3	19	3.6	25	5.1	44	4.3
Total	**11,956**	**4,307**	**82.4**	**5,516**	**82.4**	**9,823**	**82.0**	**649**	**12.4**	**959**	**14.3**	**1,608**	**13.5**	**269**	**5.2**	**256**	**3.8**	**525**	**4.4**

Source: Durkee et al. [18]

14.4.1 Socio-Demographics of Pathological Internet Users

There are a number of socio-demographic variables that have been linked with path-ological users. These include age of first exposure to the Internet, gender, Internet access at home, city residence, living in metropolitan areas, higher family income levels and migrant status [17, 19]. In addition to these factors, parental involvement, or lack thereof, appears to be a strong indicator of PIU among adolescents. Research shows that adolescents who perceive that their parents do not understand them, know what they do with their free time or do not pay attention to them have an exponentially higher risk of PIU [18].

14.4.2 Psychosocial Factors Related to Pathological Internet Use

In two extensive systematic reviews and meta-analyses of PIU [17, 19], key psycho-social and psychopathological factors related to this phenomenon were accentuated. Results showed that there were shared psychosocial traits among adult and adoles-cent pathological Internet users. These factors included loneliness, low life satisfac-tion, low well-being, low social support, low academic achievement and dysfunctional social behaviours. Adult-specific populations were linked with an insecure attachment style, lack of familial love and child maltreatment experiences. Adolescent-specific populations were associated with online social interaction, neg-ative life events, harm avoidance, low reward dependence, low emotional stability, and low conscientiousness and resourcefulness.

14.4.3 Co-morbidity

There is overwhelming evidence suggesting PIU is significantly associated with neurological complications, psychological distress and social problems. According to Block [20], 86 % of those diagnosed with PIU also meet the diagnostic criteria of another DSM-IV disorder. This notion appears to be evident in the scientific litera-ture. In an examination of adult and adolescent populations [17, 19, 21], unambigu-ously shared psychopathologies have emerged among pathological users. These include: depression, anxiety, compulsivity, sleeping disorders, attention deficit hyperactivity disorder (ADHD) and hostility. Adult-specific populations were shown to be linked with dissociative experiences, depersonalization and alcohol abuse. Adolescent-specific populations were shown to be linked with social phobia, phobic anxiety, schizophrenia, psychoticism, obsessive-compulsive disorder, affec-tive disorder, substance and alcohol use.

In a recent study involving a large and representative sample of school-based adolescents in Europe [22], results indicated a significant correlation between PIU and symptoms of depression, anxiety, conduct problems and ADHD (see Table 14.4). The correlation between PIU, conduct problems and ADHD was stronger among females, while the link between PIU and symptoms of depression and anxiety was

Table 14.4 Multivariate regression model of psychopathology, suicidal behaviours and pathological Internet use among European adolescents

	Pathological Internet use	
Psychopathology	*Coefficient*	*95% CI*
Depression	0.032	0.027–0.037
Anxiety	0.033	0.028–0.038
Emotional symptoms	−0.002	−0.017–0.013
Conduct problems	0.059	0.041–0.077
Hyperactivity and/or inattention	0.057	0.044–0.070
Peer relationship problems	−0.007	−0.024–0.009
Pro-social behaviour	−0.011	−0.026–0.003
Suicidal behaviours		
Self-injurious behaviour	0.132	0.027–0.237
Suicidal ideation	0.314	0.241–0.387
Suicide attempts	0.530	0.185–0.875

Source: Kaess et al. [22]

stronger among males. The correlation between PIU, psychopathology and suicidal behaviours was stronger in countries with a higher PIU prevalence and national suicide rates.

14.4.4 Suicidal Behaviours and Pathological Internet Use

There is currently no data on the relationship between PIU and suicidal behaviours among adult populations. The existing literature comprises limited evidence specifically assessing the liaison between PIU and suicidality among adolescent populations. Despite the ambiguity of research, there are a few studies indicating potential correlations between PIU and self-injurious behaviours (SIB) [23], suicidal ideation [24–26] and suicide attempts [27]. Results from a recent European study among adolescents support these assertions, with observations displaying significant correlations between PIU and self-injurious behaviours, suicidal ideation and suicide attempts (Table 14.4) [22].

14.5 Treatment Strategies for Pathological Internet Use

In a meta-analysis by Winkler and colleagues [28], the authors assessed and compared short- and long-term efficacy of different psychological and pharmacological treatments for PIU. In a direct comparison between cognitive behavioural therapy (CBT) and other psychological treatments, results showed CBTs superiority at reducing time spent online and depression. In regards to pharmacological treatments, escitalopram (Selective Serotonin Reuptake Inhibitor), bupropion (atypical antidepressant) and methylphenidate (Ritalin) showed to improve symptoms of PIU and reduce time spent online. The authors concluded that psychological and pharmacological interventions were highly effective for improving PIU, time spent online and symptoms of depression and anxiety.

Conclusion

In line with forgoing research, this chapter has revealed that PIU is a serious mental health condition in its own right. Results from neurobiological, epidemiological and clinical studies have consistently shown that PIU physiognomies follow similar aetiological and developmental pathways as other DSM-5 psychiatric disorders, with particular relevance to behavioural addiction. Although it is evident that PIU is a disorder that merits a decisive clinical response, the conceptual and nosological ambiguity of the condition impedes appropriate treatment. Recommendations for future research should focus on standardizing the nomenclature and diagnostic classification of PIU in order to establish a perpetual basis for impending investigations, interventions and treatments to produce constructive and purposeful outcomes.

References

1. Cooper A. Sex and the internet: a guidebook for clinicians. London: Brunner-Routledge Psychology Press; 2002.
2. Griffiths M, Wood RTA. Youth and technology: the case of gambling, video-game playing and the internet. In Derevensky JL, Gupta R, editors. Gambling problems in youth: theoretical and applied perspectives. Springer; 2004. p. 101–17.
3. Turkle S. Life on the screen. Simon and Schuster; 2011.
4. Douglas AC, Mills JE, Niang M, Stepchenkova S, Byun S, Ruffini C, Lee SK, Loutfi J, Lee J-K, Atallah M. Internet addiction: meta-synthesis of qualitative research for the decade 1996–2006. Comput Human Behav. 2008;24(6):3027–44.
5. Internet World Stats: Usage and Population Statistics. Accessed on May 12, 2015 [http://www.internetworldstats.com].
6. Biggs P, Zambrano R. Doubling digital opportunities: enhancing the inclusion of women & girls in the information society. Geneva: UNESCO; 2013. p. 66.
7. Cole JI, Suman M, Schramm P, Zhou L, Salvador A. In Dunahee M, editor. The digital future report. World internet project international report (fifth edition). University of Southern California, USA 2013. p. 181.
8. Tsitsika A, Janikian M, Schoenmakers TM, Tzavela EC, Ólafsson K, Wójcik S, Florian Macarie G, Tzavara C, Richardson C. Internet addictive behavior in adolescence: a cross-sectional study in seven European countries. Cyberpsychology, behavior, and social networking Cyberpsychol Behav Soc Netw. 2014;17(8):528–35.
9. Shaw M, Black DW. Internet addiction: definition, assessment, epidemiology and clinical management. CNS Drugs. 2008;22(5):353–65.
10. Kuss DJ, van Rooij AJ, Shorter GW, Griffiths MD, van de Mheen D. Internet addiction in adolescents: prevalence and risk factors. Comput Human Behav. 2013;29(5):1987–96.
11. Kuss DJ, Shorter GW, van Rooij AJ, Griffiths MD, Schoenmakers TM. Assessing internet addiction using the parsimonious internet addiction components model—a preliminary study. Int J Ment Health Addict. 2014;12(3):351–66.
12. Davis RA, Flett GL, Besser A. Validation of a new scale for measuring problematic internet use: implications for pre-employment screening. Cyberpsychol Behav. 2002;5(4):331–45.

13. Kim SH, Baik SH, Park CS, Kim SJ, Choi SW, Kim SE. Reduced striatal dopamine D2 receptors in people with Internet addiction. Neuroreport. 2011;22(8):407–11.
14. Hou H, Jia S, Hu S, Fan R, Sun W, Sun T, Zhang H. Reduced striatal dopamine transporters in people with internet addiction disorder. J Biomed Res Int. 2012;2012:854524.
15. Montag C, Kirsch P, Sauer C, Markett S, Reuter M. The role of the CHRNA4 gene in Internet addiction: a case-control study. J Addict Med. 2012;6(3):191–5.
16. Kuss DJ, Griffiths MD. Internet and gaming addiction: a systematic literature review of neuroimaging studies. Brain Sci. 2012;2(3):347–74.
17. Byun S, Ruffini C, Mills JE, Douglas AC, Niang M, Stepchenkova S, Lee SK, Loutfi J, Lee JK, Atallah M, et al. Internet addiction: metasynthesis of 1996–2006 quantitative research. Cyberpsychol Behav. 2009;12(2):203–7.
18. Durkee T, Kaess M, Carli V, Parzer P, Wasserman C, Floderus B, Apter A, Balazs J, Barzilay S, Bobes J, et al. Prevalence of pathological internet use among adolescents in Europe: demographic and social factors. Addiction. 2012;107(12):2210–22.
19. Kuss DJ, Griffiths MD, Karila L, Billieux J. Internet addiction: a systematic review of epidemiological research for the last decade. Curr Pharm Des. 2014;20(25):4026–52.
20. Block JJ. Issues for DSM-5: internet addiction. Am J Psychiatry. 2008;165(3):306–7.
21. Carli V, Durkee T, Wasserman D, Hadlaczky G, Despalins R, Kramarz E, Wasserman C, Sarchiapone M, Hoven CW, Brunner R, et al. The association between pathological internet use and comorbid psychopathology: a systematic review. Psychopathology. 2013;46(1):1–13.
22. Kaess M, Durkee T, Brunner R, Carli V, Parzer P, Wasserman C, Sarchiapone M, Hoven C, Apter A, Balazs J. Pathological internet use among European adolescents: psychopathology and self-destructive behaviours. Eur Child Adolesc Psychiatry. 2014;23:1093–102.
23. Lam LT, Peng Z, Mai J, Jing J. The association between internet addiction and self-injurious behaviour among adolescents. Inj Prev. 2009;15(6):403–8.
24. Park S, Hong KE, Park EJ, Ha KS, Yoo HJ. The association between problematic internet use and depression, suicidal ideation and bipolar disorder symptoms in Korean adolescents. Aust N Z J Psychiatry. 2013;47(2):153–9.
25. Kim K, Ryu E, Chon MY, Yeun EJ, Choi SY, Seo JS, Nam BW. Internet addiction in Korean adolescents and its relation to depression and suicidal ideation: a questionnaire survey. Int J Nurs Stud. 2006;43(2):185–92.
26. Fu KW, Chan WS, Wong PW, Yip PS. Internet addiction: prevalence, discriminant validity and correlates among adolescents in Hong Kong. Br J Psychiatry. 2010;196(6):486–92.
27. Lin IH, Ko CH, Chang YP, Liu TL, Wang PW, Lin HC, Huang MF, Yeh YC, Chou WJ, Yen CF. The association between suicidality and Internet addiction and activities in Taiwanese adolescents. Compr Psychiatry. 2014;55(3):504–10.
28. Winkler A, Dörsing B, Rief W, Shen Y, Glombiewski JA. Treatment of Internet addiction: a meta-analysis. Clin Psychol Rev. 2013;33(2):317–29.
29. International Telecommunications Union: ICT Statistics. 2014. http://www.ituint/en/ITU-D/Statistics/Pages/defaultaspx.
30. Johansson A, Götestam KG. Internet addiction: characteristics of a questionnaire and prevalence in Norwegian youth (12–18 years). Scand J Psychol. 2004;45(3):223–9.
31. Young K. Internet addiction: the emergence of a new clinical disorder. Cyber Psychol Behav. 1998;1(3):237–44.
32. Young K. Assessment of internet addiction. The Center for Internet Addiction Recovery Accessed on May 20, 2015. www.netaddiction.com.
33. Widyanto L, McMurran M. The psychometric properties of the internet addiction test. Cyberpsychol Behav. 2004;7(4):443–50.
34. Thatcher A, Goolam S. Development and psychometric properties of the problematic internet Use questionnaire. S Afr J Psychol. 2005;35(4):793–809.
35. Ko CH, Yen JY, Yen CF, Chen CC, Yen CN, Chen SH. Screening for Internet addiction: an empirical study on cut-off points for the Chen Internet Addiction Scale. Kaohsiung J Med Sci. 2005;21(12):545–51.

36. Morahan-Martin J, Schumacher P. Incidence and correlates of pathological Internet use among college students. Comput Human Behav. 2000;16(1):13–29.
37. Brenner V. Psychology of computer use: XLVII. Parameters of internet use, abuse and addiction: the first 90 days of the internet usage survey. Psychol Rep. 1997;80(3 Pt 1):879–82.
38. Meerkerk GJ, Van Den Eijnden RJ, Vermulst AA, Garretsen HF. The compulsive internet use scale (CIUS): some psychometric properties. Cyberpsychol Behav. 2009;12(1):1–6.
39. Caplan SE. Problematic Internet use and psychosocial well-being: development of a theory-based cognitive–behavioral measurement instrument. Comput Human Behav. 2002;18(5):553–75.
40. Caplan SE. Theory and measurement of generalized problematic internet use: a two-step approach. Comput Human Behav. 2010;26(5):1089–97.
41. Armstrong L, Phillips JG, Saling LL. Potential determinants of heavier internet usage. Int J Human Comput Stud. 2000;53(4):537–50.
42. Ceyhan E, Ceyhan AA, Gurcan A. The validity and reliability of the problematic internet usage scale. Kuram Uygul Egit Bil. 2007;7(1):387–416.
43. Kheirkhah F, Juibary AG, Gouran A. Internet addiction, prevalence and epidemiological features in Mazandaran Province, Northern Iran. Iran Red Crescent Med J. 2010;12(2):133.
44. Bakken IJ, Wenzel HG, Gotestam KG, Johansson A, Oren A. Internet addiction among Norwegian adults: a stratified probability sample study. Scand J Psychol. 2009;50(2):121–7.
45. Huang R, Lu Z, Liu J, You Y, Pan Z, Wei Z, He Q, Wang Z. Features and predictors of problematic internet use in Chinese college students. Behav Inform Technol. 2009;28(5):485–90.
46. Leung L. Net-generation attributes and seductive properties of the internet as predictors of online activities and internet addiction. Cyberpsychol Behav. 2004;7(3):333–48.
47. Siomos K, Floros G, Fisoun V, Evaggelia D, Farkonas N, Sergentani E, Lamprou M, Geroukalis D. Evolution of Internet addiction in Greek adolescent students over a two-year period: the impact of parental bonding. Eur Child Adolesc Psychiatry. 2012;21(4):211–9.
48. Siomos KE, Dafouli ED, Braimiotis DA, Mouzas OD, Angelopoulos NV. Internet addiction among Greek adolescent students. Cyberpsychol Behav. 2008;11(6):653–7.
49. Fisoun V, Floros G, Siomos K, Geroukalis D, Navridis K. Internet addiction as an important predictor in early detection of adolescent drug use experience—implications for research and practice. J Addict Med. 2012;6(1):77–84.
50. Gong J, Chen X, Zeng J, Li F, Zhou D, Wang Z. Adolescent addictive Internet use and drug abuse in Wuhan, China. Addict Res Theory. 2009;17(3):291–305.
51. Lin CH, Lin SL, Wu CP. The effects of parental monitoring and leisure boredom on adolescents' internet addiction. Adolescence. 2009;44(176):993–1004.
52. Johansson A, Gotestam KG. Internet addiction: characteristics of a questionnaire and prevalence in Norwegian youth (12–18 years). Scand J Psychol. 2004;45(3):223–9.
53. Wang L, Luo J, Bai Y, Kong J, Luo J, Gao W, Sun X. Internet addiction of adolescents in China: prevalence, predictors, and association with well-being. Addict Res Theory. 2013;21(1):62–9.
54. Li Y, Zhang X, Lu F, Zhang Q, Wang Y. Internet addiction among elementary and middle school students in China: a nationally representative sample study. Cyberpsychol Behav Soc Netw. 2014;17(2):111–6.

From Telehealth to an Interactive Virtual Clinic

Michael Krausz, John Ward, and Damon Ramsey

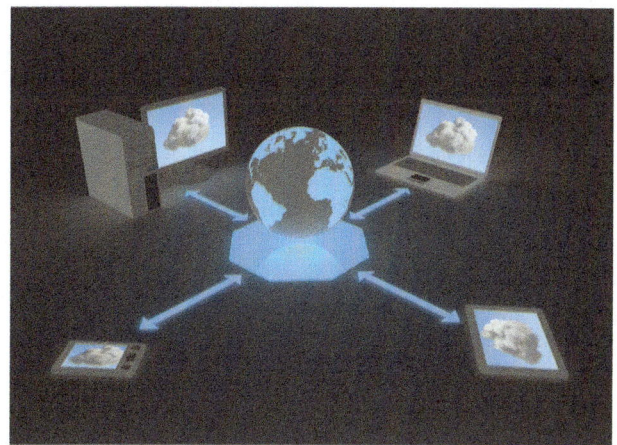

M. Krausz, MD, PhD, FRCPC
Institute of Mental Health at UBC, David Strangway Building room 430 5950 University Boulevard, Vancouver, BC V6T 1Z3, Canada
e-mail: mkrausz@mail.ubc.ca

J. Ward, PhD (✉)
Addictions & Concurrent Disorders Group, Centre for Health Evaluation and Outcome Sciences (CHÉOS), University of British Columbia,
David Strangway Bldg, 430-5950 University Blvd, Vancouver, BC V6T 1Z3, Canada
e-mail: jward@cheos.ubc.ca

D. Ramsey, MD, CCFP, MCSE
InputHealth Systems Inc., #320-638 Broughton Street, Vancouver, BC V6G 3K3, Canada
e-mail: damon@inputhealth.com
http://www.inputhealth.com

© Springer International Publishing Switzerland 2016
D. Mucic, D.M. Hilty (eds.), *e-Mental Health*,
DOI 10.1007/978-3-319-20852-7_15

Contents

15.1   Introduction 291
     15.1.1   Background 292
     15.1.2   Lack of Mental Health Service Capacity 292
     15.1.3   Problems with Quality of Care... 292
     15.1.4   Difficulties with Access and Long Waiting Times.. 292
     15.1.5   Technologies and New Strategies of Response... 293
     15.1.6   Position of a Virtual Clinic in Future Health-Care Delivery....................... 293
15.2   Vision of a Virtual Clinic (VC).. 294
     15.2.1   Building Capacity for Mental Health Services 294
     15.2.2   Quality of Care.. 295
     15.2.3   Improving Access.. 295
     15.2.4   Providing Online Resources... 295
     15.2.5   Doctor-Patient Interaction and Sustainability of Care 296
     15.2.6   Feedback and Evaluation 296
     15.2.7   Better Interaction Between Primary Care and Specialist Services 296
     15.2.8   Principles of Health-Care Delivery in the Virtual Clinic 296
     15.2.9   Advantages of a Virtual Clinic Concept from a System Perspective........... 298
15.3   A Comparison Between Virtual and Psychiatric Clinics...................................... 298
     15.3.1   Functionalities for Different Groups of Participants in the Model 298
     15.3.2   Functionality from the Patient Perspective 298
     15.3.3   Functionality from the Expert Perspective... 301
     15.3.4   Functionality for Primary Care 302
     15.3.5   Functionality for Health Authorities and Treatment Providers.................... 302
15.4   Key Components and Functionalities of a Virtual Clinic (VC)............................ 303
     15.4.1   Patient Registration 303
     15.4.2   Booking of Appointments.. 303
     15.4.3   Introduction/Engagement... 304
     15.4.4   Assessment Tools 304
     15.4.5   Videoconferencing 304
     15.4.6   Prescription and Medication Management... 304
     15.4.7   Online Treatment and Resources 304
     15.4.8   Disease-Related Modules... 305
     15.4.9   Documentation and Reporting 305
     15.4.10 Communication with Patients 305
     15.4.11 Communication Between Professionals.. 306
     15.4.12 Evaluation Section, Research Section.. 306
     15.4.13 Knowledge Exchange: Informed Decision-Making..................................... 306
     15.4.14 Interface to Integrated Web Solutions (e.g., WalkAlong) 306
     15.4.15 Interface to Providers (e.g., Capacity Check, Waiting Times, etc.)............. 306
     15.4.16 Integrated Evaluation 307
15.5   Discussion... 307
     15.5.1   Limitations 308
Conclusions.. 308
References... 309

Abstract

Access to mental health services is, due to current epidemiology, extremely limited. For some areas addressing the special needs of mental health clients, access to experts seems to be nearly impossible. In developed countries, typical explanations include a lack of funding and limited numbers of experts as well as their regional distribution. Building capacity in specialist areas and developing accessibility are two challenges for the health-care system globally.

E-health based on improving web-based technologies provides more possibilities in response. Telehealth initiatives already try to support access in remote areas. High-speed Internet coverage and the development of web-based solutions allows for a new generation of approaches – virtual mental health clinics.

This innovative approach allows for increased capacity through improved communication, more effective service delivery and improves quality of care in a patient-centered treatment model. It could redefine the role of different settings and procedures between existing physical health-care systems with its dominant role, web-based expert-patient interaction, and integrated systems, e.g., addressing frequent conditions like PTSD (PTSD coach) or mood disorders (WalkAlong) with web-based platforms.

Key elements of a virtual clinic need to build on the use of mobile communication devices, mobile health (M-health), videoconferencing (V-health), and communication with patients in an integrated manner, combined with additional online tools to improve accessibility and quality of care. Other possible features and technologies are already evolving like the use of sensor technologies, virtual reality, and gaming.

Conclusion: The web and mobile technologies offer the chance for a paradigm shift in health care towards patient empowerment, early support, and sustainable care.

15.1   Introduction

With limited resources and increasing demand, the appropriate delivery of health care becomes a complex challenge. Already today developed countries invest 10 % of their GDP into health services, while catastrophes like Ebola and HIV become global disasters with global consequences. For example, the economic impact of Ebola in West Africa could reach as high as $32.6 billion by the end of 2015 – over two times the combined GDP of the three core countries [1].

Continuation of the current pattern in health policy is not an option, and for future development – a paradigm shift is necessary. For several reasons, mental health is an area of enormous challenges, with a rapidly growing burden of disease that increased by 37.6 % between 1990 and 2010, and which could benefit from new opportunities that modern technologies are offering [2]. The concept of a virtual clinic is a core concept of web-based technologies as a key response to the crisis.

This chapter will help the reader to:

1. Understand the rationale for the emergence of virtual clinics.
2. Identify their critical components and desirable features.
3. Be aware of the potential benefits of modified service delivery and how it impacts mental health patients, providers, and commissioners.

15.1.1 Background

The structural problems of the current mental health care system are substantial. A rapidly growing burden of disease makes it the largest area in medicine, but there is minimal coverage by appropriate specialized services – with only 10 % of patients ever able to see a specialist, indicative of critical dysfunction in the standard system of care [3].

The proposed concept of a virtual mental health clinic may become a key tool and cornerstone of the paradigm shift in the delivery of mental health care. The idea is to fundamentally reorganize the interaction between patients and health-care professionals, as well as between different groups of health-care professionals especially primary care and specialist care. With a dramatic increase in the use of modern communication tools, new system solutions, and a growing readiness in the population to use web and mobile communication for health care, significant momentum may allow for real change.

15.1.2 Lack of Mental Health Service Capacity

As shown by the national comorbidity survey in the USA and other epidemiological and health-care system research, only a small minority of patients are able to access expert support or even any basic professional help [3–5].

Additionally, surveys show that primary care has to carry a huge burden of mental health care without appropriate support, training, and capacity. From a family medicine perspective, mental health expertise and support is the most critical for daily practice [6]. Moreover, there remains significant stigma attached to mental health, and patients are sometimes hesitant to mention their problems to family physicians [7]. Waiting times for direct access to psychiatry or even specialized mental health services even in metropolitan areas are unacceptably long, e.g., over 6 months for psychiatry in Vancouver.

15.1.3 Problems with Quality of Care

The quality of mental health and addiction care is often unsatisfactory. Approaches are very often generic and not based on best practice, effective interventions are not available, and polypharmacy or an ineffective use of psychopharmaca is a known problem [8]. An interesting example for research in this area is the study of the Institute of Medicine (IOM), which demonstrated the very limited overlap of best practice treatment according to existing guidelines and average treatment delivered [9].

15.1.4 Difficulties with Access and Long Waiting Times

The current health-care system use is a reflection of limited or nonexistent capacities in community mental health care. If waiting times are too long, patients – who may otherwise be able to manage their mental challenges in the community – end up in emergency rooms and acute care, at much higher cost. Such patients are also typically provided with less effective interventions. In particular, patients in remote areas with no access to mental health care may especially suffer negative consequences of this system gap. This also contributes to non-health-care-related costs in society related to absence from work and loss of productivity, police and jurisdiction, etc.

15.1.5 Technologies and New Strategies of Response

The three objectives can be identified as follows:

1. Telehealth and web-based technologies are currently being used to support services in remote areas and populations with special need. The number of apps addressing specific health issues has grown substantially and now numbers around 100,000 in total, with around 100 being specific to mental health [10].
2. Growing availability of the web and readiness to use E-health services is also documented in a recent survey by Price Waterhouse Coopers (PWC) on mobile health. This major consulting company sees web-based technologies as critical for the future development of health care [11].
3. Comparing the possibilities of emerging technologies to the level of implementation and the contribution of E-health to the current provision of health care demonstrates a significant gap that is possible to address with the concept of the virtual mental health clinic.

15.1.6 Position of a Virtual Clinic in Future Health-Care Delivery

The interplay between the following four key elements will be an important consideration for future health-care delivery.

- The existing physical health-care system, providing face-to-face services, accounts for about 90 % of current health care.
- Existing digital support services in direct connection to the physical health-care system, such as Electronic Medical Records (EMR), planning and documentation tools, financial systems, billing, etc.
- Virtual clinics are nearly nonexistent. These are web-based services catering for both professionals and patients, covered through normal health-care funding.
- Integrated web systems for disease management and knowledge exchange, providing a range of resources to clients and professionals.

The possible overlap between the current system and technology is illustrated in Fig. 15.1.

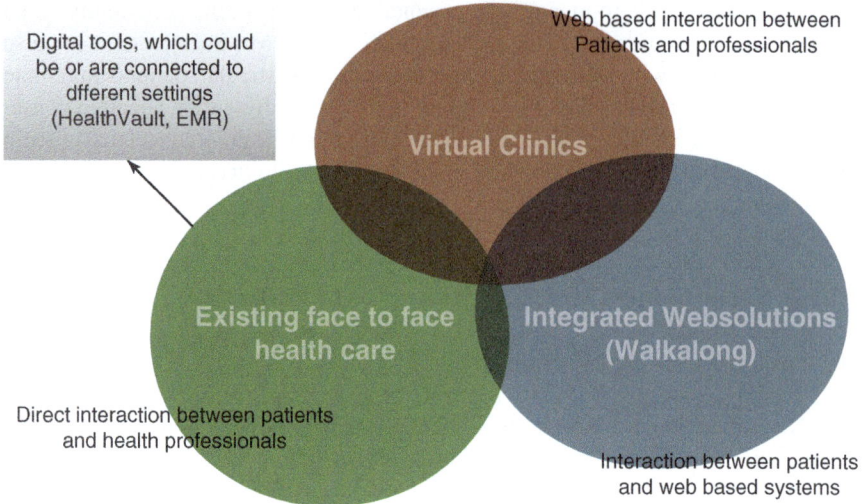

Fig. 15.1 Key components of future health care

15.2 Vision of a Virtual Clinic (VC)

The virtual clinic is an effective way of providing high-quality care, based on the needs of patients in an accessible, transparent, and dynamic manner, using existing and emerging new technologies.

The core objectives of this development are based on an overall different approach to health-care delivery: to make health-care delivery more patient centered, to empower users, and to provide an interactive and integrated framework for sustainable support across the continuum of needs.

15.2.1 Building Capacity for Mental Health Services

With very limited expertise and big problems in terms of accessibility of services, this aims to:

- Help mental health experts and physicians to focus on interaction and patient-focused activities instead of spending too much time with administrative tasks such as documentation and billing.
- Increase the flexibility of interaction through intensive use of mobile technologies and communication.
- Reducing the burden of necessary infrastructure, allowing therapeutic interaction outside of clinics and offices, more convenient for patients.
- Make it possible for mental health experts in administrative or research functions to take on a limited burden of care to address needs.

15.2.2 Quality of Care

Improvement in quality of care is a long-term, ongoing, dynamic process. The (web-based) system needs to support professional efforts in quality assurance through the following mechanisms:

- Improving the quality of assessment and screening by the provision of standardized psychometric tools and reporting mechanisms on an ongoing basis.
- Providing online resources extending the professional tool kit, as well as self-help tools.
- Providing integrated information and knowledge exchange on best practice.
- Supporting ongoing communication between doctors and patients through the use of modern communication tools and mobile devices.

15.2.3 Improving Access

Access to mental health care is one of the most critical bottlenecks in the current system. In addition to long waiting times, psychiatry and special expertise are often only available in metropolitan areas. These issues will be addressed using the following strategies:

- Web-based communication and interaction with mental health professionals, allowing patients to contact the system, and for professionals to respond in an asymmetric (asynchronous) manner whenever suitable.
- Supporting easy, ongoing communication and other services such as assessment, prescription refill, or information, without having to visit the clinic.
- Supporting direct patient-doctor interaction through videoconferencing.
- Providing effective online treatment tools at any given time.

15.2.4 Providing Online Resources

Frontline clinicians may often not be aware of existing online *resources* and consequently not recommending them to their clients. It is also complex to oversee existing solutions and new developments. An important goal of the virtual clinic is to support access to proven and effective online solutions, including:

- Online training and information.
- Online psychotherapy, which is a well-tested area with some effective solutions especially in the treatment of depression and anxiety.
- Integrated web solutions for specific populations such as WalkAlong (WalkAlong. ca) for youth with mood challenges and PTSD Coach (http://www.ptsd.va.gov/public/materials/apps/PTSDCoach.asp) for individuals with trauma experience [12, 13].

15.2.5 Doctor-Patient Interaction and Sustainability of Care

Due to workload, funding, and organization, typical physician-patient interaction is only limited to a few minutes. The virtual clinic model shall support interaction between professionals and patients over the long-term using several mechanisms:

- Long-term screening and assessment of symptoms, including feedback loops to the client.
- Questions and reminders automatically produced through the system.
- Short consultations (by email) about ongoing treatment and possible questions.

15.2.6 Feedback and Evaluation

To improve the quality of care, and adapt services to the needs of the patient, ongoing feedback loops and systematic evaluation are essential. A virtual clinic system could allow patients to rate experiences and professionals to systematically evaluate use and outcomes of their interventions, like it is already standard in other online service areas like travel.

15.2.7 Better Interaction Between Primary Care and Specialist Services

In essence any system of support needs to cover the essential domains of recovery. Primary care plays a special role, often being the main or only source of support. Its quality relies on functioning secondary and tertiary care.

Improved communication, reporting, and other mechanisms provide additional tools and support a more intense and timely collaboration between primary care and psychiatry – an especially relevant GP specialty given the enormous burden of disease in their daily practice.

With patient permission, the exchange and interpretation of assessments and information could redefine the role of experts and allow for higher quality of primary care for the mentally ill.

15.2.8 Principles of Health-Care Delivery in the Virtual Clinic

The potential strengths of the virtual clinic concept can be stated in Table 15.1, which could also be used as quality criteria.

Health-care paradigms, innovations, allocation of resources, and structural decisions appear different based on the party involved. An interesting and powerful reason to seriously consider the proposed virtual clinic approach is that it has significant advantages for the system, patients, and treatment providers.

Table 15.1 Strengths and quality criteria for the VC concept

Dimension	Function
Accessibility	Patients should be able to use mental health services without barriers. The system should be possible to use in an uncomplicated and direct manner. It should provide access and support for patients from remote areas or from marginalized populations
Increased capacity	The VC should add capacity to the existing mental health and addiction system; improving efficacy, integrating additional professionals, and using tools to optimize the diagnostic and therapeutic process, including documentation and reporting
Sustainability	The system should support mental health professionals to continuously stay in contact and monitor health outcomes, through reminders, screening and assessment, and mobile communication. Through integration with primary care and other support systems, it would be easier to create clinical pathways
Contact and communication	Through the intense use of modern mobile communication, videoconferencing, and system flexibility, the VC will be able to improve contact and enable or intensify interaction if necessary
Quality of care	It will support diagnosis and treatment according to best practice through the ongoing provision of information and links to literature and research. The integration of gold standard tools into the system will improve the quality of diagnostics and reporting to the client. The integration of online therapy and resources will increase the range of interventions
Evaluation and transparency	Ongoing feedback loops, ranking and rating, as well as quality assurance mechanisms will be part of the system to allow users and health-care providers control of the quality of care and health outcomes
Empowerment	Most of the time patients and families have to deal with problems, coping, and therapy management on their own. The professional system needs to empower and encourage them to do that in the best possible way. This includes respect for their decisions, transparency in support of informed decision-making, and acknowledgment of needs
Peer and family involvement	Family members and peers are very often the main resource for patients with mental challenges. If they want to involve them, the VC should support communication and interaction with them, including joint visits or discussions
Flexibility and adaptability	Care needs to understand and adapt to different populations and user profiles to be effective. The VC should be a learning system, providing care in the most effective way
Informed decision-making	All participants in the process should have access to necessary information, research evidence, and clinical options, as well as risks to be able to make the best possible decisions for themselves

15.2.9 Advantages of a Virtual Clinic Concept from a System Perspective

The health-care system is driven by cost. While the governance and funding structures may be different, e.g., comparing the USA, Canada, or Europe, the guiding principles and values are similar. All systems face a critical increase in costs and also growing need, based-for example-on demographic development or the growing burden of disease through mental health challenges [2]. Table 15.2 highlights several key advantages for the virtual clinic.

15.3   A Comparison Between Virtual and Psychiatric Clinics

The differences between virtual and physical psychiatric clinics are explored in Table *15.3*, using multiple dimensions of comparison.

15.3.1 Functionalities for Different Groups of Participants in the Model

The VC will be used by different parties with different needs and for different functionalities as illustrated in Fig. 15.2. Ideally it should have advantages for all users in the process.

15.3.2 Functionality from the Patient Perspective

The virtual clinic concept can provide an easy-to-use and ergonomic user interface. The system is constructed to be accessible at all times, 24 h a day. Some features may be used by patients with no direct interaction with professionals through integrated web platforms, which is preferred by certain patient populations such as young people [17]. It also allows for increased peer connectivity [18–20] and may also increase health literacy [10].

Why would a patient use it?

1. Accessibility
   An important advantage of web-based communication. In a VC, patients will be able to book appointments directly, pose questions, and access therapeutic or diagnostic resources, which otherwise would take a long time. In remote areas, patients often have no direct access to services because they are nonexistent.
2. Patient preference
   Patient preference may be especially important for younger demographics, or patients who do not want to leave their jobs to sit in a waiting room. It is easier to avoid unpleasant and stigmatized communication with access to appropriate support.

Table 15.2 Potential advantages for a virtual clinic model

Dimension	Advantage
Cost-effectiveness	The VC concept is an effective way to address overhead costs, travel times related to health care, and waiting times while improving quality of care and better health outcomes. A study from an Australian virtual clinic estimated the cost savings to be around 77 % compared to traditional treatment, without loss of efficacy. Due to the scalability of the virtual clinic model, these savings are likely to be higher in the future [14]
Avoiding ineffective use of health resources	The current approach is focused on crisis intervention and acute care. Providing mental health support online, early, and in the community could prevent the ineffective use of emergency rooms. Instead of investing in the treatment of complications and long-term consequences due to inaccessibility of care, online health platforms and virtual clinics can contribute to a more effective use of the system
Prevention and early intervention	One of the biggest problems in mental health care is the long period between first serious symptoms and a systematic/professional response. In addiction, for example, it is around 10 years [15], and this appears to be similar for most public mental illnesses [16]. Integrated web platforms and VCs can support the integration of lifestyle management, targeted prevention, and treatment in a new quality
Integration of clinical pathways along needs	The virtual clinic concept aims to connect different providers through better communication, easy referral, timely assessment, and recommendations. Access to the system is easy and encourages patients to use online treatment tools, ongoing monitoring, and other resources that go into the direction of early detection and intervention and beyond just crisis intervention
Integration with different areas of health care	The concept could function as a platform, which facilitates and integrates service provision in a transparent and collaborative way. The effectiveness of that approach depends on the readiness of different professions to change practice. Given the important role of primary care in mental health and the different professional areas involved, this may be especially important
Access to specialist	The availability and access to mental health specialists is one of the biggest problems in current service delivery. The VC concept is able to increase capacity, improve efficacy, and support timely interventions. Indeed, specialists can use Internet tools to monitor patient outcomes in order to proactively support them before a crisis develops [7]
International and transcultural options	In a virtual clinic, it may be much easier to provide services for users from different cultural backgrounds who may speak different languages. From a global health perspective, clinics may be a tool to provide health care in countries or areas with little or no infrastructure. Counseling and support can be, for instance, provided in conflict zones with international expert support for local clinicians. The potential for such a development is extremely promising
Use of resources for patients and families	The support of families and peers is critical given their role in ongoing care and crisis management for individuals with mental challenges. It is well proven that inclusion of family members into treatment is an effective psychosocial intervention, and highly underutilized

(continued)

Table 15.2 (continued)

Dimension	Advantage
Systematic evaluation	Users will be asked for informed consent on a regular basis. The system should document data on use, population, and outcomes and create performance reports whenever needed. Agglomerated data should be also possible to use for embedded trials
Development of an integrated feedback, rating, and evaluation system	Users of the clinic could be given the opportunity to rate and compare their experiences, provide suggestions for improvement, and contribute to the transparency of the process

Table 15.3 Comparison between virtual and psychiatric clinics

Function	Psychiatric clinic	Virtual clinic	Remark
Waiting times for an appointment	In Vancouver, about 6 months	Under 2 weeks	Varies across a particular region
Waiting times in the clinic	Yes	None	
Travel time	Yes	None	In some regions, long travel time with high additional cost
Standard assessments	Exception	Rule	
Mode of interaction	Face to face	Email, videoconference, chat, etc.	
Reporting	Depends	Immediately	
Regular automated follow-ups and reminders	No	Yes	
Psychotherapies	Exception	Online CBT, self-help	
Medication	Direct prescription, pharmacy waiting time, pick up	Direct prescription, medication management support	
Cost for the system		Immediate care, less loss of productivity	
Cost for the patients		No travel cost or waiting cost	
Cost for the psychiatrist	Overhead cost	License cost, no overheads	

3. Easy to navigate and user-friendly

   Good solutions are built on user expectations and are easy to navigate. Recent apps focusing on lifestyle monitoring (Nike, Apple, etc.) are fun to use, reinforcing, and engaging.

4. Availability of expertise

   Expertise is often limited. A broader network or VC helps to access specialist or people with lived experiences.

5. Additional features

   Integrated web platforms or virtual clinics provide a wealth of features which add to the expert interaction and advise from self-assessment and ongoing

VC-Expert activities

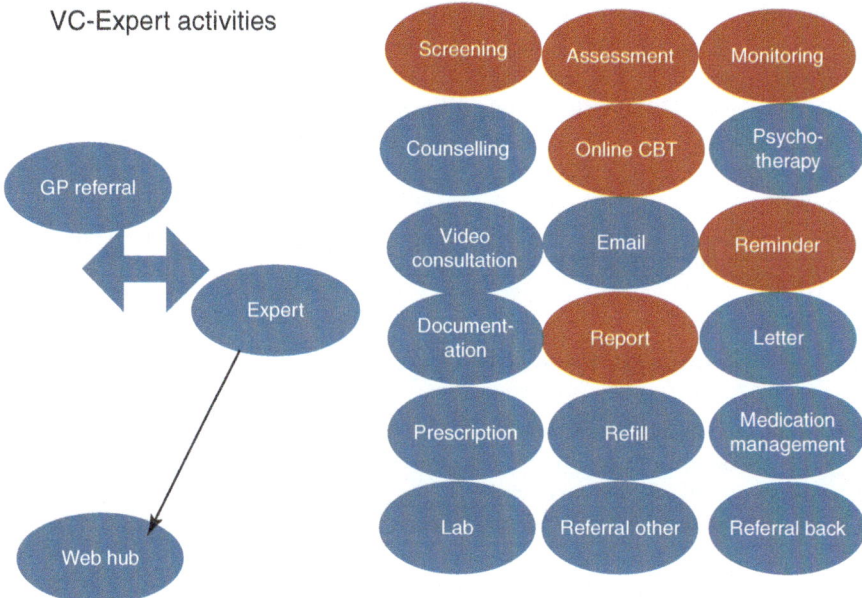

Fig. 15.2 Highlighting the various functionalities of a virtual clinic

monitoring to online therapies; easy-to-use tools expand the options for people in need.

6. Personal health record (e.g., Microsoft HealthVault https://www.healthvault.com/de/en [21])

   Only a personal health record gives users control of their records and data.

7. Privacy

Integrated Internet platforms and virtual clinics provide the option to stay anonymous and more protected.

15.3.3 Functionality from the Expert Perspective

For professionals, no office space or significant infrastructure is needed. Time-consuming processes are automated, and documentation and billing are supported. The system also improves time autonomy and flexibility in client care.

Why would an expert use it?

1. Small overheads

   Working in a VC model doesn't require administrative assistance, special rooms, or other resources.

2. Working from home, at night or in between other activities

   Given that specialists are often involved in special settings and academic environments, flexibility is crucial. The VC approach will improve flexibility of the workflow, removing the need to work specific business hours. That may also serve some patient populations better.

3. Integration of billing and documentation

   The bureaucratic burden would be reduced, so that even time-limited clinical work would be possible and useful.

4. Best range of expertise, best clinical concept

   A VC would make it easier to improve the collaboration between different levels of expertise and appropriate clinical pathways.

5. Use of agglomerated data to answer evaluation questions

Systematic data collection could answer upcoming service-related questions and improve health outcomes and quality of care.

15.3.4 Functionality for Primary Care

For referring physicians, standardized reporting and quick communication with experts, including a range of tools on mental health care, support primary care efforts and quality of care in general.

Why would a primary care physician use it?

1. Easy accessibility and communication with experts

   For primary care or emergency physicians, providing access to specialists is complicated and time-consuming. The possibilities of asynchronous communication or booked consultations could revolutionize interaction between primary care and secondary or even tertiary experts.

2. Supporting tools

   The options of an integrated web platform with assessment, monitoring, informed decision-making, etc., are useful tools already in existing practice serving the mentally ill.

3. Working from home, at night or in between other activities

   The VC approach improves flexibility of the workflow, removing the need to work specific business hours. That may also serve some patient populations better.

4. Integration of billing and documentation

   A VC system would support different aspects of medical work that are not a direct part of patient interaction, but consume enormous amount of time.

5. Effectiveness

   It would be possible to serve more patients better in a given period of time.

6. Sustainability and monitoring of clients

Automated reminders and monitoring functions allow for follow-up with necessity to intervene only in case of deterioration. Critical developments could be detected much earlier, which would support the early intervention approach.

15.3.5 Functionality for Health Authorities and Treatment Providers

The VC improves documentation, transparency of process and patient flow, and ongoing evaluation and reporting to allocate resources and improve client care.

Through integration of different components, it could help to establish and support more clinical pathways and sustainable health-care delivery beyond crisis.

Why would a health authority, treatment provider or institution use it?

1. Flexible tool with Electronic Medical Records (EMR)

   EMR systems are huge databases with limited flexibility. As part of their business model, they do not like to easily share information, and their integration into complex environments is expensive and complicated. A VC system with defined data exchange protocols can function as an interface, which remains under the control of the provider and improves functionality. The protocols are defined standards and ready to use. In the future, VC systems may also become an alternative to existing and often dysfunctional EMR systems. VC systems also reduce the dependence on certain solutions and companies and allow for choosing better solutions without loss of data and control.

2. Cost-effectiveness

   Small, flexible, organizational, and technical solutions are more functional and less expensive. Health care is a dynamic process and needs permanent development and adaptation to changing environments. The ability to change functionalities with little investment marks the superiority of this approach.

3. Quality improvement

   Quality assurance and improvement are a key domain of functional health-care systems. As already mentioned, standard assessment, monitoring of key indicators, and online resources are already available as part of integrated web platforms and apps such as WalkAlong and Mindcheck [22], for example.

4. Clinical pathways

Patients are often served by several treatment providers or institutions. Information exchange and communication is a critical component even in health authorities. VC could be tailored to specific needs, and interfaces could be created to make ongoing care more effective.

15.4 Key Components and Functionalities of a Virtual Clinic (VC)

15.4.1 Patient Registration

To use the clinic, users must register in order to benefit. After a guided tour and video explanation of the available functions, patients are asked for informed consent and other information to establish an appropriate legal framework. A picture (or avatar) should also be included to make sure that in case of a videoconference, the right person participates.

15.4.2 Booking of Appointments

The booking system should allow clients to choose their own appointments and how they interact with the system. The physician has to confirm their appointment. The booking procedures should also allow for crisis appointments in case of emergency, and participating physicians should provide a limited number of crisis consultations.

15.4.3 Introduction/Engagement

An introduction and a guided tour are critical for engagement. The whole design and atmosphere/tone of the clinic needs to support engagement. It should be warm, welcoming, and personal. A help function could support orientation.

15.4.4 Assessment Tools

The VC platform should allow for easy and flexible integration of assessments. The display and the reporting should support the use of assessments, scoring, interpretation, and ongoing long-term monitoring.

15.4.5 Videoconferencing

Videoconferencing is an important communication tool. It should allow high-quality, secure communication between doctor and patient, among professionals, between several professionals like primary care physician and expert and patient, and physician, patient, and family. High-definition video would be ideal. With two-time encryption, it is already allowed in other parts of British Columbia.

15.4.6 Prescription and Medication Management

Prescription, medication monitoring, documentation, compliance monitoring, and interpretation of side effects are key parts of the doctor-patient interaction. The clinic should support the professional side as well as the patient's side as effectively as possible. The goal is to provide high-quality information at the general and individual level, to professionals as well as patients, to make the best possible informed decisions. If this component functions well, it could contribute to better care and a reduction of polypharmacy, side effects, and noncompliance. Collaboration with pharmacies and other health professionals such as nurses, emergency settings, and acute care could also support the management of emergencies. This system should allow for an actual printed overview and history that the patient could choose to share with their support network.

15.4.7 Online Treatment and Resources

Mental health will be, and already is, the medical area with the best online treatment options. The platform should allow for integration of existing online CBT and support the interface and development of new approaches. It should provide recommendations for the use of online tools and rate them based on scientific evidence. This is an evolving area with some interventions that are well tested, like online CBT for depression and anxiety, smoking cessation, and PTSD coach, and some very good new concepts that still need evaluation. It would be invaluable if the system could contribute to the research on use and quality of online resources. Appropriate designs and evaluation strategies need to be developed.

15.4.8   Disease-Related Modules

To improve adherence to guidelines and scientific evidence in the treatment of mental illness but also physical conditions, it could be very helpful to prepare disease-related modules that could be used and recommended by experts. For example, it could contain a depression module, anxiety module, substance use module, a PTSD module, and some physical health modules like obesity, metabolic syndrome, hypertension, and sleeping disorders. These could be improved and developed over time and should include screening recommendations and tools, gold standard assessments, online resources, key facts for self-management, and online treatments and tools.

15.4.9   Documentation and Reporting

Documentation, letters, and reporting are the most time-consuming and critical areas of medicine. The support of quality documentation and reporting would be an important reason for professionals to use this system. Other than in the existing EMR systems, it needs to support patient needs and better communication between health professionals around treatment. The reporting should integrate different information sources, clinical notes, assessments, information about treatment, and medication into understandable and useful documents.

15.4.10   Communication with Patients

The support of communication between patients and therapist and patient and peers should be possible in different ways, based on the principles of easy access. It should be effective in terms of time and transparently regulated to make sure that it is used appropriately. It may also help to explore different levels of communication such as exploration and counseling in the planned session, follow-up reminders and questions, emergency advice, or questions and answers to get advice on a specific topic or general advice. In case of high volume, a moderator or administrator could help to direct users to appropriate sources. In general, it is important to discuss how communication should be organized and optimized.

15.4.11 Communication Between Professionals

Typically several professionals are involved in the treatment of complex conditions, and communication between the primary care physician and the mental health experts is especially important. Information, feedback, or advice should be shared in a defined time frame. Reports should be well structured and short. Emergency advice should be possible in a defined procedure.

15.4.12 Evaluation Section, Research Section

The evaluation section could be a separate added component, which will not be part of the basic package. It may be interesting to consider a basic and advanced version that could include a cross-sectional overview of clinic users and clinic performance (e.g., access or response times), and satisfaction levels amongst different user groups. The research tool could help set up embedded trials and evaluate specific questions like who is using what. If done in a sophisticated way, such a tool could be very helpful for timely clinical research and evaluation.

15.4.13 Knowledge Exchange: Informed Decision-Making

The availability of helpful and supporting information, links to research and evidence, and user-based input are critical and need to be updated on a regular basis. Specific links to quality Websites and a select choice of key papers, summaries, and information should be part of the different modules. The selection, presentation, and quality of content are critical in times where there is an overwhelming amount of publications.

15.4.14 Interface to Integrated Web Solutions (e.g., WalkAlong)

The virtual clinic should encourage and facilitate the use of integrated web solutions as another important setting for future health care. If possible, links should be integrated into modules but also as short recommendations in a separate spot.

15.4.15 Interface to Providers (e.g., Capacity Check, Waiting Times, etc.)

With interested providers or authorities, an interface could be defined which would allow patients to check real-time capacities, waiting times information, as well as description of services and contacts.

15.4.16   Integrated Evaluation

1. Population monitoring

    The purpose is to better understand potential users of the virtual clinic, to improve performance and adapt to the specific needs of changing populations. Data collection, based on informed consent, would happen automatically, especially using social demographic information.

2. Health outcomes

    The purpose of monitoring outcomes is to understand whether patients are improving or not using the interventions. For general monitoring, broader screening tools can be used.

3. System use and performance

    This dimension should reflect the way the VC is used by patients. Besides assessing time variables and frequencies, users should be interviewed about their experiences.

4. User satisfaction

Satisfaction is critical for efficacy and performance. Both experts and patients should be consulted with short questionnaires as well as in detailed interviews on a regular basis.

15.5   Discussion

E-Mental Health is in its early stages of development. The number of isolated health apps is increasing every week. The big technology players such as Google, Microsoft, and Apple are working on interfaces and solutions, or even their own products [23]. Big EMR companies are dominating and expanding markets in hospitals worth billions without any evidence of the positive impact they have promised for the past 25 years. The contradiction between growing possibilities, upcoming technologies as momentum, and the slow progress in addressing significant system problems in health care is becoming obvious.

In particular, two things are missing: common principles in the development of health care based on patient needs and values which guide the use of resources, structures, and decision-making. Without these, the added value to the current system is difficult to prove. The different components need to play together and interact to make a difference.

To build something significant, you need development and research capacity. Universities and private business need to take on their responsibilities. Systematic bold funding opportunities are needed to create a new sector of E-health, one that is not limited or led by EMR companies. To translate face-to-face interaction and procedures into digital formats needs expertise and capacity at universities and in development labs.

The use of a VC is flexible and provides different options in how it can be used: whether as a substitute or an addition to face-to-face interventions. The next few years will see several different models before there will be something like a mainstream approach. Some possible principles are described for consideration.

15.5.1 Limitations

The experience with the virtual clinic concept is very limited. The different, necessary components - funding models, technology, resources, professional acceptance and skills - need to be aligned, developed and implemented.

The ratio of virtual to face-to-face care is still something to explore. Virtual clinics are not a replacement for existing structures and institutions, but more of a complement which allows for capacity building in different areas of health care and makes better use of physical structures and face-to-face interactions (see Fig. 15.1). The best functionality is something which needs to be explored and may be a dynamic component based on patient needs.

The quality of existing solutions can be improved, particularly around specific engagement for target populations. User interfaces for young people may need to look different than for the elderly, for example, and navigation, media use, and platform should reflect general preferences in the use of technology.

Beyond that, the potential use of specific technologies such as virtual reality, simulation, and gaming has not been fully explored, and may well be an important direction to explore in future.

Additional costs of online resources are limited but are a factor. The involvement of private business may create a separate health market, which could contribute to developments like the Apple App Store.

Last but not least, acceptance of users is a main prerequisite for changing habits and the uptake of opportunities. The implementation of any innovation or change is a widely underestimated challenge. Even if good alternative solutions exist, it can take years until they may take over as a standard. In regard to E-Mental Health, web-based solutions need to be adapted to specific needs of a population served and to existing physical solutions and clinical pathways.

Change needs investment. Although compared to other health services E-Mental Health is inexpensive, without the support of this innovative sector nothing will happen.

Who are the change agents?

Everyone who is aware of the significant pitfalls of the current approach and its consequences. We need a coalition for a paradigm shift.

Conclusions

The web and upcoming mobile technologies are more than just gadgets: they are critical tools to change paradigms in the mental health-care system. Patient empowerment needs to be front and center to turn the development on its feet. The virtual clinic model and integrated web platforms are important web-based systems, proving it is possible that patients can control their data, have access to care, and make informed decisions. At the same time, they have the potential to improve quality, build capacity, and make treatment more effective.

Acknowledgments The authors wish to thank Bell Let's Talk for support.

References

1. World Bank Group. The economic impact of the 2014 ebola epidemic: short and medium term estimates for West Africa. 7 Oct 2014. Available online at http://www-wds.worldbank.org/external/default/WDSContentServer/WDSP/IB/2014/10/07/000456286_20141007140300/Rendered/PDF/912190WP0see0a00070385314B00PUBLIC0.pdf. Last accessed 8 Dec 2014.
2. Whiteford HA, Degenhardt L, Rehm J, Baxter AJ, Ferrari AJ, Erskine HE, et al. Global burden of disease attributable to mental and substance use disorders: findings from the Global Burden of Disease Study 2010. Lancet. 2013;382:1575–86.
3. Kessler RC, Chiu WT, Demler O, Walters EE. Prevalence, severity, and comorbidity of 12-month. Arch Gen Psychiatry. 2005;62(2005):617–28.
4. Kohn R, Saxena S, Levav I, Saraceno B. The treatment gap in mental health care. Bull World Health Organ. 2004;82:858–66.
5. Wang PS, Lane M, Olfson M, Pincus HA, Wells KB, Kessler RC. Twelve-month use of mental health services in the United States. Arch Gen Psychiatry. 2007;62:629–40.
6. Vancouver primary care stats (2014). Report by the regional Health authority Vancouver Coastal Health (VCH).
7. Andersson G, Titov N. Advantages and limitations of Internet-based interventions for common mental disorders. World Psychiatry. 2014;13:4–11.
8. Kukreja S, Kaira G, Shah N, Amresh S. Polypharmacy in psychiatry: a review. Mens Sana Monogr. 2013;11(1):82–99.
9. Institute of Medicine. Crossing the quality chiasm: a new health system for the 21st century. National Academy of Sciences; 2001. Available online at https://www.iom.edu/~/media/Files/Report%20Files/2001/Crossing-the-Quality-Chasm/Quality%20Chasm%202001%20%20report%20brief.pdf. Last accessed 31 Mar 2015.
10. NHS Confederation. The future's digital: mental health and technology. London; 2014. Available online at http://www.nhsconfed.org/~/media/Confederation/Files/Publications/Documents/the-futures-digital.pdf. Last accessed July 14, 2015
11. Price Waterhouse Cooper. Making care mobile: virtualization of health. 2014. Available online at http://www.pwc.com/ca/en/healthcare/virtual-health-making-care-mobile-canada.jhtml. Last accessed 31 Mar 2015.
12. WalkAlong [website]. Available online at https://www.walkalong.ca/. Last accessed 31 Mar 2015.
13. PTSD coach [website]. US Department of Veterans Affairs. Last updated 11 Apr 2014. Available online at http://www.ptsd.va.gov/public/materials/apps/PTSDCoach.asp. Last accessed 31 Mar 2015.
14. Klein B, Meyer D, Austin DW, Kyrios M. Anxiety online – a virtual clinic: preliminary outcomes following completion of five fully automated treatment programs for anxiety disorders and symptoms. J Med Internet Res. 2011;13(4), e89.
15. Wienberg G, Driessen M. Auf dem Weg zur vergessenen Mehrheit: Innovative Konzepte fuer die Versorgung von Menschen mit Alkoholproblemen. Psychiatrie. Verlag; 2001.
16. Goldberg D, Huxley P. Common mental disorders: a bio-social model. London: Routledge; 1992.
17. Boydell KM, Hodgins H, Pignatiello A, Edwards H, Teshma J, Willis D. Using technology to deliver mental health services to children and youth in Ontario. Toronto: Ontario Centre of Excellence for Child and Youth Mental Health. J Can Acad Child Adolesc Psychiatry. 2013;23(2):87–99.

18. Valimaki M, Hatonen H, Lahti M, Kuosmanen L, Adams CE. Information and communication technology in patient education and support for people with schizophrenia. Cochrane Database Syst Rev. 2012;(10):CD007198.
19. Muir K, Powell A, et al. Headspace evaluation report. Social policy research. Sydney: Social Policy Research Centre; 2009. Available online at http://headspace.org.au/assets/Uploads/Corporate/Publications-and-research/final-independent-evaluation-of-headspace-report.pdf. Last accessed, July 14, 2015.
20. Johnson C, Feinglos M, Pereira K, Hassell N, Blascovich J, Niollerat J, et al. Feasibility and preliminary effects of a virtual environment for adults with type 2 diabetes: pilot study. JMIR Res Protoc. 2014;3(2), e23.
21. Microsoft Healthvault [website]. Microsoft Corporation, 2015. Available online at https://www.healthvault.com/ca/en. Last accessed 31 Mar 2015.
22. Mindcheck [website]. Available online at http://mindcheck.ca/. Last accessed 31 Mar 2015.
23. Apple Health [website]. Apple Canada, 2015. Available online at: https://www.apple.com/ca/ios/whats-new/health/. Last accessed 31 Mar 2015.

The manufacturer's authorised representative in the EU is Springer
Nature Customer Service Centre GmbH, Europaplatz 3, 69115 Heidelberg,
Germany. If you have any concerns regarding our products, please
contact ProductSafety@springernature.com

Printed and bound by CPI Group (UK) Ltd, Croydon, CR0 4YY
27/04/2026
02097630-0001